Etiology, Pathophysiology and Management of Multiple Sclerosis

Etiology, Pathophysiology and Management of Multiple Sclerosis

Editor: Alfred Galswells

AMERICAN
MEDICAL PUBLISHERS
www.americanmedicalpublishers.com

AMERICAN
MEDICAL PUBLISHERS
www.americanmedicalpublishers.com

Cataloging-in-Publication Data

Etiology, pathophysiology and management of multiple sclerosis / edited by Alfred Galswells.
p. cm.
Includes bibliographical references and index.
ISBN 978-1-63927-739-1
1. Multiple sclerosis. 2. Multiple sclerosis--Etiology. 3. Multiple sclerosis--Pathophysiology.
4. Multiple sclerosis--Treatment. I. Galswells, Alfred.
RC377 .E85 2023
616.834--dc23

American Medical Publishers,
41 Flatbush Avenue,
1st Floor, New York,
NY 11217, USA

ISBN 978-1-63927-739-1 (Hardback)

Contents

Preface

Multiple sclerosis (MS) is referred as the most prevalent demyelinating disease, where the insulating covers of nerve cells in the spinal cord and brain are destroyed. This injury impairs the capability of the parts of nervous system to transmit signals. This leads to a variety of signs and symptoms such as mental, physical and occasionally psychiatric issues. Problems with coordination or sensation, double vision, muscle weakness and blindness in one eye are some of the major symptoms. The etiology of MS is unknown; but numerous risk factors have been linked to its pathogenesis, comprising a link between environmental agents and genetic vulnerability. The breakdown of myelin sheaths of neurons, creation of lesions in the central nervous system and inflammation are the three basic characteristics of MS. This book is compiled in such a manner, that it will provide in-depth knowledge about the etiology and pathophysiology of multiple sclerosis. It aims to shed light on some of the unexplored aspects of this disease. Researchers and students in this field will be assisted by this book.

All of the data presented henceforth, was collaborated in the wake of recent advancements in the field. The aim of this book is to present the diversified developments from across the globe in a comprehensible manner. The opinions expressed in each chapter belong solely to the contributing authors. Their interpretations of the topics are the integral part of this book, which I have carefully compiled for a better understanding of the readers.

At the end, I would like to thank all those who dedicated their time and efforts for the successful completion of this book. I also wish to convey my gratitude towards my friends and family who supported me at every step.

Editor

1

Characterization of Asparagine Deamidation in Immunodominant Myelin Oligodendrocyte Glycoprotein Peptide Potential Immunotherapy for the Treatment of Multiple Sclerosis

Maria-Eleni Androutsou [1], Agathi Nteli [2], Areti Gkika [2], Maria Avloniti [3], Anastasia Dagkonaki [3], Lesley Probert [3], Theodore Tselios [2,*] and Simona Golič Grdadolnik [4,*]

1 Vianex S.A., Tatoiou Str., 18th km Athens-Lamia National Road, 14671 Athens, Greece; androutsoum@vianex.gr
2 Department of Chemistry, University of Patras, 26504 Patras, Greece; anteli@upatras.gr (A.N.); areti220@gmail.com (A.G.)
3 Laboratory of Molecular Genetics, Hellenic Pasteur Institute, 127 Vasilissis Sophias Ave., 11521 Athens, Greece; m.avloniti.17.5@gmail.com (M.A.); anastaciadk16@gmail.com (A.D.); lesley.probert@gmail.com (L.P.)
4 Laboratory for Molecular Structural Dynamics, National Institute of Chemistry, Hajdrihova 19, 1001 Ljubljana, Slovenia
* Correspondence: ttselios@upatras.gr (T.T.); simona.grdadolnik@ki.si (S.G.G.);

Abstract: Mannan (polysaccharide) conjugated with a myelin oligodendrocyte glycoprotein (MOG) peptide, namely $(KG)_5MOG_{35-55}$, represents a potent and promising new approach for the immunotherapy of Multiple Sclerosis (MS). The MOG_{35-55} epitope conjugated with the oxidized form of mannan (poly-mannose) via a $(KG)_5$ linker was found to inhibit the symptoms of MOG_{35-55}-induced experimental autoimmune encephalomyelitis (EAE) in mice using prophylactic and therapeutic vaccinated protocols. Deamidation is a common modification in peptide and protein sequences, especially for Gln and Asn residues. In this study, the structural solution motif of deaminated peptides and their functional effects in an animal model for MS were explored. Several peptides based on the MOG_{35-55} epitope have been synthesized in which the Asn^{53} was replaced with Ala, Asp, or isoAsp. Our results demonstrate that the synthesized MOG peptides were formed to the deaminated products in basic conditions, and the Asn^{53} was mainly modified to Asp. Moreover, both peptides (wild type and deaminated derivative) conjugated with mannan (from *Saccharomyces cerevisiae*) independently inhibited the development of neurological symptoms and inflammatory demyelinating spinal cord lesions in MOG_{35-55}-induced EAE. To conclude, mannan conjugated with a deamidated product did not affect the efficacy of the parent peptide.

Keywords: asparagine deamidation; nuclear magnetic resonance; myelin oligodentrocyte glycoprotein; experimental autoimmune encephalomyelitis; multiple sclerosis

---

1. Introduction

Peptides and proteins play an important role in the field of medicinal chemistry and biomedical research. In the pharmaceutical industry, peptides are emerging as a novel class of therapeutic agents. To date, about 100 peptides are on the market in the USA, Europe, and Japan, as well as for diagnostics applications [1–3]. Peptides demonstrate significant advantages as potential pharmaceuticals over small molecules due to their high biological activity and high receptor specificity [4].

During the design and synthesis of peptides, one has to consider numerous interactions and behaviors of the constituting amino acids. A search of the literature revealed that in many cases, several types of impurities might be encountered in synthetic peptides. Impurities can either originate from raw materials during the manufacturing process or be formed during storage [5]. In many cases, during the characterization of synthetic peptides, detectable byproducts lack one or more amino acid residues in the desired peptide sequence. It was noticed that Met, Trp, and Cys amino acids are sensitive to oxidation. The oxidation of a Cys-containing peptide yields a disulfide bridge to form cystine; Met is converted into a sulfoxide [6]. Both transformations are reversible. Tyr and Trp in peptide sequences should be protected from sunlight, as both amino acids are at risk of photo-oxidation [7]. The rate of racemization in solid-phase peptide synthesis is common and depends on many factors, including the electron-withdrawing effect of the amino acid side chain, the temperature, the reaction solvent, and the coupling reagents [8–11]. Acetylation of amino functions could occur in acidic conditions with the treatment of trifluoroacetic acid. This reaction is reversible in mild alkaline conditions [12]. Other side-reactions in peptide synthesis address the Trp reduction by trialkyl silane and the irreversible alkylation on the Cys side chain functional group during the deprotection step [13].

Deamidation of Gln and Asn presents a frequent modification in peptide and protein sequences. This reaction is favored in neutral and mostly basic solutions. Deamidation of Asn leads to a mixture of L, D-succinimidyl, L, D-aspartyl, and L, D-iso aspartyl with the greater presence of L-iso aspartyl [14]. The new product adds to the mass of intact molecule + 0.984 Da the difference between the mass of hydroxyl (-OH) and amine (-NH_2) functional groups. The intermediate cyclic imide succinimide appears with a different molecular weight, ~17–18 Da less [15,16].

Slight modifications in the sequence can result in drastic changes in the structure and function of peptides. For example, a modified residue such as deaminated Asn could positively or negatively affect the peptide/protein potency, efficacy, and safety [17–21]. Thus, deamidation should be monitored using several analytical techniques such as LC-MS/MS analysis, capillary electrophoresis, and NMR [22].

The presented study involves the investigation of deaminated products in combination with experimental autoimmune encephalomyelitis (EAE, animal model of multiple sclerosis (MS)), the evaluation of 35–55 myelin oligodendrocyte glycoprotein (MOG_{35-55}) epitope that contains the -Asn^{53}-Gly^{54}- sequence. MOG is a glycoprotein located on the external surface of the myelin sheath [23–25]. The 35–55 epitope of rat MOG (MOG_{35-55}: H-Met^{35}-Glu-Val-Gly-Trp-Tyr-Arg-Ser-Pro-Phe-Ser-Arg-Val-Val-His-Leu-Tyr-Arg-Asn^{53}-Gly-Lys^{55}-OH) induces chronic EAE in mice of the C57BL/6 strain and is widely used for in vivo biological evaluation and immunological studies relevant to MS treatment [26–29]. The immunogenic MOG_{35-55} epitope conjugated to polysaccharide (mannan) via the $(KG)_5$ bridge at *N* terminal protected mice against EAE when administered in prophylactic and therapeutic protocols [30–37]. Combinations of different peptides from myelin proteins (including MOG peptides) have been used in clinical studies against MS [38]. Moreover, MOG_{35-55} is one of the immunodominant epitopes that, conjugated to peripheral blood monocytes, resulted in a decrease of antigen-specific T cell responses in MS patients [38]. The structure of peptides based on the Asn^{53} transformation of synthesized MOG_{35-55} peptides has been explored. Model peptides with mutations of Asn with Ala, Asp, or isoAsp were synthesized and analyzed with 2D NMR spectroscopy in neutral and basic aqueous solutions. The comparison of chemical shifts and NMR signal patterns reveals the Asn^{53} deamidation to Asp in basic conditions while it is not revealed in neutral solution. Furthermore, the modified peptide containing Asp at position 53 showed similar biological activity compared to that of the wild type peptide against EAE when the peptides are conjugated to mannan polysaccharide.

2. Results and Discussion

2.1. Design and Synthesis of Peptides Based on the Immunodominant MOG_{35-55} Epitope

MOG_{35-55} is the main immunodominant epitope of MOG protein and is of great interest in our research regarding the peptide-based EAE treatment. This epitope conjugated with the oxidized form of mannan (poly-mannose) via a $(KG)_5$ linker was found to inhibit the EAE symptoms in mice using prophylactic and therapeutic vaccinated protocols [30–34]. The conjugation reaction of $(KG)_5MOG_{35–55}$ peptide analog with oxidized mannan was performed in bicarbonate buffer solution, pH 9.0. In the basic conditions of conjugation reaction, the deamidation of Asn^{53} may occur. Model peptides were designed and synthesized (Pep 1–Pep 4), as shown in Table 1, to investigate the possibility of the formation of deaminated products during conjugation reaction. The obtained results lead to further investigation, and the $(KG)_5MOG_{35–55}$ peptides with Asn or Asp or isoAsp, respectively (Pep 5–Pep 7; human sequence) at position 53 were synthesized. A combination of reverse-phase high-performance liquid chromatography (RP-HPLC) and NMR were used to confirm the existence of deaminated products. Furthermore, it was interesting to examine how the chemically modified peptides would affect the immunological properties of the native peptide. Therefore, the rat sequence of $(KG)_5MOG_{35–55}$ (Ser^{42}) (Pep 8) and the deaminated derivative containing Asp at position 53 $(KG)_5MOG_{35–55}$ (Ser^{42}, Asp^{53}) (Pep 9) were synthesized and conjugated with the oxidized form of mannan (Con-Pep 8 and Con-Pep 9). Both conjugates were evaluated in vivo in C57BL/6 mice using the EAE animal model of MS.

Table 1. Sequence of studied peptides.

Peptide	Peptide Sequence	Abbreviation
Pep 1	H-Arg^{41}-Pro-Pro-Phe-Ser-Arg-Val-Val-His-Leu-Tyr-Arg-Asn^{53}-Gly-Lys^{55}-OH	$MOG_{41–55}$
Pep 2	H-Arg^{41}-Pro-Pro-Phe-Ser-Arg-Val-Val-His-Leu-Tyr-Arg-**Ala^{53}**-Gly-Lys^{55}-OH	$MOG_{41–55}(Ala^{53})$
Pep 3	H-Arg^{41}-Pro-Pro-Phe-Ser-Arg-Val-Val-His-Leu-Tyr-Arg-**Asp^{53}**-Gly-Lys^{55}-OH	$MOG_{41–55}(Asp^{53})$
Pep 4	H-Arg^{41}-Pro-Pro-Phe-Ser-Arg-Val-Val-His-Leu-Tyr-Arg-**isoAsp^{53}**-Gly-Lys^{55}-OH	$MOG_{41–55}(isoAsp^{53})$
Pep 5	H-Lys-Gly-Lys-Gly-Lys-Gly-Lys-Gly-Lys-Gly-Met^{35}-Glu-Val-Gly-Trp-Tyr-Arg-Pro-Pro-Phe-Ser-Arg-Val-Val-His-Leu-Tyr-Arg-**Asn^{53}**-Gly-Lys^{55}-OH	$(KG)_5MOG_{35–55}$
Pep 6	H-Lys-Gly-Lys-Gly-Lys-Gly-Lys-Gly-Lys-Gly-Met^{35}-Glu-Val-Gly-Trp-Tyr-Arg-Pro-Pro-Phe-Ser-Arg-Val-Val-His-Leu-Tyr-Arg-**Asp^{53}**-Gly-Lys^{55}-OH	$(KG)_5MOG_{35–55}(Asp^{53})$
Pep 7	H-Lys-Gly-Lys-Gly-Lys-Gly-Lys-Gly-Lys-Gly-Met^{35}-Glu-Val-Gly-Trp-Tyr-Arg-Pro-Pro-Phe-Ser-Arg-Val-Val-His-Leu-Tyr-Arg-**isoAsp^{53}**-Gly-Lys^{55}-OH	$(KG)_5MOG_{35–55}(isoAsp^{53})$
Pep 8	H-Lys-Gly-Lys-Gly-Lys-Gly-Lys-Gly-Lys-Gly-Met^{35}-Glu-Val-Gly-Trp-Tyr-Arg-**Ser^{42}**-Pro-Phe-Ser-Arg-Val-Val-His-Leu-Tyr-Arg-**Asn^{53}**-Gly-Lys^{55}-OH	$(KG)_5MOG_{35–55}$ (Ser^{42})
Pep 9	H-Lys-Gly-Lys-Gly-Lys-Gly-Lys-Gly-Lys-Gly-Met^{35}-Glu-Val-Gly-Trp-Tyr-Arg-**Ser^{42}**-Pro-Phe-Ser-Arg-Val-Val-His-Leu-Tyr-Arg-**Asp^{53}**-Gly-Lys^{55}-OH	$(KG)_5MOG_{35–55}$ (Ser^{42}, Asp^{53})
Con-Pep 8	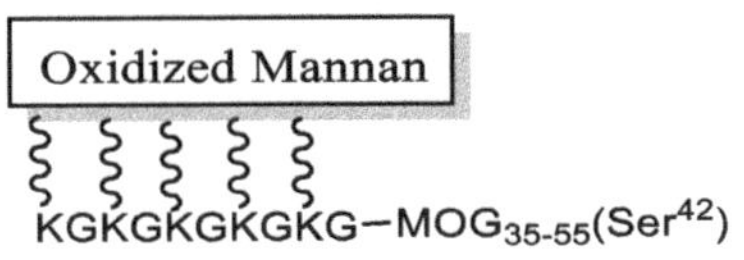	OM-$(KG)_5MOG_{35–55}$ (Ser^{42})
Con-Pep 9	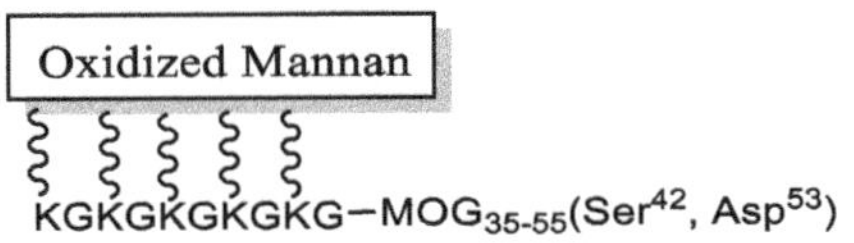	OM-$(KG)_5MOG_{35–55}$ (Ser^{42}, Asp^{53})

OG = myelin oligodendrocyte glycoprotein, KG = Lys-Gly, OM = oxidized mannan.

The Pep 1–Pep 9 peptides (Table 1) were synthesized by solid-phase peptide synthesis (SPPS) in combination with the Fmoc/tBu methodology and using acid-labile 2-chlorotrityl chloride (CLTR-Cl) resin and N^{α}-Fmoc (9-fluorenylmethyloxycarboxyl)-protected amino acids, as previously described and presented in Scheme 1 [39–46]. The first N^{α}-Fmoc protected amino acid was esterified to the CLTR-Cl resin in the presence of diisopropylethylamine (DIPEA) and followed by Fmoc deprotection. The peptide bonds were created using 1-Hydroxybenzotriazole (HOBt) and *N,N′*-Diisopropylcarbodiimide (DIC) as coupling reagents [39–46]. The final deprotection of each peptide was achieved using trifluoroacetic acid (TFA) in dichloromethane (DCM) in the presence of scavengers (Scheme 1). The synthesized peptides were further purified and identified using semi-preparative RP-HPLC and electron spray ionization mass spectrometry (ESI-MS), respectively. The purity of peptides was more than 95%, as determined by analytical RP-HPLC.

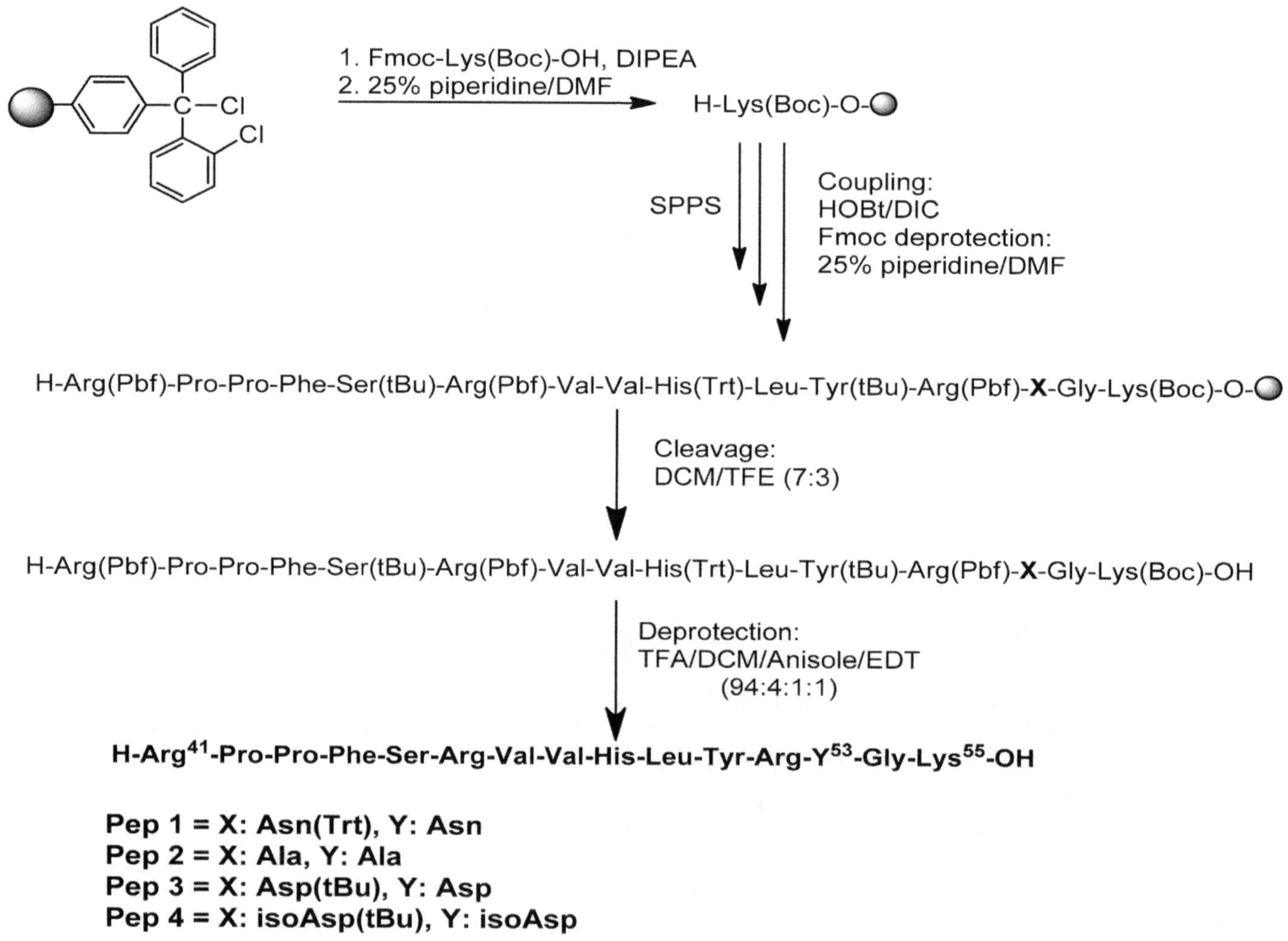

Scheme 1. Representative SPPS of model peptides (Pep 1–Pep 4). The same synthetic procedure was followed for the synthesis of Pep 5–Pep 9 peptides.

2.2. HPLC Analysis

The HPLC analysis of synthesized peptides was achieved using the analytical HPLC system (1260 Infinity, Quaternary Pump VL Agilent, Waldbronn, Germany) equipped with the Purospher RP-18 column (5 μm, Hibar 100 × 4.6 mm, Darmstadt, Germany), followed by UV detection at 214.4 nm and 254 nm. Separation was achieved by gradient elution from 18% acetonitrile (AcN) to 40% AcN over 30 min at a flow rate of 1 mL/min. The analysis demonstrated that the peptide with Asn residue at position 53 has been degraded and provided two new peaks at the right of the main peak in HPLC chromatogram after dilution in bicarbonate solution pH 9.0 (Figure 1 and Figure S1). The relative retention time of the $(KG)_5MOG_{35–55}$ (Ser^{42}) deaminated analog, based on HPLC chromatogram (Figure 1), is 1.06, and this was further investigated during the present study.

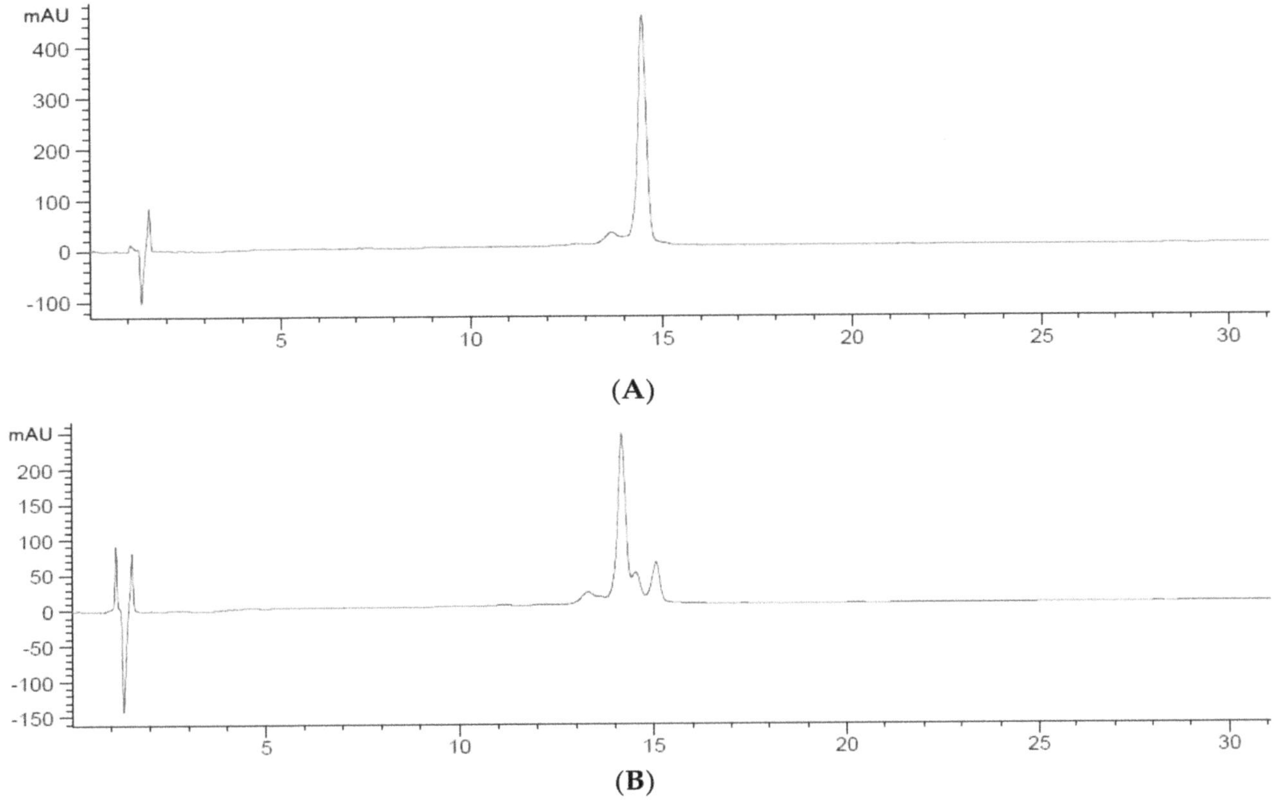

Figure 1. RP-HPLC chromatogram of $(KG)_5MOG_{35–55}$ (Ser^{42}) (Pep 8) at 214.4 nm and 48 h after dilution; (**A**) dissolved in water, (**B**) dissolved in bicarbonate buffer pH 9.0. The deaminated product was revealed as a new peak to the right of the main peak.

The possibility of deamidation of Asn was apparent since the literature has addressed studies related to this formation [14–22]. Several peptides were synthesized based on 35–55 epitope of MOG (Pep 1, Pep 5, and Pep 8); with substitution of Asn residue with Ala (Pep 2), Asp (Pep 3, Pep 6, and Pep 9), and isoAsp (Pep 4, Pep 7), and they were analyzed by HPLC and ESI-MS (Figure 1 and Figures S1–S15). It was observed that the byproduct is revealed only in Pep 1, Pep 5, and Pep 8 peptides, containing Asn^{53}, in basic conditions (carbonate buffer pH 9.0), and it was not detected in the other synthesized peptides with Ala, Asp, or isoAsp substitutions at the same position (Figures S1–S15). The deamidation formation is initiated upon dilution of the peptides in bicarbonate buffer solution and stabilizes after one day. The identified retention times in HPLC chromatograms of produced byproducts in basic conditions of peptides Pep 1, Pep 5, and Pep 8 matched the retention times of the synthesized peptides Pep 3, Pep 6, and Pep 9. This observation supports that Pep 1, Pep 5, and Pep 8 containing the Asn residue at position 53 undergo deamidation and semi-covert to the peptides Pep 3, Pep 6, and Pep 9.

2.3. NMR Analysis

The NMR chemical shift analysis of peptides 1–7 was performed to elucidate the nature of modification observed at HPLC analysis in basic conditions for peptides containing Asn at position 53. As the NMR chemical shifts are very sensitive to changes in the local chemical environment, the modifications related to Asn^{53} could also result in chemical shifts of neighboring residues. Indeed, expansions of the Total Correlated Spectroscopy (TOCSY) spectra recorded in bicarbonate buffer pH 9.0, which contain well separated ^1H α-β cross-peaks of residues 51 and 53 and α-δ cross peaks of residue 52 of all investigated peptides, came out as the most demonstrative to elucidate the modification process (Figure 2). The positions and appearance of these cross-peaks critically depend on the modification of Asn^{53} and the presence of produced byproducts. The chemical shifts of α, β and δ protons of residues 51, 52 and 53 for peptides 1 to 7, which are relevant for the position of representative cross-peaks in TOCSY, are given in Table S1.

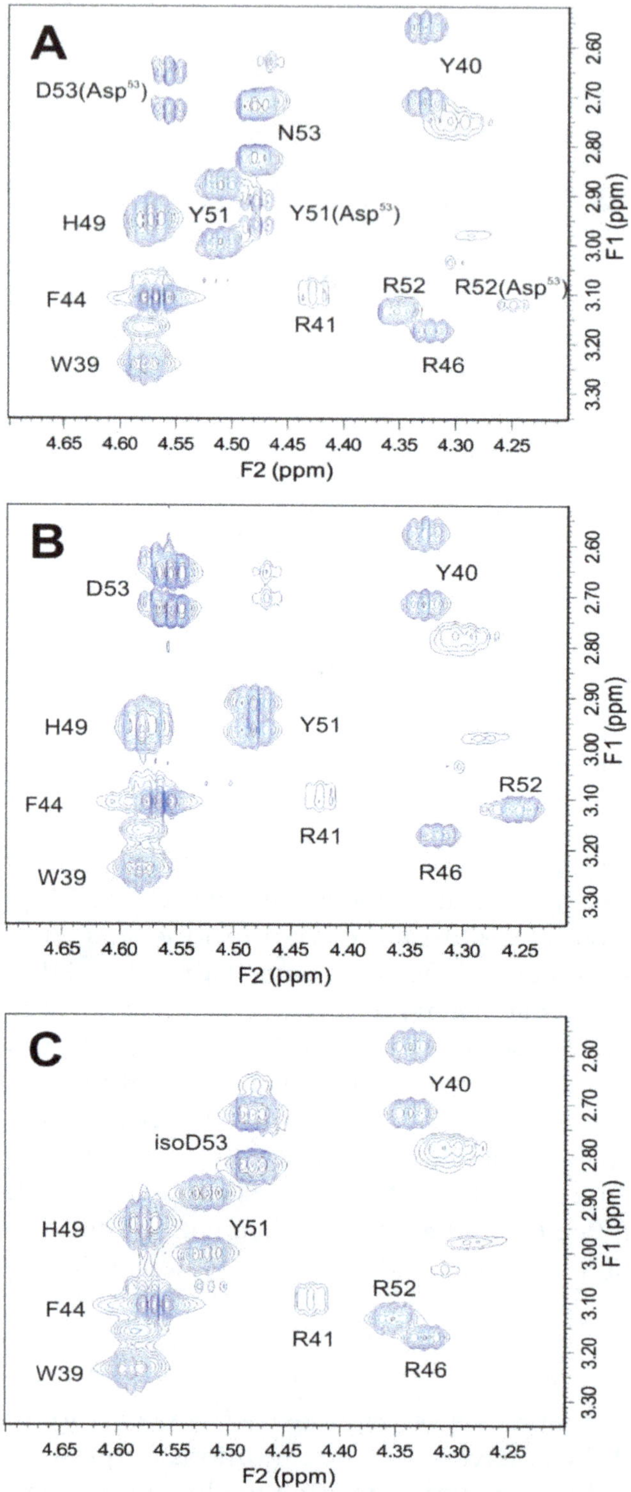

Figure 2. Expanded regions of Total Correlated Spectroscopy (TOCSY) spectra of: (**A**) $(KG)_5MOG_{35–55}$ (Pep 5), (**B**) $(KG)_5MOG_{35–55}(Asp^{53})$ (Pep 6) and (**C**) $(KG)_5MOG_{35–55}(isoAsp^{53})$ (Pep 7) recorded in bicarbonate buffer, pH 9.0.

In the expanded TOCSY spectrum of $(KG)_5MOG_{35-55}$ (Pep 5), two sets of signals were observed for residues 51, 52 and 53 (Figure 2A), indicating a modification in this peptide region. Only one set of signals was observed for the residues remote from position 53. In the spectra of $(KG)_5MOG_{35-55}(Asp^{53})$ (Pep 6) and $(KG)_5MOG_{35-55}(isoAsp^{53})$ (Pep 7), only one set of signals appeared for all residues (Figure 2B,C), indicating that these two peptides were not prone to any modification process. The comparison of cross-peak patterns in expanded TOCSY spectra of Pep 5, Pep 6, and Pep7 clearly demonstrate the type of modification at Asn^{53}. Namely, the positions of α-β cross-peaks of Asn^{53}/Asp^{53} and Tyr^{51} and α–δ cross-peaks of Arg^{52} considerably differed between Pep 6 and Pep 7 (Figure 2B, C). The positions of the additional weaker set of signals observed in expanded TOCSY region of Pep 5 (Figure 2A) were the same as the positions of the α-β cross-peaks of Asp^{53} and Tyr^{51}, and the α-δ cross-peak of Arg^{52} of Pep 6 (Figure 2B). These observations clearly indicate a partial deamidation of Asn^{53} in Pep 5 to Asp^{53}. The position of cross-peaks of the residues remote from position 53 was the same for all three peptides Pep 5, Pep 6, and Pep 7.

In the TOCSY region of the byproduct isolated via semi-preparative HPLC from $(KG)_5MOG_{35-55}$ (Pep 5) in bicarbonate buffer pH 9.0, two sets of signals appeared at the same positions as observed for Pep 5 (Table S1, Figure S16). However, the intensity ratio between the two sets of signals was different. In contrast to observations in the TOCSY spectra of Pep 5 (Figure 2A), the signals in the TOCSY spectra of byproducts corresponding to $(KG)_5MOG_{35-55}(Asp^{53})$ (Pep 6) were stronger, and the signals corresponding to Pep 5 were weaker. That means that the byproduct of Pep 5 is Pep 6, while the presence of weaker signals of Pep 5 in the spectra of byproduct was the consequence of the not totally successful separation of byproduct from Pep 5. Namely, a small amount of Pep 5 was co-eluted with its byproduct (Pep 6).

Additional confirmation for the partial deamidation of Asn^{53} was obtained by the comparison of cross-peak patterns in the corresponding expanded TOCSY spectra of the shorter model peptides MOG_{41-55}, containing Asn (Pep 1), Ala (Pep2), Asp (Pep 3), and isoAsp (Pep 4) at position 53, as recorded in bicarbonate buffer at pH 9.0 (Figure S17). Similarly to $(KG)_5MOG_{35-55}$, two sets of signals were observed only for residues 51, 52, and 53 of MOG_{41-55} (Pep 1) containing Asn at position 53 (Figure S17A). Only one set of signals was present in the spectra of Pep 2, Pep 3, and Pep 4 (Figure S17D, B and C, respectively). Moreover, the positions of the additional weaker set of cross-peaks of Pep 1 (Figure S17A) were the same as the positions of the α-β cross-peaks of Asp^{53} and Tyr^{51} and the α-δ cross peak of Arg^{52} of Pep 3 (Figure S17B), indicating partial deamidation of Asn^{53} to Asp^{53} in Pep 1.

Comparison of expanded TOCSY spectra of peptides 1 to 7 recorded in bicarbonate buffer pH 9.0, which are presented in Figure 2 and Figure S17, clearly demonstrated a modification of Pep 1 and Pep 5 due to partial deamidation of the Asn^{53} to Asp^{53}. The peptides having Asp, isoAsp, or Ala at position 53 were stable.

2.4. *In Vivo Evaluation of Con-Pep 8 and Con-Pep 9 Conjugated to Mannan*

Con-Pep 8 conjugated with the oxidized form of mannan strongly protected C57BL/6 mice against MOG-induced Experimental Autoimmune Encephalomyelitis (EAE) in prophylactic and therapeutic protocols [31]. Moreover, Con-Pep 8 strongly protected transgenic mice expressing the human *major histocompatibility complex class II* (MHC II) MS candidate susceptibility genes *DRA*0101* and *DRB1*1501* and lacking all murine MHC II molecules (DR2b.Ab° mice) against MOG-EAE with prophylactic or therapeutic applications and therapeutic administration of Con-Pep 8 in mice with ongoing MOG-EAE reduced spinal cord EAE lesions, inflammatory infiltrates, microglial activation, demyelination, and neuronal damage in DR2b.Ab° mice [47].

Administration of Con-Pep 8 [OM-$(KG)_5MOG_{35-55}$ (Ser^{42})] or Con-Pep 9 [OM-$(KG)_5MOG_{35-55}$ (Ser^{42}, Asp^{53})], conjugated to mannan in its oxidized form, in a prophylactic (vaccination) protocol both protected mice against the clinical and neuropathological symptoms of MOG-EAE.

To investigate the effect of Pep 9 on the development of MOG-EAE, we delivered Con-Pep 9 or, as a positive control, Con-Pep 8 to C57BL/6 mice in a prophylactic vaccine protocol prior to the induction of

EAE by immunization with MOG emulsified in CFA and administration of *Bordetella pertussis* toxin (MOG/CFA/PTx). As described previously, three intradermal (i.d.) injections of Con-Pep 8 in dilute soluble form and spaced at 15-day intervals prior to EAE induction protected mice against the clinical symptoms of EAE [31]. We show here that vaccination with Con-Pep 9 also strongly protected mice against the development of clinical EAE, to an equal extent as Pep 8, compared to vehicle-treated controls (Figure 3, top).

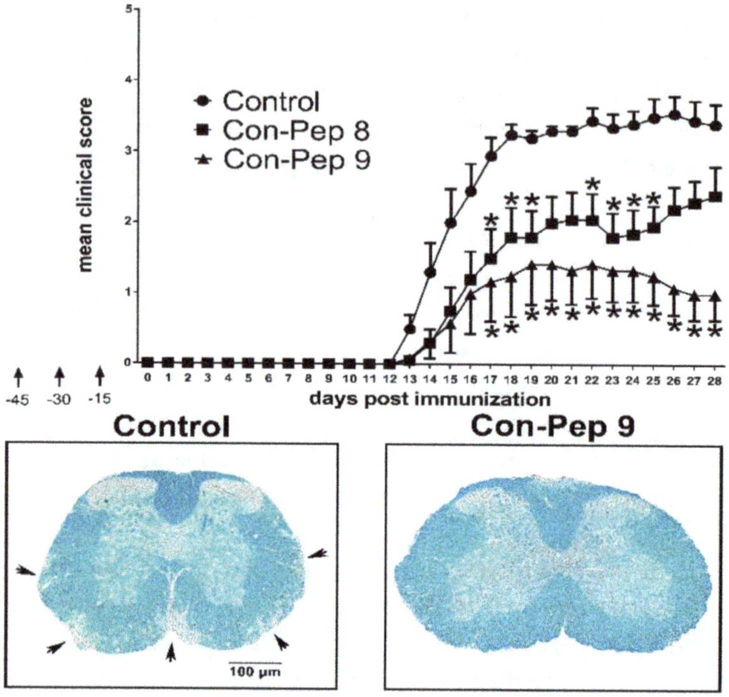

Figure 3. Administration of Con-Pep 8 and Con-Pep 9, conjugated to mannan in its oxidized form, in a prophylactic (vaccination) protocol attenuates the development of MOG-induced experimental autoimmune encephalomyelitis (EAE) in C57BL/6 mice. Top: Mean clinical scores of MOG-EAE in groups of mice vaccinated intradermally (i.d.) with dilute soluble Con-Pep 8, Con-Pep 9 or carbonate buffer pH 9.0 (disease control) at the indicated time points (arrows), prior to the induction of EAE by immunization with MOG/CFA/PTx ($n = 10$ for Con-Pep 8 and control groups, $n = 6$ for Con-Pep 9 group). Bottom: MOG-EAE vehicle control mice induces hallmark demyelinating lesions, as seen by Luxol Fast blue staining of spinal cord sections taken from mice sacrificed on day 28 post-immunization for EAE (left panel, arrows). Vaccination with either Con-Pep 8 (data not shown) or Con-Pep 9 prevented the development of spinal cord demyelination (right panel). Representative sections from three animals per group are shown. Statistical significance after comparisons between Con-Pep 8 and 9 treated with control groups of mice by 2-way ANOVA followed by Bonferroni post-hoc tests is shown (* $p \leq 0.05$).

To determine whether amelioration of the clinical symptoms of MOG-EAE by Con-Pep 9 was associated with less severe neuropathology, mice from the different groups were sacrificed 28 days after EAE induction for neuropathological analysis of spinal cord tissues. Vehicle-treated control mice showed extensive demyelination of the spinal cord white matter characteristic of this model (Figure 3, bottom left panel). As described previously [31], vaccination of mice with Con-Pep 8 protected them against the neuropathological changes of MOG-EAE (data not shown). Here we show that vaccination of mice with Con-Pep 9 also protected against the development of neuropathological changes, with Con-Pep 9-vaccinated mice showing little or no demyelination in the spinal cord (Figure 3, bottom right panel).

These results show that the administration of Con-Pep 9 as a prophylactic vaccine in mice inhibited the clinical and neuropathological features of MOG-EAE to an equal extent as Con-Pep 8.

3. Materials and Methods

3.1. Synthesis

All commercially available solvents and reagents were HPLC grade, purchased from Merck (Darmstadt, Germany), Sigma-Aldrich (Schnelldorf, Germany), Fluka (Buchs, Switzerland), and Across (Geel, Belgium), and they were used without further purification. HPLC grade water was obtained from distilled water passed through a Milli-Q water purification system (Millipore Ltd., Bedford, MA, USA). CLTR-Cl resin (1% DVB, 200–400 mesh), Fmoc-protected-amino acids and piperidine were purchased from Chemical and Biopharmaceutical Laboratories of Patras, Patras, Greece. The stated resin loading capacity was determined spectrophotometrically using a UV/Visible Spectrophotometer Varian Cary 4000. ESI-MS spectra were acquired using a Waters Micromass ZQ Electrospray Platform coupled to a MassLynx 4.1 data acquisition system (Manchester, UK). HPLC chromatograms were acquired using a 1260 Infinity, Quaternary Pump VL Agilent, (Waldbronn, Germany). The ESI-MS analysis was performed using the ion spray source in positive ion mode with the following settings: (i) capillary voltage: 3.5 kV; (ii) cone voltage: 30 V; (iii) source temperature: 80oC; (iv) desolvation temperature: 300oC; (v) desolvation gas: 300 L/h; (vi) cone gas: 50 L/h.

Peptide Synthesis

The studied peptides (Table 1) were successfully synthesized using the solid-phase peptide synthesis (SPPS) and Fmoc/tBu methodology on CLTR-Cl resin [39–46]. The first N^a-Fmoc protected amino acid, Fmoc-Lys(Boc)-OH, was esterified to the resin in the presence of DIPEA (4.5 equivalent) in DCM for 1.5 h at room temperature (RT). The remaining active site of the resin was capped using a mixture of dichloromethane (DCM) / Methanol (MeOH) / DIPEA (85/10/5; *v/v/v*) at RT. The resin was washed with *N, N*-dimethylformamide (DMF, three times × 5 mL) and isopropanol (i-PrOH; three times × 5 mL) and dried overnight under vacuum. For each peptide, 1 g CLTR-Cl resin was loaded with Fmoc-Lys(Boc)-OH (1.5 mmol), and the N^a-Fmoc group was removed with 25% piperidine in DMF (*v/v*) (Scheme 1). The second amino acid, Fmoc-Gly-OH, was added (2.5 mmol) in the presence of *N,N'*-diisopropylcarbodiimide (DIC; 2.75 mmol) and 1-hydroxybenzotriazole (HOBt; 3.75 mmol) in *N,N*-dimethylacetamide (DMAC) for 4 h, followed by Fmoc deprotection with piperidine solution; three times with 25% piperidine in DMF (*v/v*) for 5 min, 15 min and 10 min respectively The coupling and deprotection cycles were repeated for all the other remaining amino acids (Scheme 1). The coupling reaction and Fmoc deprotection were demonstrated by Kaiser test and thin-layer chromatography (TLC; eluent system: AcN/H_2O: 5/1 or 2/1; *v/v*). Then, each protected peptide was cleaved from the resin by treatment with the cleaved solution comprised of DCM/trifluoroethanol (TFE) (7/3) for 1.5 h at RT, to afford the crude side chain protected peptides. The final deprotection of the peptide was accomplished using a TFA/DCM/Anisole/Ethanodithiol (EDT) (94/4/1/1; *v/v/v/v*) solution for 5 h at RT.

The purification of each peptide was carried out on a semi-preparative reverse-phase high-performance liquid chromatography (RP-HPLC) using a Nucleosil RP-C18 column (7 μm, 250 × 4 mm, Macherey-Nagel, Duren, Germany). The separation was achieved by gradient elution from 10% AcN to 60% AcN over 45 min at a flow rate of 3 mL/min. The HPLC solvents for the analytical and semi-preparative HPLC analysis were: H_2O with 0.08% TFA, AcN with 0.08% TFA. The final products were identified using ESI-MS and NMR spectroscopy. The purity of the synthesized peptides was determined by analytical HPLC using a Purospher RP-18 column (5μm, Hibar 100 × 4.6 mm, Darmstadt, Germany) followed by UV detection at 214.4 nm. Separation was achieved by gradient elution from 18% AcN to 40% AcN over 30 min at flow rate of 1 mL/min.

The Pep 8 and Pep 9 peptides, based on the rat/mouse sequence of MOG, were conjugated with the oxidized form of mannan (poly-mannose) to Con-Pep 8 [OM-$(KG)_5MOG_{35-55}$ (Ser^{42})] and Con-Pep 9 [OM-$(KG)_5MOG_{35-55}$ (Ser^{42}, Asp^{53})] respectively as previously described [31,33,34], and they were used in the EAE animal model of MS, for further in vivo evaluation.

3.2. *NMR Spectroscopy*

The high-resolution NMR spectra were recorded on Agilent 600 MHz and Varian DirectDrive 800 MHz spectrometers (Agilent Technologies Inc., Santa Clara, CA 95051, USA) at 298 K. Cryogenic triple-resonance NMR probes were used. Ultra-precision 5 mm NMR tubes from Wilmad®were used containing peptides in a 0.7 mL aqueous solution of bicarbonate buffer (pH 9.0). The 0.1 M bicarbonate buffer solution (pH 9.0) was created using sodium bicarbonate and sodium carbonate solutions as follows: Solution A: 0.210 g Na_2CO_3 were dissolved in 10 mL D_2O; Solution B: 0.168 g $NaHCO_3$ were dissolved in 10 mL D_2O. 0.8mL of solution (A) was added to 9.6ml of solution (B), and the mixture was diluted to the final volume of 50 mL with the addition of D_2O. pH was measured with the use of a HANNA pH meter. (Calibration of pH meter was achieved with the use of calibration solutions, pH 4.0 and pH 7.0, as reported in the instruction manual).

The concentration of peptides was 1.2 mM. Water was purified with Milli-Q Water Purification System. D_2O ("100%") was purchased from Cambridge Isotope Laboratories. DSS-d_6 (0.1 mM) purchased from Sigma-Aldrich was used as an internal standard.

The proton chemical shifts of peptides 1–7 were assigned using 2D homonuclear proton experiments (Double Quantum-Filtered Correlated Spectroscopy (DQF-COSY), TOCSY, Nuclear Overhauser Effect Correlation Spectroscopy (NOESY), and Rotating-Frame Nuclear Overhauser Effect Correlation Spectroscopy (ROESY)) in combination with the 2D ^1H–^{13}C Heteronuclear Single Quantum Coherence (HSQC) experiment.

The 2D homonuclear proton spectra were acquired on a Varian DirectDrive 800 MHz spectrometer with a spectral width of 8478 Hz, 4096 data points in t_2, 4-32 scans, 512 complex points in t_1, and a relaxation delay of 1.5 s. The mixing time in TOSCY was 60 ms. The mixing times in NOESY and ROESY were 150 ms and 300 ms.

The ^1H–^{13}C HSQC was recorded on an Agilent 600 MHz spectrometer with ^1H spectral width of 6345 Hz, ^{13}C spectral width of 9498 Hz, 1024 data points in t_2, 160 scans, 128 complex points in t_1, and a relaxation delay of 1.5 s.

All data were collected in phase-sensitive mode using pulse sequences and phase-cycling routines provided in Varian/Agilent libraries of pulse programs. In the DQF-COSY and ^1H-^{13}C HSQC experiments, gradients were used for the coherence selection. The WATERGATE pulse block was used for water suppression in DQF-COSY. The residual water signal in TOCSY, NOESY, and ROESY was suppressed using excitation sculpting, and adiabatic pulses were applied for suppression of zero quantum artifacts during mixing time.

Spectra were processed and analyzed with the Felix 2007 software package (Felix NMR Inc., San Diego, CA, USA). The spectra were zero-filled twice and apodized with a squared sine-bell function shifted by $\pi/2$ in both dimensions. In the ^{13}C dimension, a linear prediction was used.

3.3. *EAE Evaluation*

3.3.1. Mice

Female C57BL/6 mice aged 24 weeks were used for the prophylactic administration of peptide conjugates. Mice were bred and maintained under specific pathogen-free conditions in the experimental animal unit of the Hellenic Pasteur Institute. All animal experiments complied with ARRIVE guidelines and were carried out in accordance with the local Ethical Committee guidelines on the use of experimental animals at the Hellenic Pasteur Institute, were approved by the national authorities and conformed to EU Directive 2010/63/EU for animal experiments. Animal experiments were performed under license number 2580/29-05-2018, entitled "Induction of experimental autoimmune encephalomyelitis (EAE) for the study of immune tolerance induced by mannan-conjugated peptides". Issued 31-05-2018 to L.P. by the Hellenic Republic Region of Attica Agricultural Economy, Veterinary and Fisheries.

3.3.2. Administration of Peptides to Mice

In a prophylactic vaccination protocol, groups of adult female C57BL/6 mice (24 week-old) were injected intradermally (i.d.) on the flanks with 100 μl carbonate buffer pH 9.0 containing Con-Pep 9 (conjugated with mannan) (n = 6) or Con-Pep 8 (conjugated with mannan) (n = 10), which has been described previously [31]; 30 μg peptide (Pep 8 or Pep 9) equivalent/injection, 700 μg mannan equivalent/injection. Three consecutive injections were performed at 15-day intervals. Control mice were injected with carbonate buffer alone (n = 10). Immunization for the induction of EAE was performed 15 days after the last i.d. injection.

3.3.3. EAE Induction

EAE was induced in vaccinated female C57BL/6 mice by subcutaneous (s.c.) tail-base injection of 38 μg of rat MOG_{35-55} (Ser^{42}) (MOG) in 100 μL saline emulsified in an equal volume of complete Freund's adjuvant (CFA), 15 days after the third vaccination injection. CFA was supplemented with 400 μg/injection of H37Ra *Mycobacterium tuberculosis* (Difco). Mice also received intraperitoneal (i.p.) injections of 200 ng of *Bordetella pertussis toxin* (PTx) (Sigma-Aldrich) at the time of immunization and 48 h later. Mice were monitored daily for the clinical signs of EAE according to the following scores: zero, normal; one, limp tail; two, hind limb weakness; three, hind limb paralysis; four, forelimb paralysis; five, moribund or dead (0.5 graduations represent intermediate scores). Mice with a score above four were euthanized and given a clinical score five for the remaining days of the experiment. All mice were allowed free access to food and water throughout the experiment.

4. Conclusions

In the present study, the deamidation of 35–55 Myelin Oligodendrocyte Glycoprotein (MOG_{35-55}) epitope that contains the -Asn^{53}-Gly^{54}- sequence was investigated via HPLC, NMR, and biological studies. The 35–55 epitope of rat MOG protein induces chronic EAE in mice of the C57BL/6 strain and is widely used as an animal model for MS for in vivo biological evaluation and immunological studies of novel therapeutics [48]. Moreover, the immunogenic $(KG)_5MOG_{35-55}$ epitope, including the $(KG)_5$ bridge in the *N*-terminal, conjugated to polysaccharide (mannan) via Schiff base, protected mice against EAE in prophylactic and therapeutic protocols [31,47]. Thus, the synthesized Pep 5 conjugated to mannan represents a potent and promising potential new therapeutic approach for the treatment of MS [31,34,36,47]. In addition to the investigation of correspondence, the unmodified form of human $(KG)_5MOG_{35-55}$ peptide, model peptides were synthesized based on the MOG_{41-55} epitope with modifications at position 53 (Pep 2–4) and studied to determine whether the deamidation reaction happens and to identify deaminated products. Furthermore, it was crucial to investigate the potency of these products and demonstrate how their presence affects the efficiency.

Deamidation may occur via several pathways, as well as peptide dilution in basic conditions. The conjugation reaction between $(KG)_5MOG_{35-55}$ peptide with mannan occurs in basic condition (pH 9.0); thus, the deamidation reaction is an unavoidable consequence (Scheme 2). Therefore, the investigation of the immunological properties of the chemically modified peptides and the demonstration of biological action of the modified form of peptide is of great importance, since the deamidation process is associated with the maintenance of action.

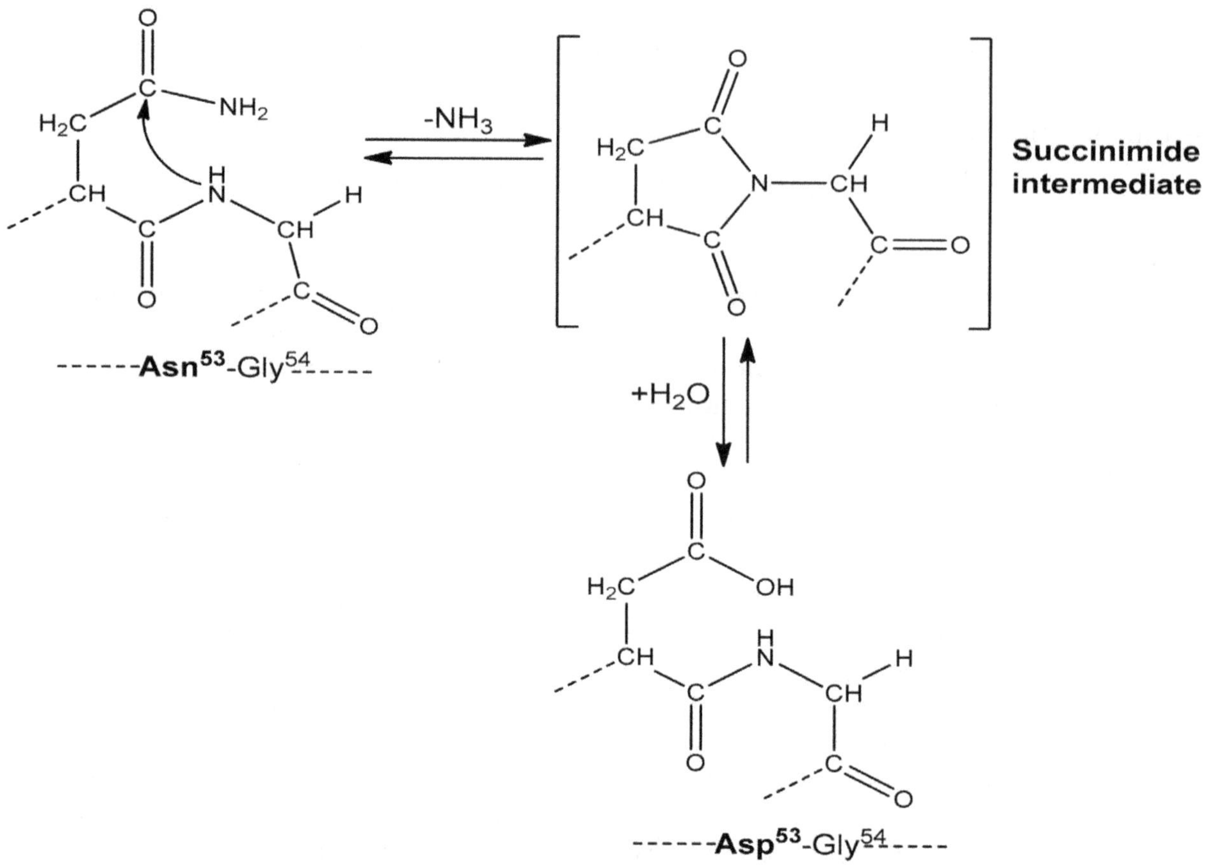

Scheme 2. The main deamidation product of -Asn^{53}-Gly^{54}- sequence in MOG peptides under basic conditions.

Our HPLC findings showed the presence of a new product when the peptide (with the -Asn^{53}-Gly^{54}- sequence) was dissolved in bicarbonate buffer solution, pH 9.0. Twenty-four hours after the dilution, the percentage of formation was almost stabilized and remained about 16% of the total. The estimated deamidation degree remained constant after three days when the analysis was repeated. The revealed new products were isolated from the mixture via HPLC and analyzed by NMR. The main NMR observations clearly indicated a partial deamidation of Asn^{53} in (KG)$_5$MOG$_{35-55}$ peptide (Pep 5) to Asp^{53}. The effect of chemically modified peptides conjugated to the oxidized form of mannan (Con-Pep 8 and Con-Pep 9) was evaluated in vivo in C57BL/6 mice using the EAE animal model of MS. The deaminated derivative containing Asp at position 53 showed similar immunological activity with the native peptide. This evidence suggests that the deaminated product did not affect the biological action of the native peptide and its efficacy while tested in the animal model for the treatment of MS.

Supplementary Materials:
Figure S1: RP-HPLC chromatogram of Pep 1 (MOG$_{41-55}$) at 214.4 nm, at time zero and 48 h after dilution; (A) dissolved in water, (B) dissolved in bicarbonate buffer pH 9.0; $t_{R\,(main\ product)}$: 7.47 min (83.1%) and $t_{R\,(byproduct)}$: 8.27 min (13.9%), Figure S2: ESI-MS spectra of Pep 1 (MOG$_{41-55}$) dissolved in bicarbonate buffer, pH 9.0; of main product (A) and byproduct (B); MW $_{theoretical\ (main\ product)}$: 1826.12 Da, Figure S3: RP-HPLC chromatogram of Pep 2 [MOG$_{41-55}$ (Ala^{53})] at 214.4 nm, at time zero and 48 h after dilution; (A) dissolved in water, (B) dissolved in bicarbonate buffer pH 9.0; $t_{R\,(main\ product)}$: 8.45 min (100%) and $t_{R\,(byproduct)}$: do not observed, Figure S4: ESI-MS spectra of Pep 2 [MOG$_{41-55}$ (Ala^{53})]; MW $_{theoretical\ (main\ product)}$: 1783.11 Da, Figure S5: RP-HPLC chromatogram of Pep 3 [MOG$_{41-55}$ (Asp^{53})] at 214.4 nm, at time zero and 48 h after dilution; (A) dissolved in water, (B) dissolved in bicarbonate buffer pH 9.0; $t_{R\,(main\ product)}$: 8.3 min (100%) and $t_{R\,(byproduct)}$: do not observed; (C) RP-HPLC chromatogram after co-injection of MOG$_{41-55}$ (Pep 1) (dissolved in bicarbonate buffer) and MOG$_{41-55}$ (Asp^{53}) (Pep 3) (dissolved in water) at 214.4 nm, Figure S6: ESI-MS spectra of Pep 3 [MOG$_{41-55}$ (Asp^{53})]; MW $_{theoretical\ (main\ product)}$: 1827.12 Da, Figure S7: RP-HPLC chromatogram of Pep 4 [MOG$_{41-55}$ (isoAsp^{53})] at 214.4 nm, dissolved in water; $t_{R\,(main\ product)}$: 7.6 min (100%), Figure S8:

ESI-MS spectra of Pep 4 [$MOG_{41–55}$ ($isoAsp^{53}$)]; MW $_{theoretical\ (main\ product)}$: 1827.12 Da, Figure S9: RP-HPLC chromatogram of Pep 5 [$(KG)_5MOG_{35–55}$] at 214.4 nm, at time zero and 48 h after dilution; (A) dissolved in water, (B) dissolved in bicarbonate buffer pH 9.0; $t_{R\ (main\ product)}$: 13.3 min (88.6%) and $t_{R\ (byproduct)}$: 13.9 min (11.4%), Figure S10: ESI-MS spectra of Pep 5 [$(KG)_5MOG_{35–55}$] dissolved in bicarbonate buffer, pH 9.0; of main product (A) and byproduct (B). MW $_{theoretical\ (main\ product)}$: 3518.1 Da, Figure S11: RP-HPLC chromatogram of Pep 6 [$(KG)_5MOG_{35–55}(Asp^{53})$] at 214.4 nm, at 48 h after dilution; (A) dissolved in water, (B) dissolved in bicarbonate buffer pH 9.0; $t_{R\ (main\ product)}$: 13.8 min, Figure S12: RP-HPLC chromatogram of Pep 7 [$(KG)_5MOG_{35–55}(isoAsp^{53})$] at 214.4 nm, at 48 h after dilution; (A) dissolved in water, (B) dissolved in bicarbonate buffer pH 9.0; $t_{R\ (main\ product)}$: 13.3 min, Figure S13: RP-HPLC chromatogram of co-injection [$(KG)_5MOG_{35–55}(Asn^{53})$-$(KG)_5MOG_{35–55}(Asp^{53})$] at 214.4 nm, at 48 h after dilution in bicarbonate buffer pH 9.0; $t_{R\ (pep\ 5)}$: 13.3 min, $t_{R\ (pep\ 6)}$: 13.9 min, Figure S14: RP-HPLC chromatogram of Pep 8 [$(KG)_5MOG_{35–55}(Ser^{42})$] at 214.4 nm, at time zero after dilution; (A) dissolved in water, (B) dissolved in bicarbonate buffer pH 9.0, Figure S15: ESI-MS spectra of Pep 8 [$(KG)_5MOG_{35–55}(Ser^{42})$] dissolved in bicarbonate buffer, pH 9.0; of main product (A) and byproduct (B); MW $_{theoretical\ (main\ product)}$: 3508.07 Da; MW $_{theoretical\ (by\ product)}$: 3509.06 Da, Figure S16: Expanded regions of TOCSY spectra of: (A) $(KG)_5MOG_{35–55}$ (Pep 5) and (B) isolated byproduct, after semipreparative-HPLC purification, $(KG)_5MOG_{35–55}(Asp^{53})$ (Pep 6) of $(KG)_5MOG_{35–55}$ (Pep 5) recorded in bicarbonate buffer, pH 9.0, Figure S17: Expanded regions of TOCSY spectra of: (A) $MOG_{41–55}$ (Pep 1), (B) $MOG_{41–55}(Asp^{53})$ (Pep 3), (C) $MOG_{41–55}(isoAsp^{53})$ (Pep 4) and (D) $MOG_{41–55}(Ala^{53})$ (Pep 2) recorded in bicarbonate buffer, pH 9.0, Table S1: Chemical shifts in ppm of α, β protons of residues 51 and 53 and α, δ protons of residue 52 for peptides 1 to 7 in bicarbonate buffer (pH 9.0) referenced according to DSS-d_6. These chemical shifts define the position of representative cross-peaks in expanded TOCSY spectra (Figure 2, Figures S16 and S17) relevant for the explanation of degradation of peptides containing Asn at position 53.

Author Contributions: All authors contributed equally. M.-E.A., A.N. and A.G. carried out the synthesis and HPLC analysis of MOG peptides; L.P. designed and analyzed the EAE experiments; M.A. and A.D. carried out the EAE experiments; T.T. designed the MOG peptides and analyzed the HPLC chromatograms; S.G.G. designed and studied the NMR experiments; All authors analyzed the data; T.T. and S.G.G. wrote the paper together with all co-authors. All authors have read and agreed to the published version of the manuscript.

Acknowledgments: AmbioPharm in USA for observations during early stability studies and pharmaceutical company Vianex SA in Greece for their continuous support for Multiple Sclerosis research studies. We recorded NMR spectra on NMR spectrometers of Slovenian NMR Centre at National Institute of Chemistry.

Abbreviations

MOG	Myelin Oligodendrocyte Glycoprotein
MS	Multiple Sclerosis
EAE	Experimental Autoimmune Encephalomyelitis
SPPS	Solid Phase Peptide Synthesis
RP-HPLC	Reverse Phase-High Performance Liquid Chromatography
ESI-MS	Electron Spray Ionization-Mass Spectrometry
DQF-COSY	Double Quantum-Filtered Correlated Spectroscopy
TOCSY	Total Correlated Spectroscopy
NOESY	Nuclear Overhauser Effect Correlation Spectroscopy
ROESY	Rotating-Frame Nuclear Overhauser Effect Correlation Spectroscopy
HSQC	Heteronuclear Single Quantum Coherence

References

1. Kaspar, A.A.; Reichert, J.M. Future directions for peptide therapeutics. *Drug. Discov. Today* **2013**, *18*, 807–817. [CrossRef]
2. Lau, L.J.; Dunn, K.M. Therapeutic peptides: Historical perspectives, current development trends, and future directions. *Bioorg. Med. Chem.* **2017**, *26*, 2700–2707. [CrossRef]
3. Fosgerau, K.; Hoffmann, T. Peptide therapeutics: Current status and future directions. *Drug. Discov. Today* **2014**, *20*, 122–128. [CrossRef] [PubMed]
4. Vlieghe, P.; Lisowski, V.; Martinez, J.; Khrestchatisky, M. Synthetic therapeutic peptides: Science and market. *Drug. Discov. Today* **2010**, *15*, 40–56. [CrossRef] [PubMed]
5. Currier, J.; Galley, L.; Wenschuh, H.; Morafo, V.; Ratto-Kim, S.; Gray, C.; Maboko, L.; Hoelscher, M.; Marovich, M.; Cox, J. Peptide impurities in commercial synthetic peptides and their implications for vaccine trial assessment. *Clin. Vac. Immunol.* **2008**, *15*, 267–276. [CrossRef] [PubMed]
6. Vogt, W. Oxidation of methionyl residues in proteins: Tools, targets, and reversal. *Free Radic. Biol. Med.* **1995**, *18*, 93–105. [CrossRef]

7. Posadaz, A.; Biasutti, A.; Casale, C.; Sanz, J.; Amat-Guerri, F.; García, N. A Rose Bengal-sensitized photooxidation of the dipeptides L-tryptophyl-L-phenylalanine, L-tryptophyl-L-tyrosine and L-tryptophyl-L-tryptophan: Kinetics, mechanism and photoproducts. *Photochem. Photobiol.* **2004**, *80*, 132–138. [CrossRef]
8. Katritzky, A.R.; Haase, D.N.; Johnson, J.V.; Chung, A. Benzotriazole-assisted solid-phase assembly of Leu-enkephalin, amyloid beta segment 34-42, and other "difficult" peptide sequences. *J. Org. Chem.* **2009**, *74*, 2028–2032. [CrossRef]
9. Angell, Y.; Alsina, J.; Albericio, F.; Barany, G. Practical protocols for stepwise solid-phase synthesis of cysteine-containing peptides. *J. Pept. Res.* **2002**, *60*, 292–299. [CrossRef]
10. Angeletti, R.H.; Bibbs, L.; Bonewald, L.F.; Fields, G.B.; Kelly, J.W.; McMurray, J.S.; Moore, W.T.; Weintraub, S.T. 1997. Analysis of racemization during "standard" solid phase peptide synthesis: A multicenter study. In *Techniques in Protein Chemistry VIII*; Marshak, D.R., Ed.; Academic Press, Inc.: San Diego, CA, USA, 1997; pp. 875–890.
11. Han, Y.; Albericio, F.; Barany, G. Occurrence and Minimization of Cysteine Racemization during Stepwise Solid-Phase Peptide Synthesis. *J. Org. Chem.* **1997**, *7*, 4307–4312. [CrossRef]
12. Vommina, V.V.; Narendra, N. Protection Reactions. In *Amino Acids, Peptides and Proteins in Organic Chemistry. In Protection Reactions, Medicinal Chemistry, Combinatorial Synthesis*; Hughes, A.B., Ed.; Wiley-VCH Verlag GmbH & Co.: Weinheim, Germany, 2011; Volume 4; pp. 1–97.
13. Yang, Y. Peptide Oxidation/Reduction Side Reactions. In *Side Reactions in Peptide Synthesis*; Elsevier Inc.: Amsterdam, The Netherlands, 2015; pp. 217–233.
14. Yang, H.; Zubarev, R. Mass spectrometric analysis of asparagine deamidation and aspartate isomerization in polypeptides. *Electrophoresis* **2010**, *31*, 1764–1772. [CrossRef] [PubMed]
15. Ouellette, D.; Chumsae, C.; Clabbers, A.; Radziejewski, C.; Correia, I. Comparison of the *in vitro* and *in vivo* stability of a succinimide intermediate observed on a therapeutic IgG1 molecule. *mAbs* **2013**, *5*, 432–444. [CrossRef] [PubMed]
16. Zhang, J.; Yip, H.; Katta, V. Identification of isomerization and racemization of aspartate in the Asp-Asp motifs of a therapeutic protein. *Anal. Biochem.* **2011**, *410*, 234–243. [CrossRef]
17. Machado, Y.; Rabasa, Y.; Montesinos, R.; Cremata, J.; Besada, V.; Fuentes, D.; Castillo, A.; de la Luz, K.; Vázquez, A.; Himly, M. Physicochemical and biological characterization of 1E10 Anti-Idiotype vaccine. *BMC Biotechnol.* **2011**, *11*, 112.
18. Cacia, J.; Keck, R.; Presta, L.G.; Frenz, J. Isomerization of an aspartic acid residue in thecomplementarity-determining regions of a recombinant antibody to human IgE: Identification and effect on binding affinity. *Biochemistry* **1996**, *35*, 1897–1903. [CrossRef] [PubMed]
19. Xie, M.; Shahrokh, Z.; Kadkhodayan, M.; Henzel, W.J.; Powell, M.F.; Borchardt, R.T.; Schowen, R.L. Asparagine deamidation in recombinant human lymphotoxin: Hindrance by three-dimensional structures. *J. Pharm. Sci.* **2003**, *92*, 869–880. [CrossRef] [PubMed]
20. Stevenson, C.L.; Friedman, A.R.; Kubiak, T.M.; Donlan, M.E.; Borchardt, R.T. Effect of secondary structure on the rate of deamidation of several growth hormone releasing factor analogs. *Int. J. Pept. Protein Res.* **1993**, *42*, 497–503. [CrossRef]
21. Di Salvo, M.L.; Delle Fratte, S.; Maras, B.; Bossa, F.; Wright, H.T.; Schirch, V. Deamidation of asparagine residues in a recombinant serine hydroxy methyltransferase. *Arch. Biochem. Biophys.* **1999**, *372*, 271–279. [CrossRef]
22. Huang, L.; Lu, J.; Wroblewski, V.J.; Beals, J.M.; Riggin, R.M. In vivo deamidation characterization of monoclonal antibody by LC/MS/MS. *Anal. Chem.* **2005**, *77*, 1432–1439. [CrossRef]
23. Kerlero de Rosbo, N.; Milo, R.; Lees, M.B.; Burger, D.; Bernard, C.C.; Ben-Nun, A. Reactivity to myelin antigens in multiple sclerosis. Peripheral blood lymphocytes respond predominantly to myelin oligodendrocyte glycoprotein. *J. Clin. Investig.* **1993**, *92*, 2602–2608. [CrossRef]
24. Linington, C.; Berger, T.; Perry, L.; Werth, S.; Hinze-Selch, D.; Zhang, Y.; Lu, H.C.; Lassmann, H.; Wekerle, H. T cells specific for the myelin oligodendrocyte glycoprotein mediate an unusual autoimmune inflammatory response in the central nervous system. *Eur. J. Immunol.* **1993**, *23*, 1364–1372. [CrossRef] [PubMed]
25. Amor, S.; Groome, N.; Linington, C.; Morris, M.M.; Dornmair, K.; Gardinier, M.V.; Matthieu, J.M.; Baker, D. Identification of epitopes of myelin oligodendrocyte glycoprotein for the induction of experimental allergic encephalomyelitis in SJL and Biozzi AB/H mice. *J. Immunol.* **1994**, *153*, 4349–4356. [PubMed]

26. Ichikawa, M.; Johns, T.G.; Liu, J.; Bernard, C.C. Analysis of the fine B cell specificity during the chronic/relapsing course of a multiple sclerosis-like disease in Lewis rats injected with the encephalitogenic myelin oligodendrocyte glycoprotein peptide 35–55. *J. Immunol.* **1996**, *157*, 919–926. [PubMed]
27. Constantinescu, C.S.; Farooqi, N.; O'Brien, K.; Gran, B. Experimental autoimmune encephalomyelitis (EAE) as a model for multiple sclerosis (MS). *Br. J. Pharmacol.* **2011**, *164*, 1079–1106. [CrossRef] [PubMed]
28. Bittner, S.; Afzali, A.M.; Wiendl, H.; Meuth, S.G. Myelin oligodendrocyte glycoprotein (MOG35–55) induced experimental autoimmune encephalomyelitis (EAE) in C57BL/6 mice. *J. Vis. Exp.* **2014**, *86*, e51275.
29. Stromnes, I.M.; Goverman, J.M. Active induction of experimental allergic encephalomyelitis. *Nat. Protoc.* **2006**, *1*, 1810–1819. [CrossRef]
30. Tselios, T.; Aggelidakis, M.; Tapeinou, A.; Tseveleki, V.; Kanistras, I.; Gatos, D.; Matsoukas, J. Rational design and synthesis of altered peptide ligands based on Human myelin oligodendrocyte glycoprotein 35-55 epitope: Inhibition of chronic experimental autoimmune encephalomyelitis in mice. *Molecules* **2014**, *19*, 17968–17984. [CrossRef]
31. Tseveleki, V.; Tselios, T.; Kanistras, I.; Koutsoni, O.; Karamita, M.; Vamvakas, S.S.; Apostolopoulos, V.; Dotsika, E.; Matsoukas, J.; Lassmann, H.; et al. Mannan-conjugated myelin peptides prime non-pathogenic Th1 and Th17 cells and ameliorate experimental autoimmune encephalomyelitis. *Exp. Neurol.* **2014**, *267*, 254–267. [CrossRef]
32. Tapeinou, A.; Matsoukas, M.T.; Simal, C.; Tselios, T. Review cyclic peptides on a merry-go-round; towards drug design. *Biopolymers* **2015**, *104*, 453–461. [CrossRef]
33. Day, S.; Tselios, T.; Androutsou, M.E.; Tapeinou, A.; Frilligou, I.; Stojanovska, L.; Matsoukas, J.; Apostolopoulos, V. Mannosylated Linear and Cyclic Single Amino Acid Mutant Peptides Using a Small 10 Amino Acid Linker Constitute Promising Candidates Against Multiple Sclerosis. *Front. Immunol.* **2015**, *6*, 136. [CrossRef]
34. Tapeinou, A.; Androutsou, M.E.; Kyrtata, K.; Vlamis-Gardikas, A.; Apostolopoulos, V.; Matsoukas, J.; Tselios, T. Conjugation of a peptide to mannan and its confirmation by tricine sodium dodecyl sulfate-polyacrylamide gel electrophoresis. *Anal. Biochem.* **2015**, *485*, 43–45. [CrossRef] [PubMed]
35. Tapeinou, A.; Giannopoulou, E.; Simal, C.; Hansen, B.E.; Kalofonos, H.; Apostolopoulos, V.; Vlamis-Gardikas, A.; Tselios, T. Design, synthesis and evaluation of an anthraquinone derivative conjugated to myelin basic protein immunodominant (MBP85-99) epitope: Towards selective immunosuppression. *Eur. J. Med. Chem.* **2018**, *143*, 621–631. [CrossRef] [PubMed]
36. Androutsou, M.E.; Tapeinou, A.; Vlamis-Gardikas, A.; Tselios, T. Myelin Oligodendrocyte Glycoprotein and Multiple Sclerosis. *Med. Chem.* **2018**, *14*, 120–128. [CrossRef] [PubMed]
37. Yannakakis, M.P.; Simal, C.; Tzoupis, H.; Rodi, M.; Dargahi, N.; Prakash, M.; Mouzaki, A.; Platts, J.A.; Apostolopoulos, V.; Tselios, T. Design and Synthesis of Non-Peptide Mimetics Mapping the Immunodominant Myelin Basic Protein (MBP83-96) Epitope to Function as T-Cell Receptor Antagonists. *Int. J. Mol. Sci.* **2017**, *18*, 1215. [CrossRef] [PubMed]
38. Lutterotti, A.; Yousef, S.; Sputtek, A.; Stürner, K.; Stellmann, J.P.; Breiden, P.; Reinhardt, S.; Schulze, C.; Bester, M.; Heesen, C.; et al. Antigen-Specific Tolerance by Autologous Myelin Peptide-Coupled Cells: A Phase 1 Trial in Multiple Sclerosis. *Sci. Transl. Med.* **2013**, *5*, 188ra75. [CrossRef]
39. Emmanouil, M.; Tseveleki, V.; Triantafyllakou, I.; Nteli, A.; Tselios, T.; Probert, L. A Cyclic Altered Peptide Analogue Based on Myelin Basic Protein 87–99 Provides Lasting Prophylactic and Therapeutic Protection Against Acute Experimental Autoimmune Encephalomyelitis. *Molecules* **2018**, *2*, 304. [CrossRef]
40. Tselios, T.; Daliani, I.; Deraos, S.; Thymianou, S.; Matsoukas, E.; Troganis, A.; Gerothanassis, I.; Mouzaki, A.; Mavromoustakos, T.; Probert, L.; et al. Treatment of experimental allergic encephalomyelitis (eae) by a rationally designed cyclic analogue of myelin basic protein (mbp) epitope 72–85. *Bioorg. Med. Chem. Lett.* **2000**, *10*, 2713–2717. [CrossRef]
41. Tselios, T.; Apostolopoulos, V.; Daliani, I.; Deraos, S.; Grdadolnik, S.; Mavromoustakos, T.; Melachrinou, M.; Thymianou, S.; Probert, L.; Mouzaki, A.; et al. Antagonistic effects of human cyclic MBP(87–99) altered peptide ligands in experimental allergic encephalomyelitis and human t-cell proliferation. *J. Med. Chem.* **2002**, *45*, 275–283. [CrossRef]

42. Matsoukas, J.; Apostolopoulos, V.; Kalbacher, H.; Papini, A.M.; Tselios, T.; Chatzantoni, K.; Biagioli, T.; Lolli, F.; Deraos, S.; Papathanassopoulos, P.; et al. Design and synthesis of a novel potent myelin basic protein epitope 87-99 cyclic analogue: Enhanced stability and biological properties of mimics render them a potentially new class of immunomodulators. *J. Med. Chem.* **2005**, *48*, 1470–1480. [CrossRef]
43. Mantzourani, E.D.; Platts, J.A.; Brancale, A.; Mavromoustakos, T.M.; Tselios, T.V. Molecular dynamics at the receptor level of immunodominant myelin basic protein epitope 87–99 implicated in multiple sclerosis and its antagonists altered peptide ligands: Triggering of immune response. *J. Mol. Graph. Model.* **2007**, *26*, 471–481. [CrossRef]
44. Mantzourani, E.D.; Mavromoustakos, T.M.; Platts, J.A.; Matsoukas, J.M.; Tselios, T.V. Structural requirements for binding of myelin basic protein (mbp) peptides to mhc ii: Effects on immune regulation. *Curr. Med. Chem.* **2005**, *12*, 1521–1535. [CrossRef] [PubMed]
45. Friligou, I.; Rizzolo, F.; Nuti, F.; Tselios, T.; Evangelidou, M.; Emmanouil, M.; Karamita, M.; Matsoukas, J.; Chelli, M.; Rovero, P.; et al. Divergent and convergent synthesis of polymannosylated dibranched antigenic peptide of the immunodominant epitope mbp(83–99). *Bioorg. Med. Chem.* **2013**, *21*, 6718–6725. [CrossRef] [PubMed]
46. Ieronymaki, M.; Androutsou, M.E.; Pantelia, A.; Friligou, I.; Crisp, M.; High, K.; Penkman, K.; Gatos, D.; Tselios, T. Use of the 2-chlorotrityl chloride resin for microwave-assisted solid phase peptide synthesis. *Biopolymers* **2015**, *104*, 506–514. [CrossRef] [PubMed]
47. Dagkonaki, A.; Avloniti, M.; Evangelidou, M.; Papazian, I.; Kanistras, I.; Tseveleki, V.; Lampros, F.; Tselios, T.; Jensen, L.T.; Möbius, W.; et al. Mannan-$MOG_{35–55}$ reverses experimental autoimmune encephalomyelitis, inducing a peripheral type 2 myeloid response, reducing CNS inflammation and preserving axons in spinal cord lesions. *Front. Immunol.* **2020**, accepted for publication.
48. Mendel, I.; de Rosbo, N.K.; Ben-Nun, A. A myelin oligodendrocyte glycoprotein peptide induces typical chronic experimental autoimmune encephalomyelitis in H-2b mice: Fine specificity and T cell receptor V beta expression of encephalitogenic T cells. *Eur. J. Immunol.* **2015**, *25*, 1951–1959. [CrossRef]

2

Relationship between Fatigue and Physical Activity in a Polish Cohort of Multiple Sclerosis Patients

Michalina Rzepka [1], Mateusz Toś [1], Michał Boroń [2], Katarzyna Gibas [1] and Ewa Krzystanek [1,*]

1 Department of Neurology, Faculty of Medical Sciences in Katowice, Medical University of Silesia, 40-752 Katowice, Poland; michalina.rzepka93@gmail.com (M.R.); mateusz.tos@sum.edu.pl (M.T.); kgibas@sum.edu.pl (K.G.)

2 Department of Gynecology and Obstetrics, Faculty of Medical Sciences in Katowice, Medical University of Silesia, 40-752 Katowice, Poland; michal.boron123@gmail.com

* Correspondence: ekrzystanek@sum.edu.pl

Abstract: *Background and objectives:* Fatigue is one of the most common and disabling symptoms of multiple sclerosis (MS). It can be defined as a subjective lack of physical and mental energy. The aim of this study was to evaluate the frequency and severity of fatigue in patients with MS and its relationship with overall physical activity and disease-related disability. *Materials and Methods:* The study included 100 patients with a clinical relapsing-remitting form of MS. Patients with severe depression were excluded. Neurological impairment was rated using the Expanded Disability Status Scale (EDSS). Fatigue was assessed using the Modified Fatigue Impact Scale (MFIS) and the Fatigue Severity Scale (FSS), with FSS scores greater than 36 indicating patients with fatigue. Physical activity was evaluated with the International Physical Activity Questionnaire (IPAQ) and categorized on three levels: low, moderate, and high, using standard metabolic equivalents (MET). *Results:* The average FSS and MFIS scores were (mean ± SD) 31.3 ± 15.2 and 30.1 ± 17.0, respectively. The mean EDSS score was 2.5 ± 1.5. 42%. Patients were classified as fatigued based on FSS. Fatigued patients had higher mean EDSS scores than non-fatigued (3.0 ± 1.6 vs. 2.2 ± 1.4, respectively, $p = 0.002$). Low, moderate, and high levels of physical activity were reported in 35%, 20%, and 45% of patients, respectively. Higher scores of fatigue in FSS and MFIS were inversely correlated with the intensity of physical activity ($r = -0.38$, $p < 0.001$ and $r = -0.33$, $p < 0.001$, respectively). *Conclusions:* In patients with MS, fatigue is a common symptom. Patients with lower physical activity and greater MS-related disability have a higher severity of fatigue, which negatively affects cognitive, psychosocial, and physical functioning.

Keywords: multiple sclerosis; fatigue; physical activity; disability; professional activity

1. Introduction

Multiple sclerosis (MS) is a chronic, inflammatory-demyelinating disease of the central nervous system [1]. There are over 2 million people suffering from MS worldwide and approximately 40,000–60,000 in Poland [2,3]. Moreover, it is one of the main causes of disability among young people [4,5]. Multifocal cerebral damage is characterized by a large variety of symptoms, such as paresis, sensation deficits, or balance disorders, which are often accompanied by mental and cognitive disorders or excessive fatigue [6].

Fatigue occurs in many pathological conditions, whereas MS belongs to neurological diseases most often accompanied by fatigue. It is defined as a subjective feeling of a lack of energy to start and sustain any activity, which is unrelated to depression or muscle weakness. In contrast to tiredness, fatigue is characterized by longer duration, lack of improvement after rest, intensification under the influence of heat, and the peak of intensity occurring in the morning. Until now, no clear cause of fatigue has been found. It is believed that pathophysiology is complex and multifactorial. In many neurological disorders, fatigue is perceived as one of the most disabling symptoms, which has a strong impact on every aspect of the patients' life, e.g., quality of life or social and professional functioning [7–13]. For clinicians, it is important to understand the relationship of fatigue with the progress of MS and its association with patients' physical performance.

Therefore, the objective of this study was to assess the prevalence and severity of fatigue among patients with MS and its relationship with overall physical activity and disease-related disability.

2. Materials and Methods

The study involved 100 Polish patients with a relapsing-remitting form of MS (RRMS), treated in the Neurological Outpatient Clinic and Department of Neurology of our institution from December 2016 to March 2018. All participants had to have confirmed diagnosis of RRMS, according to the 2010 Revised McDonald criteria [14]. The exclusion criterion was severe depression, determined with Beck's Depression Inventory (BDI). The study was performed in compliance with the Declaration of Helsinki. Ethics committee approval was not required as this was a questionnaire-based survey, which did not fulfil the criteria of a medical experiment. All participants gave their oral informed consent before providing any information to the questionnaire.

In the first part of the questionnaire, we collected demographic and socioeconomic data (gender, age, educational level, marital status, place of residence, smoking, profession), as well as basic clinical information (comorbidities, duration of MS, first symptoms, course of the disease, present and previous treatment, and number of relapses).

Fatigue was assessed using two scales: The Fatigue Severity Scale (FSS) [15] and the Modified Fatigue Impact Scale (MFIS) [16]. The International Physical Activity Questionnaire (IPAQ) [17] was used to assess physical activity and BDI was used to evaluate depressive disorders [18,19].

The FSS is the most common tool used to assess severity of fatigue, through nine items concerning various aspects of fatigue over the last week. Higher scoring indicates greater severity of fatigue, with a maximum score of 63. A score above 36 is considered abnormal and indicates fatigue [8–10,15,20]. In this study, we have implemented this cut-off to identify participants with fatigue and to assess the overall incidence of fatigue in patients with MS.

The MFIS consists of three subscales, which assess impact of fatigue on physical (F-1, 9 items), cognitive (F-2; 10 items), and psychosocial functioning (F-3; 2 items) over the last four weeks [16]. The respondent answers the question by determining the frequency of specific disorders. The result ranges from 21 to 105 points. The higher the value of the result, the greater the effect of fatigue on the patient's functioning [7,16,21–23].

The Polish version of the IPAQ short-form consists of seven questions to indirectly evaluate physical activity throughout the last week prior to the survey [18,24]. Questions concern physical activity related to everyday life, work, and leisure. Physical activity was expressed as a standard metabolic equivalent (MET) of the task (unit of work/kg body weight/hour) in MET-min/week [25]. Depending on the result, patients were categorized to three groups of different levels of physical activity: low (below 600 MET-min/week), moderate (600–1499 MET-min/week), or high (at least 1500 MET-min/week) [18,24].

BDI was used to evaluate possible exclusion criteria: the presence and severity of depressive symptoms. It was a self-administered questionnaire containing 21 questions covering a period of the past 2 weeks. Higher scoring indicated greater severity of depression with the maximum score of 63, and scores of 30 or greater indicate severe depression [18,19,26].

To quantify disability and neurological impairment, the Expanded Disability Status Scale (EDSS) was used [27]. The EDSS scores range from 0 (no disability) to 10 (death due to MS) in 0.5-unit increments. Higher scores indicate greater disability, with scores from 1.0 to 4.5 assigned to patients who are able to walk without any aid and scores from 5.0 to 9.5 assigned to patients with different levels of walking impairment. This assessment was performed by an experienced neurologist, who was certified in administering the scale.

Statistical analysis was performed with the Statistica 13.0 software (TIBCO Software Inc., Palo Alto, CA, USA) [28]. For assessing distribution, we used the Shapiro-Wilk test. The between-group comparisons were performed with a *t*-test, chi-squared test, Mann-Whitney U test, or ANOVA, with post-hoc pairwise comparisons performed using Dunn's multiple comparison test. Correlations were assessed using the Pearson correlation coefficients or the Spearman correlation coefficients. Significance was determined at the level of $p < 0.05$.

3. Results

3.1. Fatigue—General Results

The study group consisted of 100 patients with RRMS; 78 women and 22 men, aged 38.8 ± 9.8 years (mean ± SD), with an age range of 19–65 years. The average FSS score was 31.3 ± 15.2 points, and 42 patients (42%) had scores greater than 36. Patients with fatigue had a higher mean score of EDSS than patients without fatigue (3.0 ± 1.6 vs. 2.2 ± 1.4, respectively, $p = 0.002$) and a longer mean duration of the disease than those without fatigue (9.6 ± 5.2 years vs. 7.1 ± 6.9, respectively, $p = 0.003$). Demographic, socioeconomic, and clinical data of the studied group are summarized in Table 1.

Table 1. Demographic, socioeconomic, and clinical characteristics of the studied patients with relapsing-remitting multiple sclerosis (MS), categorized as fatigued and non-fatigued based on Fatigue Severity Scale (FSS) scores.

Characteristics	Whole Group ($n = 100$)	Fatigued ($n = 42$)	Non-Fatigued ($n = 58$)	p
Gender n (%)				
Women	78 (78%)	85.7%	72.4%	0.110 *
Men	22 (22%)	14.2%	27.6%	
Age (years) (mean ± SD)	38.8 ± 9.8	41.0 ± 9.4	37.3 ± 9.9	0.071 †
Marital status n (%)				
Single	40 (40%)	33.3%	44.8%	0.247 *
In relationship	60 (60%)	55.2%	44.8%	
Place of residence n (%)				
Rural areas	12 (12%)	14.3%	10.3%	
Town (population):				
up to 50,000	18 (18%)	14.3%	20.7%	0.616 *
50,000–99,999	18 (18%)	14.3%	20.7%	
100,000 and more	52 (52%)	57.1%	48.3%	
Smoking n (%)				
Yes	12 (12%)	4.8%	17.2%	0.058 *
No	88 (88%)	95.2%	82.8%	
Education n (%)				
Vocational	12 (12%)	19.0%	6.9%	
Secondary	32 (32%)	42.9%	24.1%	0.007 *
Higher	56 (56%)	38.1%	69.0%	
Duration of the disease (years) (mean ± SD)	8.19 ± 6.34	9.6 ± 5.2	7.1 ± 6.9	0.003 ‡
EDSS (mean ± SD)	2.5 ± 1.5	3.0 ± 1.6	2.2 ± 1.4	0.002 ‡
MET (mean ± SD)	2234 ± 2865	1294 ± 2317	2860 ± 3038	<0.001 ‡
MFIS total score (mean ± SD)	30.0 ± 17.0	42.4 ± 13.0	21.2 ± 13.7	<0.001 †
MFIS physical score (mean ± SD)	14.1 ± 8.4	19.9 ± 6.4	10.0 ± 7.1	<0.001 ‡
MFIS cognitive score (mean ± SD)	13.2 ± 8.0	18.6 ± 7.0	9.4 ± 6.3	<0.001 †
MFIS psychosocial score (mean ± SD)	2.8 ± 2.0	4.1 ± 1.4	1.8 ± 1.7	<0.001 ‡

Fatigued and non-fatigued patients were categorized based on FFS, where scores up to 36 indicated non-fatigue. Multiple sclerosis (MS); Fatigue Severity Scale (FSS); Metabolic equivalent (MET) estimated with International Physical Activity Questionnaire (IPAQ); Modified Fatigue Impact Scale (MFIS); Expanded Disability Status Scale (EDSS); standard deviation (SD); *p*—values of statistical significance for comparisons of fatigued and non-fatigued patients; *—chi-squared test; †—student's *t*-test; ‡—Mann–Whitney U test.

3.2. Fatigue and Physical Activity

According to the IPAQ, 35% of subjects had low (below 600 MET-min/week), 20% moderate (600–1499 MET-min/week), and 45% high (above 1500 MET-min/week) levels of physical activity over the previous 7 days. The average level of physical activity measured with MET was significantly lower in patients with fatigue than in those without (mean ± SD; 1294 ± 2317 vs. 2860 ± 3038, respectively, $p < 0.001$) (Table 1), and overall FSS scores were inversely correlated with levels of physical activity ($r = -0.38$, $p < 0.001$) (Table 2). Similar results were found in the total MFIS score ($r = -0.33$, $p < 0.001$) and in physical and psychosocial subscales of the MFIS ($r = -0.36$, and $r = -0.36$, $p < 0.001$, respectively). Subjects who were more physically active also had lower levels of fatigue in the MFIS cognitive score ($r = -0.25$, $p = 0.012$) (Table 2 and Figure 1).

Table 2. Correlations of demographic, socioeconomic, and clinical characteristics with fatigue scores in studied patients with relapsing-remitting MS.

Characteristics		FSS Score	MFIS Total Score	MFIS Physical Score	MFIS Psychosocial Score	MFIS Cognitive Score
Age	R	0.17 *	0.27 †	0.32 *	0.38 *	0.18 †
	p	0.09	0.00	0.00	0.00	0.09
Place of residence	R	0.00 *	0.02 *	−0.02 *	0.02 *	0.03 *
	p	0.97	0.84	0.88	0.86	0.76
Smoking	R	−0.04 *	−0.02 *	0.01 *	0.02 *	−0.11 *
	p	0.70	0.86	0.95	0.83	0.28
Education	R	−0.21 *	−0.23 *	−0.21 *	−0.28 *	−0.21 *
	p	0.04	0.02	0.03	0.01	0.03
Duration of the disease	R	0.30 *	0.27 *	0.37 *	0.37 *	0.29 *
	p	0.00	0.00	0.00	0.00	0.00
IPAQ (MET)	R	−0.38 *	−0.33 *	−0.36 *	−0.36 *	−0.25 *
	p	0.00	0.00	0.00	0.00	0.01
EDSS	R	0.36 *	0.45 *	0.49 *	0.54 *	0.29 *
	p	0.00	0.00	0.00	0.00	0.00

Fatigue Severity Scale (FSS); Modified Fatigue Impact Scale (MFIS); Metabolic equivalent (MET) estimated with International Physical Activity Questionnaire (IPAQ); Expanded Disability Status Scale (EDSS); *—Spearman's rank correlation coefficient; †—Pearson correlation coefficient.

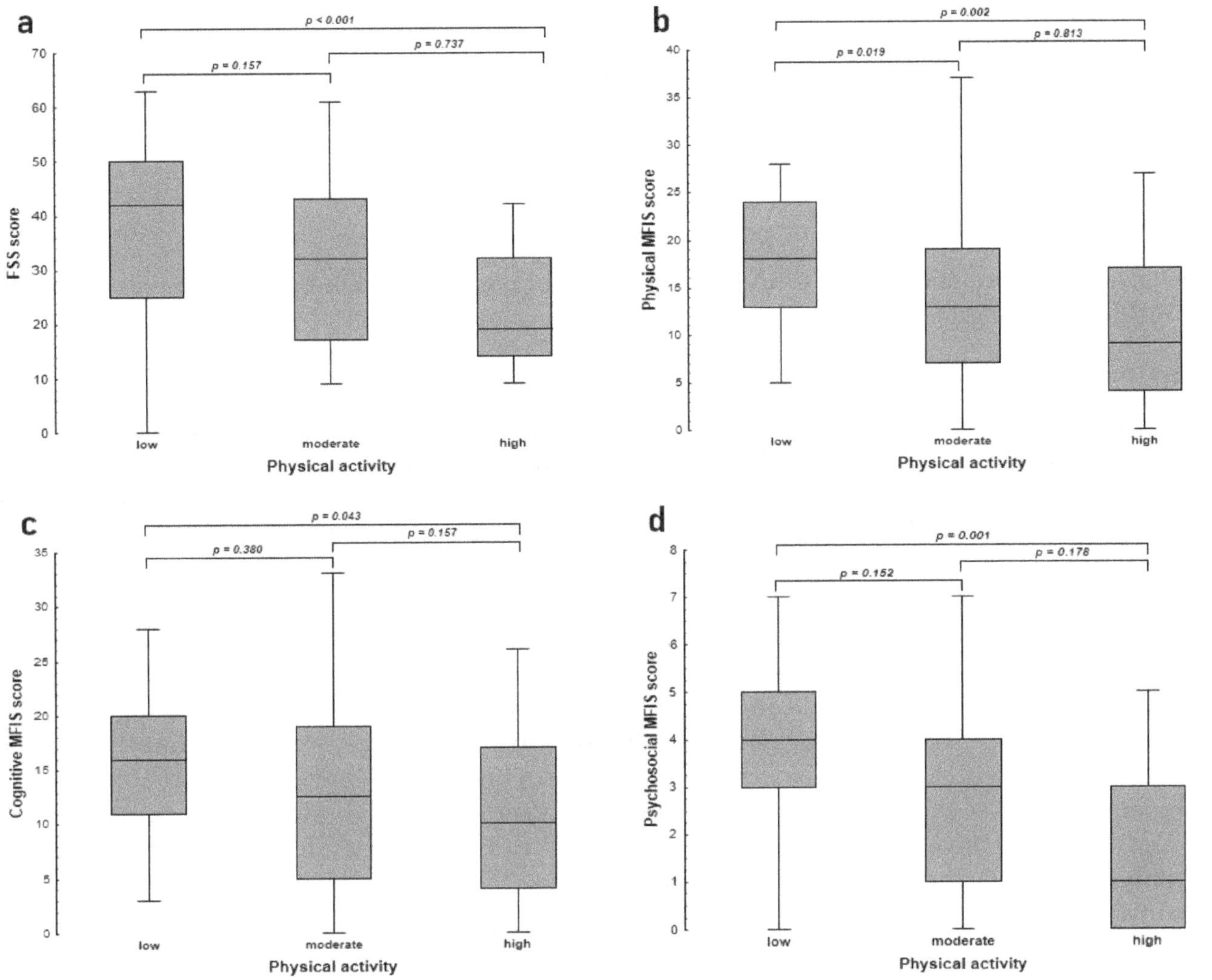

Figure 1. Intensity of fatigue in three groups of patients with MS categorized by their level of physical activity: low ($n = 35$), moderate ($n = 20$), and high ($n = 45$). Engagement in physical activities (low, moderate, and high) assessed with the International Physical Activity Questionnaire (IPAQ). Intensity of fatigue assessed with the Fatigue Severity Scale (FSS) (**a**) and the Modified Fatigue Impact Scale (MFIS) (**b–d**). Higher scores in fatigue scales represent greater fatigue perceived. Between-group comparisons were performed with ANOVA ($p < 0.05$ in each scale) and presented pairwise comparisons performed with the post-hoc Dunn's multiple comparison test. The central line of the box represents the median score; the top and bottom of the box represent the 1st and 3rd quartiles; and the ends of the whiskers represent the minimum and maximum values.

3.3. Fatigue and Disability

Mean EDSS scores were higher in patients with fatigue than in those without (3.0 ± 1.6 vs. 2.2 ± 1.4, respectively, $p = 0.002$) (Table 1). Greater neurological disability assessed with EDSS was associated with higher levels of fatigue, measured with FSS, and higher impact of fatigue on patients' functioning, measured with all MFIS scores (Table 2).

3.4. Fatigue and Disease Duration

Patients with fatigue had MS longer than those without (9.6 ± 5.2 vs. 7.1 ± 6.9 years, respectively, $p = 0.003$) (Table 1). Duration of MS was positively correlated with the impact of fatigue on a patient's life, measured with MFIS total physical, psychosocial, and cognitive scores (Table 2).

3.5. Fatigue and Professional Status

Among professionally active patients (overall 62%), a higher proportion of participants was categorized as non-fatigued based on the FSS score than those not professionally active (68% vs. 47%, respectively, $p = 0.044$). Moreover, professionally active patients had overall lower MFIS total scores than those who were non-active (27.5 ± 17.4 vs. 34.3 ± 15.7, respectively, $p = 0.046$).

3.6. Fatigue and Gender, Place of Residence, or Smoking

No significant correlations were found between severity or impact of fatigue and patients' gender, place of residence, or cigarette smoking.

4. Discussion

Our study showed that the prevalence of fatigue among Polish patients with a relapsing-remitting form of MS, who were not substantially disabled or limited in their functioning (mean EDSS of 2.5 ± 1.5), is quite high (42%). According to Lobentanz et al., for 60.3% of patients with MS, fatigue is one of the three most troublesome symptoms of the disease, and for 64.1%, it significantly affects work and family life [29]. Many investigators proved that fatigue has a significant impact on quality of life [30–33]. Similar results to ours have been reported in other studies. Runia et al. found the occurrence of fatigue in 46.5% of patients with clinically isolated syndrome (CIS) [34]. Simpson et al. examined almost 300 patients, mostly with low levels of disability (median EDSS 1.5), detecting fatigue in 41.3% [35]. However, in many publications, the prevalence of fatigue is higher, on average between 55–80% [8,13,29,30,36]. The differences between the results may be due to the fact that the authors included MS patients with a progressive form of the disease, thus with a longer duration of the disease and a higher level of disability [8,13,29,30]. We should consider that both methods of fatigue testing (the FSS and the MFIS) have some limitations, which may be also the reason for some underestimation. The FSS only determines the severity of fatigue, whereas the MFIS measures the impact of fatigue on a patient's life. Grading in MFIS subscales (physical, cognitive, and psychosocial fatigue) does not take into account a possible severity of deficits contributing to observed limitations [37].

The analysis showed that patients with higher neurological disability, according to the EDSS, were significantly more fatigued. We also found that a higher level of fatigue occurs in patients with a longer duration of the disease. Many other studies reported similar conclusions [29,38–42]. Interestingly, some studies confirmed correlation between fatigue and higher disability, but not with the disease duration [35]. This can be explained by the heterogeneous course of MS and the fact that the primary progressive form has a worse course than the relapsing-remitting form. The course of the disease may be mild and neurological disability may not correlate with the disease duration.

This study confirmed a negative correlation between the level of fatigue and intensity of physical activity. The more physically active the patient, the lower the level of fatigue. These results were found in the total MFIS score for all subscales and in FSS score, as well. According to the World Health Organization (WHO), physical activity is defined as any skeletal muscle activity exerted by an individual resulting in energy expenditure [43]. The recommended intensity of physical activity for people with chronic conditions refers to moderate aerobic activity (50–70% of maximum heart rate) of at least 150 min a week or vigorous aerobic activity (70–85% of maximum heart rate) of at least 75 min a week, or a combination of both each week [43]. It was challenging to provide a more detailed recommendation for exercise, since, in our research, intensity of physical activity was measured by a self-reported questionnaire. Over the years, many studies have confirmed that higher physical activity improves fatigue [20,35,44–52], although the pathophysiology of fatigue in MS is multifactorial and still not fully understood. Langeskov-Christensen's study shows that exercise can alleviate fatigue on both the primary and secondary pathways [44]. It is still unknown which exercises have the most beneficial effect on fatigue. According to Latimer-Cheung et al., exercise of moderate intensity performed twice a week is effective in improving mobility and fatigue in MS patients with mild to moderate disability [53].

Moreover, it seems that resistance training with the use of weights or aerobic training may be most effective for reduction of fatigue [53]. The positive effect may be the result of aerobic capacity and muscle strength improvement, although there are studies demonstrating that aerobic training does not reduce fatigue [54]. It should be noted that, when recommending physical activity, exercises ought to be individually adjusted to the patient's abilities. Inconsistency about the best type of physical activity between studies makes it difficult to draw meaningful recommendations for exact type of exercise or training [21,48–50,54].

Adequate physical activity has a positive impact on the health of patients with chronic diseases [55]. It has been proven that properly selected exercises improve the physical and mental condition in patients with chronic fatigue syndrome (CFS) and are often implemented together with the other forms of therapy [56–61]. However, some researches question the clinical efficacy of graded-exercise-related therapy (GET) [62], while other sources even report deterioration after GET [63,64]. Among several patients with myalgic encephalomyelitis/chronic fatigue syndrome (ME/CFS), the post-exertional "malaise" (PEM) was observed, which can be defined as a 'pathological inability to produce sufficient energy on demand'. Excessive activity can lead to PEM, so it is essential to find a balance between rest and activity for PEM prevention [61,65,66]. In our study, we did not observe such a phenomenon, nor did we determine the optimum level of activity. Interestingly, Janson et al. compared ME/CFS with MS and reported significantly more functional limitation and more severe symptoms in ME/CSF patients than those with MS [67].

Interestingly, more physically active patients were also mostly professionally active. We showed a marked reduction in fatigue in the professionally active group compared to unemployed or pensioners. Similar conclusions are confirmed by other studies [8,13,35]. On the other hand, it should be noted that chronic fatigue is one of the main causes of unemployment among patients with MS [68–70].

Our results confirmed previous observations, that the incidence and level of fatigue is not different between genders in patients with MS [8,13,22,34,71–73]. However, some studies indicate that fatigue may be more frequent or more severe in women [7,35]. The explanation of gender differences requires further research.

This study has several limitations. It was based on a self-report questionnaire, which entails the risk of a reporting bias and some associated confounding factors. The study group might not be representative of the entire population of MS patients (e.g., a higher prevalence of women, only the relapsing-remitting course of the disease, average low disability). We also did not investigate the differences in the effect of physical activity on fatigue and the type of exercise. Taking into consideration the limitations of this study, further research is needed.

Fatigue, due to its high prevalence and significant impact on the quality of life, is a crucial problem among patients with MS. In clinical practice, we often observe insufficient effectiveness of pharmacological treatment. To effectively reduce the occurrence of fatigue, further research should be performed to understand its etiology. It is also important to identify other factors that can reduce fatigue. It seems that physical involvement associated with professional activities may represent protective measures for fatigue in MS patients or contribute to a decrease of its level, despite a long duration of illness. The specific impact of physical activity could contribute to the creation of new recommendations and thus to the improvement of a patient's quality of life.

5. Conclusions

In patients with MS, fatigue is a common symptom. Patients with lower physical activity and greater MS-related disability have a higher severity of fatigue, which negatively affects cognitive, psychosocial, and physical functioning. Fatigue is more severe in MS patients with longer disease duration and higher levels of disability.

Author Contributions: Conceptualization, E.K., M.R. and M.B.; methodology, E.K., M.R. and M.B.; software, M.T.; validation, M.T. and E.K.; formal analysis, M.T.; investigation, M.R., M.B. and M.T.; resources, E.K.; data curation, M.T.; writing—original draft preparation, M.R., K.G., M.B., M.T. and E.K.; writing—review and editing, E.K.;

visualization, M.R., K.G. and M.T.; supervision, E.K.; project administration, E.K. and M.R.; All authors have read and agreed to the published version of the manuscript.

Acknowledgments: We thank all the patients who agreed to participate in this research.

References

1. Reich, D.S.; Lucchinetti, C.F.; Calabresi, P.A. Multiple sclerosis. *N. Engl. J. Med.* **2018**, *378*, 169–180. [CrossRef] [PubMed]
2. Atlas of MS 2013: Mapping Multiple Sclerosis around the World. London: Multiple Sclerosis International Federation. 2013. Available online: http://www.msif.org/about-ms/publications-and-resources/ (accessed on 19 July 2020).
3. Lad, S.P.; Chapman, C.H.; Vaninetti, M.; Steinman, L.; Green, A.; Boakye, M. Socioeconomic trends in hospitalization for multiple sclerosis. *Neuroepidemiology* **2010**, *35*, 93–99. [CrossRef] [PubMed]
4. Compston, A.; Coles, A. Multiple sclerosis. *Lancet* **2008**, *372*, 1502–1517. [CrossRef]
5. Guzik, A.; Kwolek, A. The prevalence and distribution of Multiple Sclerosis in Poland and around the world. *Przegląd Med. Uniw. Rzesz. Nar. Inst. Leków Warszawie* **2015**, *1*, 55–62.
6. Garczyński, W. Obraz Kliniczny Chorych na Stwardnienie Rozsiane w Kontekście Rehabilitacji Opartej na Objawach. In *Horyzonty Współczesnej Fizjoterapii*; Wydawnictwo WSEiT: Poznań, Poland, 2016; pp. 129–143.
7. Krajewski, S.; Dobek, A.; Zawadka-Kunikowska, M.; Kowalewski, M.; Jakimiec, R.; Kunikowski, K. Zespół przewlekłego zmęczenia problem osób chorych na stwardnienie rozsiane, Hygeia Public Health 2014, 49, 519–525. *Hygeia Public Health* **2014**, *49*, 519–525.
8. Łabuz-Roszak, B.; Kubicka-Baczyk, K.; Pierzchała, K.; Machowska-Majchrzak, A.; Skrzypek, M. Fatigue and its association with sleep disorders, depressive symptoms and anxiety in patients with multiple sclerosis. *Neurol. Neurochir. Pol.* **2012**, *46*, 309–317. [CrossRef] [PubMed]
9. Brola, W.; Fudala, M. Current opinions of pathogenesis and treatment of fatigue syndrome in multiple sclerosis. *Aktualności Neurol.* **2011**, *11*, 23–28.
10. Losy, J. Zmęczenie w stwardnieniu rozsianym. *Farm. Psychiatry Neurol.* **2005**, *3*, 279–282.
11. Ziemssen, T. Multiple sclerosis beyond EDSS: Depression and fatigue. *J. Neurol. Sci.* **2009**, *77* (Suppl. 1), 37–41. [CrossRef]
12. Brenner, P.; Piehl, F. Fatigue and depression in multiple sclerosis: Pharmacological and non-pharmacological interventions. *Acta Neurol. Scand.* **2016**, *134* (Suppl. 200), 47–54. [CrossRef]
13. Lerdal, A.; Celius, E.G.; Krupp, L.; Dahl, A.A. A prospective study of patterns of fatigue in multiple sclerosis. *Eur. J. Neurol.* **2007**, *14*, 1338–1343. [CrossRef] [PubMed]
14. Polman, C.H.; Reingold, S.C.; Banwell, B.; Clanet, M.; Cohen, J.A.; Filippi, M.; Fujihara, K.; Havrdova, E.; Hutchinson, M.; Kappos, L.; et al. Diagnostic criteria for multiple sclerosis: 2010 revisions to the McDonald criteria. *Ann. Neurol.* **2011**, *69*, 292–302. [CrossRef] [PubMed]
15. Krupp, L.B.; LaRocca, N.G.; Muir-Nash, J.; Steinberg, A.D. The fatigue severity scale. Application to patients with multiple sclerosis and systemic lupus erythematosus. *Arch. Neurol.* **1989**, *46*, 1121–1123. [CrossRef] [PubMed]
16. Gruszczak, A.; Bartosik-Psujek, H.; Pocińska, K.; Stelmasiak, Z. Validation analysis of selected psychometric features of Polish version of Modified Fatigue Impact Scale–preliminary findings. *Neurol. Neurochir. Pol.* **2009**, *43*, 148–154.
17. Craig, C.L.; Marshall, A.L.; Sjostrom, M.; Bauman, A.; Booth, M.L.; Ainsworth, B.E.; Pratt, M.; Ekelund, U.; Yngve, A.; Sallis, J.F.; et al. International Physical Activity Questionnaire: 12-country reliability and validity. *Med. Sci Sports Exerc.* **2003**, *35*, 1381–1395. [CrossRef]
18. Beck, A.T.; Ward, C.H.; Mendelson, M.; Mock, J.; Erbaugh, J. An inventory for measuring depression. *Arch. Gen. Psychiatry* **1961**, *4*, 561–571. [CrossRef]
19. Benedict, R.H.; Fishman, I.; McClellan, M.M.; Bakshi, R.; Weinstock-Guttman, B. Validity of the Beck Depression Inventory-Fast Screen in multiple sclerosis. *Mult. Scler.* **2003**, *9*, 393–396. [CrossRef]
20. Pasiut, S.; Juda, K.; Mirek, E.; Szymura, J. Wpływ rehabilitacji na poziom odczuwanego zmęczenia u pacjentów ze stwardnieniem rozsianym. *Fizjoterapia* **2015**, *23*, 3–10. [CrossRef]

21. Coghe, G.; Corona, F.; Marongiu, E.; Fenu, G.; Frau, J.; Lorefice, L.; Crisafulli, A.; Galli, M.; Concu, A.; Marrosu, M.G.; et al. Fatigue, as measured using the Modified Fatigue Impact Scale, is a predictor of processing speed improvement induced by exercise in patients with multiple sclerosis: Data from a randomized controlled trial. *J. Neurol.* **2018**, *265*, 1328–1333. [CrossRef]
22. Brola, W.; Fudala, M. Problem zmęczenia w stwardnieniu rozsianym. *Przegląd Med. Uniw. Rzesz.* **2010**, *2*, 237–243.
23. Téllez, N.; Río, J.; Tintoré, M.; Nos, C.; Galán, I.; Montalban, X. Does the Modified Fatigue Impact Scale offer a more comprehensive assessment of fatigue in MS? *Mult. Scler.* **2005**, *11*, 198–202. [CrossRef] [PubMed]
24. Biernat, E.; Stupnicki, R.; Gajewski, A.K. Międzynarodowy Kwestionariusz Aktywności Fizycznej (IPAQ)—Wersja polska. *Wych. Fiz. Sport.* **2007**, *51*, 47–54.
25. Mendes, M.A.; da Silva, I.; Ramires, V.; Reichert, F.; Martins, R.; Ferreira, R.; Tomasi, E. Metabolic equivalent of task (METs) thresholds as an indicator of physical activity intensity. *PLoS ONE* **2018**, *13*, e0200701. [CrossRef] [PubMed]
26. Nagaraj, K.; Taly, A.B.; Gupta, A.; Prasad, C.; Christopher, R. Depression and sleep disturbances in patients with multiple sclerosis and correlation with associated fatigue. *J. Neurosci. Rural. Pract.* **2013**, *4*, 387–391. [CrossRef] [PubMed]
27. Kurtzke, J.F. Rating neurologic impairment in multiple sclerosis: An expanded disability status scale (EDSS). *Neurology* **1983**, *33*, 1444–1452. [CrossRef] [PubMed]
28. Stanisz, A. *Accessible Statistics Course Using Statistica PL Examples from Medicine*; StatSoft Polska: Kraków, Poland, 2006.
29. Lobentanz, I.S.; Asenbaum, S.; Vass, K.; Sauter, C.; Klösch, G.; Kollegger, H.; Kristoferitsch, W.; Zeitlhofer, J. Factors influencing quality of life in multiple sclerosis patients: Disability, depressive mood, fatigue and sleep quality. *Acta Neurol. Scand.* **2004**, *110*, 6–13. [CrossRef]
30. Nagaraj, K.; Taly, A.B.; Gupta, A.; Prasad, C.; Christopher, R. Prevalence of fatigue in patients with multiple sclerosis and its effect on the quality of life. *J. Neurosci. Rural. Pract.* **2013**, *4*, 278–282. [CrossRef]
31. Janardhan, V.; Bakshi, R. Quality of life in patients with multiple sclerosis: The impact of fatigue and depression. *J. Neurol. Sci.* **2002**, *205*, 51–58. [CrossRef]
32. Göksel Karatepe, A.; Kaya, T.; Günaydn, R.; Demirhan, A.; Ce, P.; Gedizlioğlu, M. Quality of life in patients with multiple sclerosis: The impact of depression, fatigue, and disability. *Int. J. Rehabil. Res.* **2011**, *34*, 290–298. [CrossRef]
33. Łabuz-Roszak, B.; Kubicka-Baczyk, K.; Pierzchała, K.; Horyniecki, M.; Machowska-Majchrzak, A.; Augustyńska-Mutryn, D.; Kosałka, K.; Michalski, K.; Pyszak, D.; Wach, J. Quality of life in multiple sclerosis—Association with clinical. *Psychiatr. Pol.* **2013**, *3*, 433–442.
34. Runia, T.F.; Jafari, N.; Siepman, D.A.; Hintzen, R.Q. Fatigue at time of CIS is an independent predictor of a subsequent diagnosis of multiple sclerosis. *J. Neurol. Neurosurg. Psychiatry* **2015**, *86*, 543–546. [CrossRef] [PubMed]
35. Simpson, S., Jr.; Tan, H.; Otahal, P.; Taylor, B.; Ponsonby, A.L.; Lucas, R.M.; Blizzard, L.; Valery, P.C.; Lechner-Scott, J.; Shaw, C.; et al. Anxiety, depression and fatigue at 5-year review following CNS demyelination. *Acta Neurol. Scand.* **2016**, *134*, 403–413. [CrossRef] [PubMed]
36. Kister, I.; Bacon, T.E.; Chamot, E.; Salter, A.R.; Cutter, G.R.; Kalina, J.T.; Herbert, J. Natural history of multiple sclerosis symptoms. *Int. J. MS Care* **2013**, *15*, 146–158. [CrossRef]
37. Patejdl, R.; Penner, I.K.; Noack, T.K.; Zettl, U.K. Multiple sclerosis and fatigue: A review on the contribution of inflammation and immune-mediated neurodegeneration. *Autoimmun. Rev.* **2016**, *15*, 210–220. [CrossRef]
38. Patrick, E.; Christodoulou, C.; Krupp, L.B. New York State MS Consortium. Longitudinal correlates of fatigue in multiple sclerosis. *Mult. Scler.* **2009**, *15*, 258–261. [CrossRef] [PubMed]
39. Braga, D.M.; Prado, G.F.; Bichueti, D.B.; Oliveira, E.M. Positive correlation between functional disability, excessive daytime sleepiness, and fatigue in relapsing-remitting multiple sclerosis. *Arq. Neuropsiquiatr.* **2016**, *74*, 433–438. [CrossRef] [PubMed]
40. Pittion-Vouyovitch, S.; Debouverie, M.; Guillemin, F.; Vandenberghe, N.; Anxionnat, R.; Vespignani, H. Fatigue in multiple sclerosis is related to disability, depression and quality of life. *J. Neurol. Sci.* **2006**, *243*, 39–45. [CrossRef]

41. Colosimo, C.; Millefiorini, E.; Grasso, M.G.; Vinci, F.; Fiorelli, M.; Koudriavtseva, T.; Pozzilli, C. Fatigue in MS is associated with specific clinical features. *Acta Neurol. Scand.* **1995**, *92*, 353–355. [CrossRef]
42. Iriarte, J.; Carreño, M.; Castro, P. Fatigue and functional system involvement in multiple sclerosis. *Neurologia* **1996**, *11*, 210–215.
43. World Health Organization. Global Recommendations on Physical Activity for Health. 2010. Available online: http://apps.who.int/iris/bitstream/10665/44399/1/9789241599979_eng.pdf (accessed on 26 November 2020).
44. Langeskov-Christensen, M.; Bisson, E.J.; Finlayson, M.L.; Dalgas, U. Potential pathophysiological pathways that can explain the positive effects of exercise on fatigue in multiple sclerosis: A scoping review. *J. Neurol. Sci.* **2017**, *373*, 307–320. [CrossRef]
45. Andreasen, A.K.; Stenager, E.; Dalgas, U. The effect of exercise therapy on fatigue in multiple sclerosis. *Mult. Scler.* **2011**, *17*, 1041–1054. [CrossRef] [PubMed]
46. Petajan, J.H.; Gappmaier, E.; White, A.T.; Spencer, M.K.; Mino, L.; Hicks, R.W. Impact of aerobic training on fitness and quality of life in multiple sclerosis. *Ann. Neurol.* **1996**, *39*, 432–441. [CrossRef] [PubMed]
47. Pilutti, L.A.; Greenlee, T.A.; Motl, R.W.; Nickrent, M.S.; Petruzzello, S.J. Effects of exercise training on fatigue in multiple sclerosis: A meta-analysis. *Psychosom. Med.* **2013**, *75*, 575–580. [CrossRef] [PubMed]
48. Mostert, S.; Kesselring, J. Effects of a short-term exercise training program on aerobic fitness, fatigue, health perception and activity level of subjects with multiple sclerosis. *Mult. Scler.* **2002**, *8*, 161–168. [CrossRef] [PubMed]
49. Bansi, J.; Bloch, W.; Gamper, U.; Riedel, S.; Kesselring, J. Endurance training in MS: Short-term immune responses and their relation to cardiorespiratory fitness, health-related quality of life, and fatigue. *J. Neurol.* **2013**, *260*, 2993–3001. [CrossRef]
50. Ozkul, C.; Guclu-Gunduz, A.; Irkec, C.; Fidan, I.; Aydin, Y.; Ozkan, T.; Yazici, G. Effect of combined exercise training on serum brain-derived neurotrophic factor, suppressors of cytokine signaling 1 and 3 in patients with multiple sclerosis. *J. Neuroimmunol.* **2018**, *316*, 121–129. [CrossRef]
51. Edwards, T.; Pilutti, L.A. The effect of exercise training in adults with multiple sclerosis with severe mobility disability: A systematic review and future research directions. *Mult. Scler. Relat. Disord.* **2017**, *16*, 31–39. [CrossRef]
52. Opara, J.; Szwejkowski, W.; Brola, W. Aktualne kierunki rehabilitacji w stwardnieniu rozsianym. *Aktual. Neurol.* **2009**, *9*, 140–146.
53. Latimer-Cheung, A.E.; Pilutti, L.A.; Hicks, A.L.; Martin Ginis, K.A.; Fenuta, A.M.; MacKibbon, K.A.; Motl, R.W. Effects of exercise training on fitness, mobility, fatigue, and health-related quality of life among adults with multiple sclerosis: A systematic review to inform guideline development. *Arch. Phys. Med. Rehabil.* **2013**, *94*, 1800–1828.e3. [CrossRef]
54. Heine, M.; Verschuren, O.; Hoogervorst, E.L.; van Munster, E.; Hacking, H.G.; Visser-Meily, A.; Twisk, J.W.; Beckerman, H.; de Groot, V.; Kwakkel, G.; et al. Does aerobic training alleviate fatigue and improve societal participation in patients with multiple sclerosis? A randomized controlled trial. *Mult. Scler.* **2017**, *23*, 1517–1526. [CrossRef]
55. Blair, S.N.; Morris, J.N. Healthy hearts–and the universal benefits of being physically active: Physical activity and health. *Ann. Epidemiol.* **2009**, *19*, 253–256. [CrossRef] [PubMed]
56. Fulcher, K.Y.; White, P.D. Randomised controlled trial of graded exercise in patients with the chronic fatigue syndrome. *BMJ* **1997**, *314*, 1647–1652. [CrossRef] [PubMed]
57. Clark, L.V.; White, P.D. The role of deconditioning and therapeutic exercise in chronic fatigue syndrome (CFS). *J. Ment. Health* **2005**, *14*, 237–252. [CrossRef]
58. Kim, D.Y.; Lee, J.S.; Park, S.Y.; Kim, S.J.; Son, C.G. Systematic review of randomized controlled trials for chronic fatigue syndrome/myalgic encephalomyelitis (CFS/ME). *J. Transl. Med.* **2020**, *18*, 7. [CrossRef]
59. Avellaneda Fernández, A.; Pérez Martín, A.; Izquierdo Martínez, M.; Arruti Bustillo, M.; Barbado Hernández, F.J.; de la Cruz Labrado, J.; Díaz-Delgado Peñas, R.; Gutiérrez Rivas, E.; Palacín Delgado, C.; Rivera Redondo, J.; et al. Chronic fatigue syndrome: Aetiology, diagnosis and treatment. *BMC Psychiatry* **2009**, *9* (Suppl. 1), S1. [CrossRef]
60. Wallman, K.E.; Morton, A.R.; Goodman, C.; Grove, R. Exercise prescription for individuals with chronic fatigue syndrome. *Med. J. Aust.* **2005**, *183*, 142–143. [CrossRef]

61. Rowe, P.C.; Underhill, R.A.; Friedman, K.J.; Gurwitt, A.; Medow, M.S.; Schwartz, M.S.; Speight, N.; Stewart, J.M.; Vallings, R.; Rowe, K.S. Myalgic Encephalomyelitis/Chronic Fatigue Syndrome Diagnosis and Management in Young People: A Primer. *Front. Pediatrics* **2017**, *5*, 121. [CrossRef]
62. Larun, L.; Brurberg, K.G.; Odgaard-Jensen, J.; Price, J.R. Exercise therapy for chronic fatigue syndrome. *Cochrane Database Syst. Rev.* **2019**, *10*, CD003200. [CrossRef]
63. Bjørkum, T.; Wang, C.E.; Waterloo, K. Patients' experience with treatment of chronic fatigue syndrome. *Tidsskr. Nor. Laegeforen.* **2009**, *129*, 1214–1216. [CrossRef]
64. Twisk, F.N.; Maes, M. A review on cognitive behavorial therapy (CBT) and graded exercise therapy (GET) in myalgic encephalomyelitis (ME)/chronic fatigue syndrome (CFS): CBT/GET is not only ineffective and not evidence-based, but also potentially harmful for many patients with ME/CFS. *Neuro. Endocrinol. Lett.* **2009**, *30*, 284–299.
65. Twisk, F.N. Objective Evidence of Post-exertional "Malaise" in Myalgic Encephalomyelitis and Chronic Fatigue Syndrome. *J. Sports Med. Doping Stud.* **2015**, *5*, 159. [CrossRef]
66. Carruthers, B.M.; van de Sande, M.I.; De Meirleir, K.L.; Klimas, N.G.; Broderick, G.; Mitchell, T.; Staines, D.; Powles, A.C.; Speight, N.; Vallings, R.; et al. Myalgic encephalomyelitis: International Consensus Criteria. *J. Intern. Med.* **2011**, *270*, 327–338. [CrossRef] [PubMed]
67. Jason, L.A.; Ohanian, D.; Brown, A.; Sunnquist, M.; McManimen, S.; Klebek, L.; Fox, P.; Sorenson, M. Differentiating Multiple Sclerosis from Myalgic Encephalomyelitis and Chronic Fatigue Syndrome. *Insights Biomed.* **2017**, *2*, 11. [CrossRef]
68. Smith, M.M.; Arnett, P.A. Factors related to employment status changes in individuals with multiple sclerosis. *Mult. Scler.* **2005**, *11*, 602–609. [CrossRef] [PubMed]
69. Krupp, L.B. Fatigue in multiple sclerosis: Definition, pathophysiology and treatment. *CNS Drugs* **2003**, *17*, 225–234. [CrossRef] [PubMed]
70. Jackson, M.F.; Quaal, C.; Reeves, M.A. Effects of multiple sclerosis on occupational and career patterns. *Axone* **1991**, *13*, 16–22.
71. Mills, R.J.; Young, C.A.; Pallant, J.F.; Tennant, A. Development of a patient reported outcome scale for fatigue in multiple sclerosis: The Neurological Fatigue Index (NFI-MS). *Health Qual. Life Outcomes* **2010**, *8*, 22. [CrossRef]
72. Flachenecker, P.; Kümpfel, T.; Kallmann, B.; Gottschalk, M.; Grauer, O.; Rieckmann, P.; Trenkwalder, C.; Toyka, K.V. Fatigue in multiple sclerosis: A comparison of different rating scales and correlation to clinical parameters. *Mult. Scler.* **2002**, *8*, 523–526. [CrossRef]
73. Iriarte, J.; Subirá, M.L.; Castro, P. Modalities of fatigue in multiple sclerosis: Correlation with clinical and biological factors. *Mult. Scler.* **2000**, *6*, 124–130. [CrossRef]

3

Blood Neurofilament Light Chain: The Neurologist's Troponin?

Simon Thebault [1,*], Ronald A. Booth [2] and Mark S. Freedman [1,*]

1 Department of Medicine and the Ottawa Hospital Research Institute, The University of Ottawa, Ottawa, ON K1H8L6, Canada
2 Department of Pathology and Laboratory Medicine, Eastern Ontario Regional Laboratory Association and Ottawa Hospital Research Institute, University of Ottawa & The Ottawa Hospital, Ottawa, ON K1H8L6, Canada; rbooth@eorla.ca
* Correspondence: sthebault@toh.ca (S.T.); mfreedman@toh.ca (M.S.F.)

Abstract: Blood neurofilament light chain (NfL) is a marker of neuro-axonal injury showing promising associations with outcomes of interest in several neurological conditions. Although initially discovered and investigated in the cerebrospinal fluid (CSF), the recent development of ultrasensitive digital immunoassay technologies has enabled reliable detection in serum/plasma, obviating the need for invasive lumbar punctures for longitudinal assessment. The most evidence for utility relates to multiple sclerosis (MS) where it serves as an objective measure of both the inflammatory and degenerative pathologies that characterise this disease. In this review, we summarise the physiology and pathophysiology of neurofilaments before focusing on the technological advancements that have enabled reliable quantification of NfL in blood. As the test case for clinical translation, we then highlight important recent developments linking blood NfL levels to outcomes in MS and the next steps to be overcome before this test is adopted on a routine clinical basis.

Keywords: neurofilament light chain; biomarkers; multiple sclerosis

---

1. Neurofilament Structure and Function

Neurofilaments are neuronal-specific heteropolymers conventionally considered to consist of a triplet of light (NfL), medium (NfM) and heavy (NfH) chains according to their molecular mass [1]. More recent discoveries show that α-Internexin in the central nervous system [2] and peripherin in the peripheral nervous system [3] can also be included in neurofilament heteropolymers. These five proteins co-assemble into the 10 nM intermediate filaments in different combinations and concentrations depending on the type of neuron, location in the axon and stage of development [4].

Each of the neurofilament proteins consists of an amino-terminal domain that is thought to regulate the formation of oligomers [5], a central helical rod domain, and a variable carboxy-terminal domain. The chain-specific C-terminal domains are the main determinants of differences in molecular mass and phosphorylation between subunits. Following synthesis and assembly in the neuron cell body, tetramers of neurofilament proteins are transported bidirectionally along axons by the microtubular apparatus prior to forming a continuously overlapping array that runs parallel to axons. Once formed, in the healthy state, they are remarkably stable for months to years [6].

In mature myelinated axons, neurofilaments are the single most abundant protein [7]. They perform key roles as part of the neuroaxonal scaffold to resist external pressures, determine axonal diameter, indirectly moderate conduction velocity, and act as an attachment for organelles and other proteins [4]. Beyond their primary structural role in axons, mounting evidence indicates that a unique pool of synaptic neurofilament proteins serves dynamic functions beyond static structural support [8].

Changes in neurofilament phosphorylation may be involved in long term potentiation that underpins memory [9] and NMDA receptor stability is dependent on a synaptic scaffold of neurofilament proteins.

2. Neurofilament Pathophysiology

Damage to central nervous system (CNS) neurons and physiologic turnover causes neurofilament release. This translates to elevated levels in the cerebrospinal fluid (CSF) and eventually blood, where the concentration reflects the rate of release from neurons (Figure 1, where we focus on NfL). Physiologic degradation of neurofilaments within neurons is proposed to be a combination of ubiquitin-mediated proteasomal and apophagocytotic pathways [10]. Based on the trafficking of other proteins degraded in the CNS, it is likely that partially degraded fragments of neurofilaments drain directly into CSF and blood via multiple routes. These include direct drainage into CSF and blood via arachnoid granulations as well as lymphatic drainage into the subarachnoid spaces and perivascular spaces [11,12]. Several studies have demonstrated strong correlations between blood and CSF NfL, with r values typically ranging from 0.7 to 8 (e.g., [13]). However, our understanding of the kinetics of neurofilament release, distribution and metabolism is incomplete.

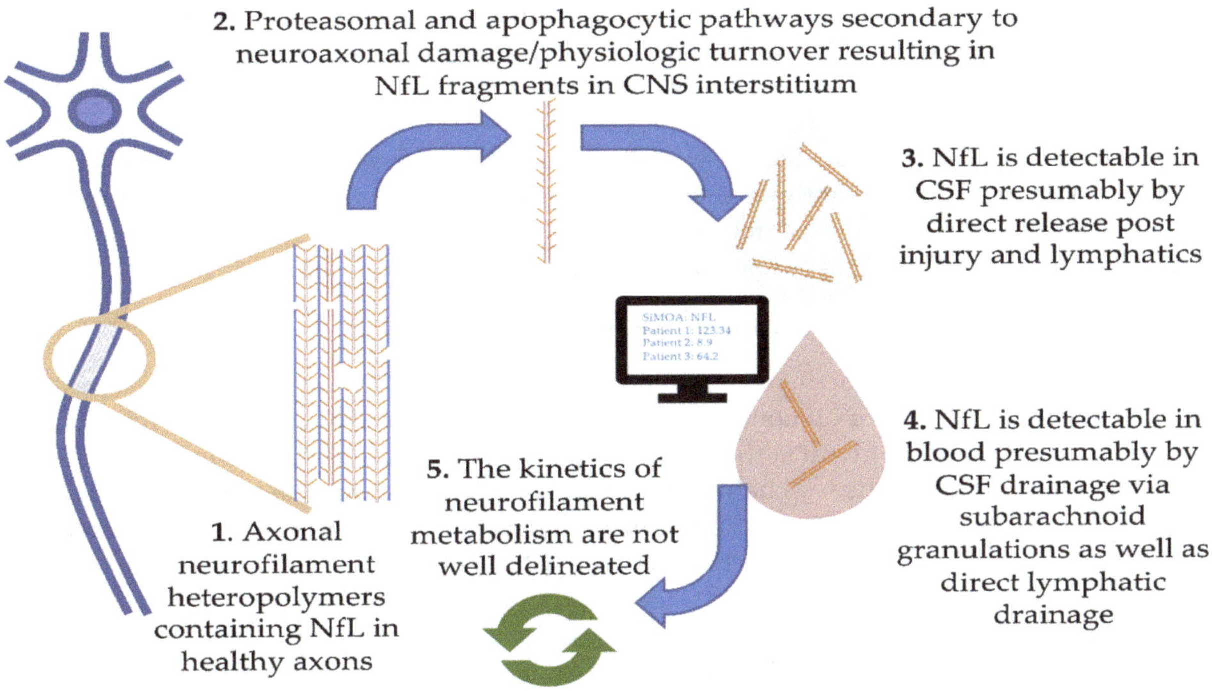

Figure 1. Pathophysiology of neurofilament light chain in blood and cerebrospinal fluid (CSF).

Blood–brain barrier permeability itself may be a confounder; neurofilament quotient in blood compared to CSF could be selectively increased following periods of inflammation such as that seen in MS relapse, positively skewing blood NfL levels. Two recent studies on this topic in MS patients present conflicting results [14,15].

Once NfL enters the blood, the half-life is a key consideration with implications on the frequency of disease activity monitoring. In a longitudinal study of NfL levels before and after intrathecal catheter insertion, NfL in both CSF and serum peaked at 1-month post-surgery, returning to baseline after 6 to 9 months [16]. In longitudinally sampled MS patients around the time of relapse, levels increasing 5 months before, peaking at clinical onset, and recovery within 4–5 months [17]. Therefore, quarterly measurement is likely sufficient, a frequency that our group is currently investigating in longitudinal prospective studies of serum NfL.

Age is the principal physiologic covariate of NfL levels. Levels in healthy controls increase by 2.2% per year [18,19]. Furthermore, an inflection point is observable above the age of 60, after which both sNfL levels, as well as the inter-individual variability in levels, increase greatly [20]. It is speculated that these changes are attributable to both aging itself as well as the accumulation of subclinical comorbidities. Other factors outside of neurological disease itself that may alter neurofilament levels include BMI [21] as well as vascular risk factors [22].

Although the primary focus of this review is the pathophysiologic relevance of NfL concentrations as they relate to neurological diseases such as MS, the vital role of neurofilaments is underlined by various human mutations that interfere with their function and homeostasis. Mutations of gigaxonin, a key component in the ubiquitin-dependent intermediate filament degradation, results in the pathological aggregation of neurofilaments in neurons and a severe neurodegenerative condition called giant axonal neuropathy [23]. Mutations in the neurofilament light chain gene itself result in axonal forms of hereditary motor sensory polyneuropathy [24] and variants of the heavy neurofilament subunit are associated with the development of amyotrophic lateral sclerosis [25].

Intriguingly there is evidence that autoimmunity can be directed against neurofilament proteins themselves [26–30]. CSF from MS patients contain anti-NfL antibodies [26] and these antibodies co-localise with neurons in human MS pathological lesions [27]. The pathogenic potential of anti-NfL antibodies is a topic of debate as the neurofilament light chain is intracellular and presumably not amenable to immune surveillance or targeting in the healthy state. However, intrathecally transferred anti-NfL antibodies in rodent models of experimental autoimmune encephalomyelitis (EAE) results in disability progression [28]. Anti-NfL antibody concentration also appears to correlate with MRI tissue damage, particularly lower brain volumes [29]. Following effective treatment of MS with natalizumab, anti-NfL antibody concentrations decrease [30]. Although the pathogenic potential of antibodies directed against an intracellular antigen such as NfL remains debatable, these circulating antibodies could also have important and unexplored implications on neurofilament metabolism in the periphery as well as interference in NfL assays which are antibody-based immunoassays.

3. Measurement of Blood Levels of Neurofilament Light Chain

Of the family of neurofilament proteins, neurofilament light chain (NfL) has gained the most interest as a candidate marker of outcomes in neurological diseases. This was not without contention. While the neurofilament light chain is the most abundant and soluble of the neurofilament proteins, phosphorylated neurofilament heavy chain (NfH) was initially thought to be more resistant to protease activity [31–33]. NfL was thought to be unstable in vitro [34] and initial research focused on NfH quantified by enzyme-linked immunosorbent assay (ELISA) or electrochemiluminescence (ECL) as a biomarker of axonal damage in MS [35,36]. However, in 2013, a comparative study of NfL and NfH found both proteins showed equivalent stability after several days at room temperature and through freeze–thaw cycles [37]. Moreover, although some of the differences observed may correspond to analytical methodologies, this study found that NfL levels were higher than NfH and NfL was a better discriminator of MS patients from controls.

Initial studies looking at NfL in association with neurological disease outcomes focused on CSF measurements. Although CSF is "closer" to the CNS pathologies (e.g., MS) and NfL concentration is approximately 500-fold higher, the inconvenient and invasive lumbar puncture required severely limits its clinical utility as a frequent serial biomarker. Concentrations in the blood however were too low to be reliably measured with conventional immunoassays such as ELISA or ECL assays. It was not until recently, with the development of the Single-Molecule Assay (SiMoA), that analytical methods become sufficiently sensitive to measure the single-digit picogram per milliliter levels present in blood [38]. This SiMoA technology, similar to other immunoassays, is based on fluorescent microbeads coated with high-affinity capture antibodies that bind NfL followed secondly by a fluorescently labelled detector antibody [39]. The increased analytical sensitivity of the SiMoA assay is due to its unique method of detection. Assay beads with captured NfL and fluorescent detector antibody, are loaded onto an assay disk containing >200,000 microwells capable of holding only a single bead. At high analyte concentration, the total fluorescence can be captured in the traditional manner (analog) and correlated to the analyte concentration. At low analyte concentrations, rather than detecting total fluorescence, a digital image is captured that enumerates individual fluorescent microwells in a binary fashion, effectively lowering the limit of quantitation to the femtomolar range. Although there are several neurofilament assays in development based on other technologies, including widely used chemiluminescent-based assay [40], the data we present here were exclusively generated using the SiMoA platform.

4. Blood NfL in Neurological Diseases

As a neuron-specific marker of neurological injury, elevated NfL levels can be found in a variety of conditions that involve neuroaxonal injury in both the central and peripheral nervous system (reviewed by Khalil et al., 2018 [41]). In purely neurodegenerative diseases, NfL could serve as both a prognostic marker of decline but also an efficacy biomarker of experimental therapies. In a meta-analysis of Alzheimer's disease, frontotemporal and amyotrophic lateral sclerosis [42], plasma NfL levels were elevated in patients compared to controls with utility in differentiating neurodegenerative conditions from non-neurodegenerative mimics. However, due to a lack of specificity to any particular flavor of neurodegeneration, its role as a diagnostic marker is limited. The exception to this is in amyotrophic lateral sclerosis where the uniquely rapid neurodegeneration that characterises this condition results in blood NfL levels several times higher than both controls and other forms of neurodegeneration, and hence may play are role in diagnosis.

In more indolent neurodegenerative processes, early prognostication is an important clinical role. In a study of carriers and non-carriers of autosomal dominant Alzheimer's disease, the trajectory of NfL in affected individuals compared to controls became segregated during their 30's, long before clinical onset [43]. Conversely, in Parkinson's, a condition characterised by particularly slow neurodegeneration, differences between controls and patients are especially small, and the separation NfL trajectories only become apparent after the age of 70 [44] at which point marked disability is usually apparent. Meanwhile, for more acute neuronal injury, neurofilament may also have utility in stroke and traumatic brain injury prognostication. Following a stroke, blood NfL takes several hours to rise, limiting their utility in the hyperacute setting, however, the presence of elevated NfL may have utility in diagnosing subacute strokes as well as in the prognostication of outcomes [45,46]. Similarly, following traumatic brain injury, the extent of NfL increase acutely is predictive of the severity of injury, and while NfL decreases over time, it remains elevated relative to controls several years after the injury. Of recent topical interest, NfL was found to be subtly elevated in the serum of mild-moderate COVID-19 patients [47]. While some have used this evidence to bolster theories of direct neuronal invasion by the virus, these subtle differences could also be attributed to cerebral hypoxia induced by the respiratory virus.

5. Blood NfL in MS

Multiple sclerosis is the most common neurological autoimmune disease, known for its varied clinical presentations and unpredictable clinical course [48]. Over the last few decades, there has been a dramatic expansion in the number of immunosuppressive therapies on offer to prevent damaging bouts of focal inflammation and demyelination that characterise this condition. However, a victim of its own success, objective disease monitoring biomarkers are lacking, and adjuncts that can help neurologists track and personalise treatments are sorely needed. Regular MRI scanning remains the gold standard means of detecting sub-clinical inflammatory lesions [49,50], but this costly and inconvenient test has a number of shortcomings. It is poorly predictive of future activity (Ontaneda and Fox, 2017), lacks sensitivity [51], tends to be focused mainly on the brain (leaving out the spinal cord and optic nerves) and entails a large degree of technical variation and subjective interpretation. Notable examples of fluid biomarkers that are already in clinical use in MS include oligoclonal bands [52] (now part of MS diagnostic criteria), antibodies against aquaporin-4 [53] and myelin oligodendrocyte protein [54] (which define pathologically discrete disease entities which previously fell under the umbrella of MS), as well as serological assays for JC virus [55] (pre-immunosuppression risk stratification). However, as of yet, no fluid biomarker has established clinical use in routine disease monitoring and prediction. As a result of this unmet need, associations of blood neurofilament have been intensely studied in MS. In the last two years, more than 200 studies have contributed to a groundswell of evidence associating NfL with outcomes related to disease activity, progression, treatment response and prognosis.

As a cross-sectional measure in groups of MS patients, the strongest evidence links high NfL levels with inflammatory endpoints such as relapses and MRI lesions [19,56–61]. This is perhaps counter-intuitive, as one might expect this neuroaxonal protein to associate most strongly with outcomes to neurodegeneration and disease progression. However, axonal damage and loss are hallmarks of demyelinating MS lesions even early-on [62], presumably reflected in a transient marked elevation of NfL.

Other than inflammatory disease activity, an interrelated facet of MS pathology is neurodegeneration and progressive disability accrual. Conveniently, this facet of MS pathology is also objectified with NfL measurement. Patients with progressive MS have higher levels than age and sex matched patients with relapsing disease [63]. Associations can be found between high blood NfL levels and poorer disease progression outcomes including disability scores, conversion to a secondary progressive phenotype, MRI atrophy, and measures of cognitive function [13,18,57,61,64–69].

Several groups have also studied the longitudinal significance of blood NfL as a serial disease monitoring/treatment response measure in prospective cohorts from clinical trials. Studies exploring the relationship of NfL kinetics with clinical relapse showed elevations beginning approximately 5 months prior to relapse with a peak at clinical onset and recovery within 4–5 months of remission [17]. When profiled longitudinally, "peaks" of NfL (more than three standard deviations above steady-state) were associated with nearly 80% of MRI and clinical disease activity.

In response to treatment, often related to the availability of retrospective sample sets from well-characterised groups of patients involved in seminal studies, longitudinal NfL reductions have been reported for most established treatments for relapsing MS. These include injectable therapies [18,56,59,70], dimethyl fumarate [71], fingolimod [61,70,72], natalizumab [73], rituximab [74], ocrelizumab [75], ofatumumab [76], alemtuzumab [17] and hematopoietic stem cell transplantation [13]. Encouragingly, reductions in NfL seen after different treatments broadly fall in line with the perceived hierarchy of treatment efficacies, with the greatest reductions seen following the most intensive treatments. Accordingly, in a recent Swedish cohort study of more than 1000 patients receiving one of 6 treatments, the largest reductions in plasma levels were seen following alemtuzumab (48%), and the smallest reduction for teriflunomide (7%), with the other agents falling in the middle [56].

For secondary progressive MS, reductions in NfL have been shown following siponimod [77], ocrelizumab [78] and natalizumab [79]. In primary progressive disease, reductions were seen following fingolimod [80] and ocrelizumab [78]. Given the lack of useful biomarkers otherwise for progressive types of MS, NfL is increasingly seen as an important secondary endpoint in phase 2 and 3 studies of treatments [81].

Many groups have shown the value of NfL in the prediction of future relapses, MRI disease activity, disability worsening, MRI brain and spine atrophy and poorer cognitive outcomes [18,19,59,60,82–84]. In a 5-year longitudinal study of more than 1200 Swiss MS patients, high age-adjusted NfL was associated with increased risk of relapse and new MRI activity in the following year [63]. Even in patients who met criteria for "no evidence of disease activity" [85], higher NfL was independently associated with increased risk of clinical and/or MRI disease activity in the next year, indicating that NfL is capable of predicting subclinical disease activity otherwise not captured. NfL may also have utility in long term prediction, with 2 separate studies finding an association of early NfL measurements with clinical and MRI disease outcomes more than a decade later [86,87].

While NfL is the closest blood-based disease monitoring marker to clinical translation in MS, there are also other promising candidates that may provide additional information. For instance, glial fibrillary acidic protein (GFAP) is a marker of astrocytic turnover or damage that may serve more as a marker of disease progression [88]. Although not a fluid biomarker, ocular coherence tomography (OCT) peripapillary retinal nerve fibre layer thickness also seems to be useful as a biomarker for the prediction of disability progression [89]. Thus, NfL may represent the first of several fluid biomarkers with relevance in MS monitoring and prediction; one-day multimodal composite indices could be used to most accurately objectify different components of an individual patient's disease and inform treatment decisions.

6. Conclusions

Measurement of a convenient objective blood marker of neuronal injury in patients is an appealing prospect for neurologists. Analogous to the cardiologist's troponin, neurofilament light chain is a structural axonal protein that can be detected in the blood at elevated levels in a variety of neurological disease states which can be followed longitudinally. Enabled by recent advancements in assay technologies, many consider this test to be on the verge of clinical translation in a number of different settings. Given its neuron-specific nature, but lack of disease specificity, on its own it is not a helpful diagnostic marker. However, in defined neurological conditions that require monitoring, in particular MS where we have treatments to offer, NfL is rapidly gaining traction.

It seems likely that MS will represent the test case for the clinical translation of blood NfL, where it will be a greatly-needed adjunct to clinical and MRI assessment. While we already know that elevated NfL is concerning and low NfL is reassuring, a number of challenges remain before this test is ready for widespread adoption. Foremost amongst them is the need for age-adjusted normative datasets and cutoff values so that physicians can better interpret individual patient results. Key elements of neurofilament kinetics in the blood, such as blood half-life, need to be delineated to inform optimal testing frequency in clinical practice. Additionally, the ongoing efforts of multisite validation efforts will be important in standardising measurement between clinical laboratories and ensuring that any concerns of analytical validity are allayed. Nonetheless, many are optimistic that NfL could represent the first of its kind in neurology: a broadly-applicable protein biomarker that objectively reflects underlying pathology which can be harnessed to improve patient outcomes.

Author Contributions: S.T.: conceptualization, literature review and writing—original draft preparation, reviewing and editing, R.A.B. and M.S.F.: conceptualization, writing—reviewing and editing, supervision. All authors have read and agreed to the published version of the manuscript.

References

1. Fuchs, E.; Cleveland, D.W. A structural scaffolding of intermediate filaments in health and disease. *Science* **1998**, *279*, 514–519. [CrossRef] [PubMed]
2. Yuan, A.; Rao, M.V.; Sasaki, T.; Chen, Y.; Kumar, A.; Veeranna; Liem, R.K.H.; Eyer, J.; Peterson, A.C.; Julien, J.P.; et al. α-internexin is structurally and functionally associated with the neurofilament triplet proteins in the mature CNS. *J. Neurosci.* **2006**, *26*, 10006–10019. [CrossRef] [PubMed]
3. Yuan, A.; Sasaki, T.; Kumar, A.; Peterhoff, C.M.; Rao, M.V.; Liem, R.K.; Julien, J.P.; Nixon, R.A. Peripherin is a subunit of peripheral nerve neurofilaments: Implications for differential vulnerability of cns and peripheral nervous system axons. *J. Neurosci.* **2012**, *32*, 8501–8508. [CrossRef] [PubMed]
4. Yuan, A.; Rao, M.V.; Veeranna; Nixon, R.A. Neurofilaments and neurofilament proteins in health and disease. *Cold Spring Harb. Perspect. Biol.* **2017**, *9*, a018309. [CrossRef] [PubMed]
5. Ching, G.Y.; Liem, R.K.H. Roles of head and tail domains in α-internexin's self-assembly and coassembly with the neurofilament triplet proteins. *J. Cell Sci.* **1998**, *111*, 321–333.
6. Millecamps, S.; Gowing, G.; Corti, O.; Mallet, J.; Julien, J.P. Conditional NF-L transgene expression in mice for in vivo analysis of turnover and transport rate of neurofilaments. *J. Neurosci.* **2007**, *27*, 4947–4956. [CrossRef]
7. Fliegner, K.H.; Liem, R.K.H. Cellular and Molecular Biology of Neuronal Intermediate Filaments. *Int. Rev. Cytol.* **1991**, *131*, 109–167. [CrossRef]
8. Bragina, L.; Conti, F. Expression of Neurofilament Subunits at Neocortical Glutamatergic and GABAergic Synapses. *Front. Neuroanat.* **2018**, *12*, 74. [CrossRef]

9. Hashimoto, R.; Nakamura, Y.; Komai, S.; Kashiwagi, Y.; Tamura, K.; Goto, T.; Aimoto, S.; Kaibuchi, K.; Shiosaka, S.; Takeda, M. Site-specific phosphorylation of neurofilament-L is mediated by calcium/calmodulin-dependent protein kinase II in the apical dendrites during long-term potentiation. *J. Neurochem.* **2000**, *75*, 373–382. [CrossRef]
10. Bomont, P. Degradation of the Intermediate Filament Family by Gigaxonin. *Methods Enzymol.* **2016**, *569*, 215–231. [CrossRef]
11. Carare, R.O.; Bernardes-Silva, M.; Newman, T.A.; Page, A.M.; Nicoll, J.A.R.; Perry, V.H.; Weller, R.O. Solutes, but not cells, drain from the brain parenchyma along basement membranes of capillaries and arteries: Significance for cerebral amyloid angiopathy and neuroimmunology. *Neuropathol. Appl. Neurobiol.* **2008**, *34*, 131–144. [CrossRef] [PubMed]
12. Gafson, A.R.; Barthélemy, N.R.; Bomont, P.; Carare, R.O.; Durham, H.D.; Julien, J.-P.; Kuhle, J.; Leppert, D.; Nixon, R.A.; Weller, R.O.; et al. Neurofilaments: Neurobiological foundations for biomarker applications. *Brain* **2020**, *143*, 1975–1998. [CrossRef] [PubMed]
13. Thebault, S.; Tessier, D.; Lee, H.; Bowman, M.; Bar-Or, A.; Arnold, D.L.; Atkins, H.; Tabard-Cossa, V.; Freedman, M.S. High Serum Neurofilament Light Chain normalises after Haematopoietic Stem Cell Transplant for MS. *Neurol. Neuroimmunol. Neuroinflamm.* **2019**, *6*, e598. [CrossRef] [PubMed]
14. Kalm, M.; Boström, M.; Sandelius, Å.; Eriksson, Y.; Ek, C.J.; Blennow, K.; Björk-Eriksson, T.; Zetterberg, H. Serum concentrations of the axonal injury marker neurofilament light protein are not influenced by blood-brain barrier permeability. *Brain Res.* **2017**, *1668*, 12–19. [CrossRef]
15. Uher, T.; McComb, M.; Galkin, S.; Srpova, B.; Oechtering, J.; Barro, C.; Tyblova, M.; Bergsland, N.; Krasensky, J.; Dwyer, M.; et al. Neurofilament levels are associated with blood–brain barrier integrity, lymphocyte extravasation, and risk factors following the first demyelinating event in multiple sclerosis. *Mult. Scler. J.* **2020**, 1–12. [CrossRef]
16. Bergman, J.; Dring, A.; Zetterberg, H.; Blennow, K.; Norgren, N.; Gilthorpe, J.; Bergenheim, T.; Svenningsson, A. Neurofilament light in CSF and serum is a sensitive marker for axonal white matter injury in MS. *Neurol. Neuroimmunol. Neuroinflamm.* **2016**, *3*, e271. [CrossRef]
17. Akgün, K.; Kretschmann, N.; Haase, R.; Proschmann, U.; Kitzler, H.H.; Reichmann, H.; Ziemssen, T. Profiling individual clinical responses by high-frequency serum neurofilament assessment in MS. *Neurol. Neuroimmunol. NeuroInflamm.* **2019**, *6*, 1–12. [CrossRef]
18. Disanto, G.; Barro, C.; Benkert, P.; Naegelin, Y.; Schädelin, S.; Giardiello, A.; Zecca, C.; Blennow, K.; Zetterberg, H.; Leppert, D.; et al. Serum Neurofilament light: A biomarker of neuronal damage in multiple sclerosis. *Ann. Neurol.* **2017**, *81*, 857–870. [CrossRef]
19. Barro, C.; Benkert, P.; Disanto, G.; Tsagkas, C.; Amann, M.; Naegelin, Y.; Leppert, D.; Gobbi, C.; Granziera, C.; Yaldizli, Ö.; et al. Serum neurofilament as a predictor of disease worsening and brain and spinal cord atrophy in multiple sclerosis. *Brain* **2018**, *141*, 2382–2391. [CrossRef]
20. Khalil, M.; Pirpamer, L.; Hofer, E.; Voortman, M.M.; Barro, C.; Leppert, D.; Benkert, P.; Ropele, S.; Enzinger, C.; Fazekas, F.; et al. Serum neurofilament light levels in normal aging and their association with morphologic brain changes. *Nat. Commun.* **2020**, *11*, 1–9. [CrossRef]
21. Manouchehrinia, A.; Piehl, F.; Hillert, J.; Kuhle, J.; Alfredsson, L.; Olsson, T.; Kockum, I. Confounding effect of blood volume and body mass index on blood neurofilament light chain levels. *Ann. Clin. Transl. Neurol.* **2020**, *7*, 139–143. [CrossRef] [PubMed]
22. Korley, F.K.; Goldstick, J.; Mastali, M.; Van Eyk, J.E.; Barsan, W.; Meurer, W.J.; Sussman, J.; Falk, H.; Levine, D. Serum NfL (Neurofilament Light Chain) Levels and Incident Stroke in Adults with Diabetes Mellitus. *Stroke* **2019**, *50*, 1669–1675. [CrossRef] [PubMed]
23. Bomont, P.; Cavalier, L.; Blondeau, F.; Hamida, C. Ben; Belal, S.; Tazir, M.; Demir, E.; Topaloglu, H.; Korinthenberg, R.; Tüysüz, B.; et al. The gene encoding gigaxonin, a new member of the cytoskeletal BTB/kelch repeat family, is mutated in giant axonal neuropathy. *Nat. Genet.* **2000**, *26*, 370–374. [CrossRef] [PubMed]
24. Mersiyanova, I.V.; Perepelov, A.V.; Polyakov, A.V.; Sitnikov, V.F.; Dadali, E.L.; Oparin, R.B.; Petrin, A.N.; Evgrafov, O.V. A new variant of Charcot-Marie-Tooth disease type 2 is probably the result of a mutation in the neurofilament-light gene. *Am. J. Hum. Genet.* **2000**, *67*, 37–46. [CrossRef] [PubMed]

25. Figlewicz, D.A.; Krizus, A.; Martinoli, M.G.; Meininger, V.; Dib, M.; Rouleau, G.A.; Julien, J.P. Variants of the heavy neurofilament subunit are associated with the development of amyotrophic lateral sclerosis. *Hum. Mol. Genet.* **1994**, *3*, 1757–1761. [CrossRef]
26. Silber, E.; Semra, Y.K.; Gregson, N.A.; Sharief, M.K. Patients with progressive multiple sclerosis have elevated antibodies to neurofilament subunit. *Neurology* **2002**, *58*, 1372–1381. [CrossRef]
27. Sádaba, M.C.; Tzartos, J.; Paíno, C.; García-Villanueva, M.; Álvarez-Cermeño, J.C.; Villar, L.M.; Esiri, M.M. Axonal and oligodendrocyte-localized IgM and IgG deposits in MS lesions. *J. Neuroimmunol.* **2012**, *247*, 86–94. [CrossRef]
28. Puentes, F.; van der Star, B.J.; Boomkamp, S.D.; Kipp, M.; Boon, L.; Bosca, I.; Raffel, J.; Gnanapavan, S.; van der Valk, P.; Stephenson, J.; et al. Neurofilament light as an immune target for pathogenic antibodies. *Immunology* **2017**, *152*, 580–588. [CrossRef]
29. Eikelenboom, M.J.; Petzold, A.; Lazeron, R.H.C.; Silber, E.; Sharief, M.; Thompson, E.J.; Barkhof, F.; Giovannoni, G.; Polman, C.H.; Uitdehaag, B.M.J. Multiple sclerosis: Neurofilament light chain antibodies are correlated to cerebral atrophy. *Neurology* **2003**, *60*, 219–223. [CrossRef]
30. Amor, S.; van der Star, B.J.; Bosca, I.; Raffel, J.; Gnanapavan, S.; Watchorn, J.; Kuhle, J.; Giovannoni, G.; Baker, D.; Malaspina, A.; et al. Neurofilament light antibodies in serum reflect response to natalizumab treatment in multiple sclerosis. *Mult. Scler. J.* **2014**, *20*, 1355–1362. [CrossRef]
31. Schlaepfer, W.W.; Lee, C.; Lee, V.M.; Zimmerman, U.-J.P. An Immunoblot Study of Neurofilament Degradation In Situ and During Calcium-Activated Proteolysis. *J. Neurochem.* **1985**, *44*, 502–509. [CrossRef] [PubMed]
32. Goldstein, M.E.; Sternberger, N.H.; Sternberger, L.A. Phosphorylation protects neurofilaments against proteolysis. *J. Neuroimmunol.* **1987**, *14*, 149–160. [CrossRef]
33. Pant, H.C. Dephosphorylation of neurofilament proteins enhances their susceptibility to degradation by calpain. *Biochem. J.* **1988**, *256*, 665–668. [CrossRef] [PubMed]
34. Koel-Simmelink, M.J.A.; Teunissen, C.E.; Behradkia, P.; Blankenstein, M.A.; Petzold, A. The neurofilament light chain is not stable in vitro. *Ann. Neurol.* **2011**, *69*, 1065–1066. [CrossRef] [PubMed]
35. Petzold, A.; Keir, G.; Green, A.J.E.; Giovannoni, G.; Thompson, E.J. A specific ELISA for measuring neurofilament heavy chain phosphoforms. *J. Immunol. Methods* **2003**, *278*, 179–190. [CrossRef]
36. Leppert, D.; Petzold, A.; Regeniter, A.; Schindler, C.; Mehling, M.; Anthony, D.C.; Kappos, L.; Lindberg, R.L.P. Neurofilament heavy chain in CSF correlates with relapses and disability in multiple sclerosis. *Neurology* **2011**, *76*, 1206–1213.
37. Kuhle, J.; Plattner, K.; Bestwick, J.P.; Lindberg, R.L.; Ramagopalan, S.V.; Norgren, N.; Nissim, A.; Malaspina, A.; Leppert, D.; Giovannoni, G.; et al. A comparative study of CSF neurofilament light and heavy chain protein in MS. *Mult. Scler. J.* **2013**, *19*, 1597–1603. [CrossRef]
38. Kuhle, J.; Barro, C.; Andreasson, U.; Derfuss, T.; Lindberg, R.; Sandelius, Å.; Liman, V.; Norgren, N.; Blennow, K.; Zetterberg, H. Comparison of three analytical platforms for quantification of the neurofilament light chain in blood samples: ELISA, electrochemiluminescence immunoassay and Simoa. *Clin. Chem. Lab. Med.* **2016**, *54*, 1655–1661. [CrossRef]
39. Wilson, D.H.; Rissin, D.M.; Kan, C.W.; Fournier, D.R.; Piech, T.; Campbell, T.G.; Meyer, R.E.; Fishburn, M.W.; Cabrera, C.; Patel, P.P.; et al. The Simoa HD-1 Analyzer: A Novel Fully Automated Digital Immunoassay Analyzer with Single-Molecule Sensitivity and Multiplexing. *J. Lab. Autom.* **2016**, *21*, 533–547. [CrossRef]
40. Carvalho, T. Siemens Healthineers, Novartis Partner to Develop NfL Diagnostic Test. 2020. Available online: https://multiplesclerosisnewstoday.com/news-posts/2020/09/21/siemens-healthineers-novartis-partner-to-develop-new-nfl-diagnostic-test-for-ms/ (accessed on 28 October 2020).
41. Khalil, M.; Teunissen, C.E.; Otto, M.; Piehl, F.; Sormani, M.P.; Gattringer, T.; Barro, C.; Kappos, L.; Comabella, M.; Fazekas, F.; et al. Neurofilaments as biomarkers in neurological disorders. *Nat. Rev. Neurol.* **2018**, *14*, 577–589. [CrossRef]
42. Forgrave, L.M.; Ma, M.; Best, J.R.; DeMarco, M. The diagnostic performance of neurofilament light chain in CSF and blood for Alzheimer's disease, frontotemporal dementia, and amyotrophic lateral sclerosis: A systematic review and meta-analysis. *Alzheimer's Dement. Diagnosis Assess. Dis. Monit.* **2019**, *11*, 730–743. [CrossRef] [PubMed]

43. Quiroz, Y.T.; Zetterberg, H.; Reiman, E.M.; Chen, Y.; Su, Y.; Fox-Fuller, J.T.; Garcia, G.; Villegas, A.; Sepulveda-Falla, D.; Villada, M.; et al. Plasma neurofilament light chain in the presenilin 1 E280A autosomal dominant Alzheimer's disease kindred: A cross-sectional and longitudinal cohort study. *Lancet Neurol.* **2020**, *19*, 513–521. [CrossRef]
44. Wilke, C.; dos Santos, M.C.T.; Schulte, C.; Deuschle, C.; Scheller, D.; Verbelen, M.; Brockmann, K.; von Thaler, A.K.; Sünkel, U.; Roeben, B.; et al. Intraindividual Neurofilament Dynamics in Serum Mark the Conversion to Sporadic Parkinson's Disease. *Mov. Disord.* **2020**, *35*, 1233–1238. [CrossRef] [PubMed]
45. Nielsen, H.H.; Soares, C.B.; Høgedal, S.S.; Madsen, J.S.; Hansen, R.B.; Christensen, A.A.; Madsen, C.; Clausen, B.H.; Frich, L.H.; Degn, M.; et al. Acute Neurofilament Light Chain Plasma Levels Correlate With Stroke Severity and Clinical Outcome in Ischemic Stroke Patients. *Front. Neurol.* **2020**, *11*. [CrossRef] [PubMed]
46. O'Connell, G.C.; Alder, M.L.; Smothers, C.G.; Still, C.H.; Webel, A.R.; Moore, S.M. Diagnosis of ischemic stroke using circulating levels of brain-specific proteins measured via high-sensitivity digital ELISA. *Brain Res.* **2020**, *1739*. [CrossRef]
47. Ameres, M.; Brandstetter, S.; Toncheva, A.A.; Kabesch, M.; Leppert, D.; Kuhle, J.; Wellmann, S. Association of neuronal injury blood marker neurofilament light chain with mild-to-moderate COVID-19. *J. Neurol.* **2020**. [CrossRef]
48. Confavreux, C.; Vukusic, S. The clinical course of multiple sclerosis. *Handb. Clin. Neurol.* **2014**, *122*, 343–369. [CrossRef]
49. Igra, M.S.; Paling, D.; Wattjes, M.P.; Connolly, D.J.A.; Hoggard, N. Multiple sclerosis update: Use of MRI for early diagnosis, disease monitoring and assessment of treatment related complications. *Br. J. Radiol.* **2017**, *90*, 20160721. [CrossRef]
50. Wattjes, M.P.; Steenwijk, M.D.; Stangel, M. MRI in the Diagnosis and Monitoring of Multiple Sclerosis: An Update. *Clin. Neuroradiol.* **2015**, *25*, 157–165. [CrossRef]
51. Wattjes, M.P.; Rovira, À.; Miller, D.; Yousry, T.A.; Sormani, M.P.; De Stefano, N.; Tintoré, M.; Auger, C.; Tur, C.; Filippi, M.; et al. Evidence-based guidelines: MAGNIMS consensus guidelines on the use of MRI in multiple sclerosis—Establishing disease prognosis and monitoring patients. *Nat. Rev. Neurol.* **2015**, *11*, 597–606. [CrossRef]
52. Freedman, M.S.; Thompson, E.J.; Deisenhammer, F.; Giovannoni, G.; Grimsley, G.; Keir, G.; Öhman, S.; Racke, M.K.; Sharief, M.; Sindic, C.J.M.; et al. Recommended standard of cerebrospinal fluid analysis in the diagnosis of multiple sclerosis: A consensus statement. *Arch. Neurol.* **2005**, *62*, 865–870. [CrossRef] [PubMed]
53. Lennon, V.A.; Wingerchuk, D.M.; Kryzer, T.J.; Pittock, S.J.; Lucchinetti, C.F.; Fujihara, K.; Nakashima, I.; Weinshenker, B.G. A serum autoantibody marker of neuromyelitis optica: Distinction from multiple sclerosis. *Lancet* **2004**, *364*, 2106–2112. [CrossRef]
54. Waters, P.; Woodhall, M.; O'Connor, K.C.; Reindl, M.; Lang, B.; Sato, D.K.; Jurynczyk, M.; Tackley, G.; Rocha, J.; Takahashi, T.; et al. MOG cell-based assay detects non-MS patients with inflammatory neurologic disease. *Neurol. Neuroimmunol. NeuroInflamm.* **2015**, *2*, e89. [CrossRef] [PubMed]
55. Subramanyam, M.; Goelz, S.; Natarajan, A.; Lee, S.; Plavina, T.; Scanlon, J.V.; Sandrock, A.; Bozic, C. Risk of Natalizumab-Associated Progressive Multifocal Leukoencephalopathy. *N. Engl. J. Med.* **2012**, *366*, 1870–1880.
56. Delcoigne, B.; Manouchehrinia, A.; Barro, C.; Benkert, P.; Michalak, Z.; Kappos, L.; Leppert, D.; Tsai, J.A.; Plavina, T.; Kieseier, B.C.; et al. Blood neurofilament light levels segregate treatment effects in multiple sclerosis. *Neurology* **2020**, *94*, e1201–e1212. [CrossRef]
57. Novakova, L.; Zetterberg, H.; Sundström, P.; Axelsson, M.; Khademi, M.; Gunnarsson, M.; Malmeström, C.; Svenningsson, A.; Olsson, T.; Piehl, F.; et al. Monitoring disease activity in multiple sclerosis using serum neurofilament light protein. *Neurology* **2017**, *89*, 2230–2237. [CrossRef]
58. Bittner, S.; Steffen, F.; Uphaus, T.; Muthuraman, M.; Fleischer, V.; Salmen, A.; Luessi, F.; Berthele, A.; Klotz, L.; Meuth, S.G.; et al. Clinical implications of serum neurofilament in newly diagnosed MS patients: A longitudinal multicentre cohort study. *EBioMedicine* **2020**, *56*, 1–13. [CrossRef]
59. Varhaug, K.N.; Barro, C.; Bjørnevik, K.; Myhr, K.M.; Torkildsen, Ø.; Wergeland, S.; Bindoff, L.A.; Kuhle, J.; Vedeler, C. Neurofilament light chain predicts disease activity in relapsing-remitting MS. *Neurol. Neuroimmunol. NeuroInflamm.* **2018**, *5*, e422. [CrossRef]

60. Siller, N.; Kuhle, J.; Muthuraman, M.; Barro, C.; Uphaus, T.; Groppa, S.; Kappos, L.; Zipp, F.; Bittner, S. Serum neurofilament light chain is a biomarker of acute and chronic neuronal damage in early multiple sclerosis. *Mult. Scler. J.* **2018**. [CrossRef]
61. Kuhle, J.; Kropshofer, H.; Haering, D.A.; Kundu, U.; Meinert, R.; Barro, C.; Dahlke, F.; Tomic, D.; Leppert, D.; Kappos, L. Blood neurofilament light chain as a biomarker of MS disease activity and treatment response. *Neurology* **2019**, *92*, E1007–E1015. [CrossRef]
62. Bitsch, A.; Schuchardt, J.; Bunkowski, S.; Kuhlmann, T.; Brück, W. Acute axonal injury in multiple sclerosis. Correlation with demyelination and inflammation. *Brain* **2000**, *123*, 1174–1183. [CrossRef] [PubMed]
63. Yaldizli, O. Value of serum neurofilament light chain levels as a biomarker of suboptimal treatment response in MS clinical practice. *ECTRIMS Online Library*, 10 December 2018.
64. Ferraro, D.; Guicciardi, C.; De Biasi, S.; Pinti, M.; Bedin, R.; Camera, V.; Vitetta, F.; Nasi, M.; Meletti, S.; Sola, P. Plasma neurofilaments correlate with disability in progressive multiple sclerosis patients. *Acta Neurol. Scand.* **2020**, *141*, 16–21. [CrossRef] [PubMed]
65. Högel, H.; Rissanen, E.; Barro, C.; Matilainen, M.; Nylund, M.; Kuhle, J.; Airas, L. Serum glial fibrillary acidic protein correlates with multiple sclerosis disease severity. *Mult. Scler. J.* **2020**, *26*, 210–219. [CrossRef] [PubMed]
66. Filippi, P.; Vestenická, V.; Siarnik, P.; Sivakova, M.; Čopíková-Cudráková, D.; Belan, V.; Hanes, J.; Novák, M.; Kollar, B.; Turcani, P. Neurofilament light chain and MRI volume parameters as markers of neurodegeneration in multiple sclerosis. *Neuro Endocrinol. Lett.* **2020**, *41*, 17–26. [PubMed]
67. Mattioli, F.; Bellomi, F.; Stampatori, C.; Mariotto, S.; Ferrari, S.; Monaco, S.; Mancinelli, C.; Capra, R. Longitudinal serum neurofilament light chain (sNfL) concentration relates to cognitive function in multiple sclerosis patients. *J. Neurol.* **2020**. [CrossRef]
68. Bridel, C.; van Wieringen, W.N.; Zetterberg, H.; Tijms, B.M.; Teunissen, C.E.; Alvarez-Cermeño, J.C.; Andreasson, U.; Axelsson, M.; Bäckström, D.C.; Bartos, A.; et al. Diagnostic Value of Cerebrospinal Fluid Neurofilament Light Protein in Neurology. *JAMA Neurol.* **2019**, *76*, 1035. [CrossRef]
69. Jakimovski, D.; Zivadinov, R.; Ramanthan, M.; Hagemeier, J.; Weinstock-Guttman, B.; Tomic, D.; Kropshofer, H.; Fuchs, T.A.; Barro, C.; Leppert, D.; et al. Serum neurofilament light chain level associations with clinical and cognitive performance in multiple sclerosis: A longitudinal retrospective 5-year study. *Mult. Scler. J.* **2019**. [CrossRef]
70. Reinert, M.C.; Benkert, P.; Wuerfel, J.; Michalak, Z.; Ruberte, E.; Barro, C.; Huppke, P.; Stark, W.; Kropshofer, H.; Tomic, D.; et al. Serum neurofilament light chain is a useful biomarker in pediatric multiple sclerosis. *Neurol. Neuroimmunol. Neuroinflamm.* **2020**, *7*. [CrossRef]
71. Sejbaek, T.; Nielsen, H.H.; Penner, N.; Plavina, T.; Mendoza, J.P.; Martin, N.A.; Elkjaer, M.L.; Ravnborg, M.H.; Illes, Z. Dimethyl fumarate decreases neurofilament light chain in CSF and blood of treatment naïve relapsing MS patients. *J. Neurol. Neurosurg. Psychiatry* **2019**, *90*, 1324–1330. [CrossRef]
72. Piehl, F.; Kockum, I.; Khademi, M.; Blennow, K.; Lycke, J.; Zetterberg, H.; Olsson, T. Plasma neurofilament light chain levels in patients with MS switching from injectable therapies to fingolimod. *Mult. Scler. J.* **2017**. [CrossRef]
73. Gunnarsson, M.; Malmeström, C.; Axelsson, M.; Sundström, P.; Dahle, C.; Vrethem, M.; Olsson, T.; Piehl, F.; Norgren, N.; Rosengren, L.; et al. Axonal damage in relapsing multiple sclerosis is markedly reduced by natalizumab. *Ann. Neurol.* **2011**, *69*, 83–89. [CrossRef] [PubMed]
74. de Flon, P.; Laurell, K.; Sundström, P.; Blennow, K.; Söderström, L.; Zetterberg, H.; Gunnarsson, M.; Svenningsson, A. Comparison of plasma and cerebrospinal fluid neurofilament light in a multiple sclerosis trial. *Acta Neurol. Scand.* **2019**, *139*, 462–468. [CrossRef] [PubMed]
75. Cross, A. Ocrelizumab treatment reduced levels of neurofilament light chain and numbers of B cells in the cerebrospinal fluid of patients with relapsing multiple sclerosis in the OBOE study S56.008. *Neurology* **2019**, *92*, 52.
76. Hauser, S.L.; Bar-Or, A.; Cohen, J.A.; Comi, G.; Correale, J.; Coyle, P.K.; Cross, A.H.; de Seze, J.; Leppert, D.; Montalban, X.; et al. Ofatumumab versus Teriflunomide in Multiple Sclerosis. *N. Engl. J. Med.* **2020**, *383*, 546–557. [CrossRef]
77. Kuhle, J.; Kropshofer, H.; Barro, C.; Meinert, R.; Haring, D.A.; Leppert, D.; Tomic, D.; Dahlke, F.; Kuhle, J.; Kropshofer, H.; et al. Siponimod Reduces Neurofilament Light Chain Blood Levels in Secondary Progressive Multiple Sclerosis Patients. *Neurology* **2018**, *90* (Suppl. 15), S8.006.

78. Bar-Or, A. Blood neurofilament light levels are lowered to a healthy donor range in patients with RMS and PPMS following ocrelizumab treatment. *ECTRIMS Online Library*, 9 December 2019.
79. Kapoor, R.; Sellebjerg, F.; Hartung, H.-P.; Arnold, D.L.; Freedman, M.S.; Jeffery, D.; Miller, A.; Edwards, K.R.; Singh, C.M.; Chang, I.; et al. Natalizumab reduced serum levels of neurofilament light chain in secondary progressive multiple sclerosis patients from the phase 3 ASCEND study. *Mult. Scler. J.* **2018**, *24*, 988. [CrossRef]
80. Kuhle, J.; Kropshofer, H.; Haring, D.A.; Barro, C.; Dahlke, F.; Leppert, D.; Tomic, D. Neurofilament light levels in the blood of patients with secondary progressive MS are higher than in primary progressive MS and may predict brain atrophy in both MS subtypes. *Mult. Scler. J.* **2018**, *24*, 111. [CrossRef]
81. Kapoor, R.; Smith, K.E.; Allegretta, M.; Arnold, D.L.; Carroll, W.; Comabella, M.; Furlan, R.; Harp, C.; Kuhle, J.; Leppert, D.; et al. Serum neurofilament light as a biomarker in progressive multiple sclerosis. *Neurology* **2020**. [CrossRef]
82. Kuhle, J.; Nourbakhsh, B.; Grant, D.; Morant, S.; Barro, C.; Yaldizli, Ö.; Pelletier, D.; Giovannoni, G.; Waubant, E.; Gnanapavan, S. Serum neurofilament is associated with progression of brain atrophy and disability in early MS. *Neurology* **2017**, *88*, 826–831. [CrossRef]
83. Jakimovski, D.; Kuhle, J.; Ramanathan, M.; Barro, C.; Tomic, D.; Hagemeier, J.; Kropshofer, H.; Bergsland, N.; Leppert, D.; Dwyer, M.G.; et al. Serum neurofilament light chain levels associations with gray matter pathology: A 5-year longitudinal study. *Ann. Clin. Transl. Neurol.* **2019**, *6*, 1757–1770. [CrossRef]
84. Manouchehrinia, A.; Stridh, P.; Khademi, M.; Leppert, D.; Barro, C.; Michalak, Z.; Benkert, P.; Lycke, J.; Alfredsson, L.; Kappos, L.; et al. Plasma neurofilament light levels are associated with risk of disability in multiple sclerosis. *Neurology* **2020**, *94*, e2457–e2467. [CrossRef] [PubMed]
85. Lublin, F.D. Disease activity free status in MS. *Mult. Scler. Relat. Disord.* **2012**, *1*, 6–7. [CrossRef] [PubMed]
86. Thebault, S.; Abdoli, M.; Fereshtehnejad, S.M.; Tessier, D.; Tabard-Cossa, V.; Freedman, M.S. Serum neurofilament light chain predicts long term clinical outcomes in multiple sclerosis. *Sci. Rep.* **2020**, *10*, 1–11. [CrossRef] [PubMed]
87. Chitnis, T.; Gonzalez, C.; Healy, B.C.; Saxena, S.; Rosso, M.; Barro, C.; Michalak, Z.; Paul, A.; Kivisakk, P.; Diaz-Cruz, C.; et al. Neurofilament light chain serum levels correlate with 10-year MRI outcomes in multiple sclerosis. *Ann. Clin. Transl. Neurol.* **2018**, 1478–1491. [CrossRef]
88. Novakova, L.; Axelsson, M.; Khademi, M.; Zetterberg, H.; Blennow, K.; Malmeström, C.; Piehl, F.; Olsson, T.; Lycke, J. Cerebrospinal fluid biomarkers as a measure of disease activity and treatment efficacy in relapsing-remitting multiple sclerosis. *J. Neurochem.* **2017**, *141*, 296–304. [CrossRef]
89. Bsteh, G.; Hegen, H.; Teuchner, B.; Amprosi, M.; Berek, K.; Ladstätter, F.; Wurth, S.; Auer, M.; Di Pauli, F.; Deisenhammer, F.; et al. Peripapillary retinal nerve fibre layer as measured by optical coherence tomography is a prognostic biomarker not only for physical but also for cognitive disability progression in multiple sclerosis. *Mult. Scler. J.* **2019**, *25*, 196–203. [CrossRef]

4

Monoclonal Antibodies in Multiple Sclerosis: Present and Future

Natalia V. Voge and Enrique Alvarez *

Rocky Mountain Multiple Sclerosis Center at the University of Colorado, Department of Neurology, University of Colorado School of Medicine, Academic Office 1, Mail Stop B-185, 12631 East 17th Avenue, Aurora, CO 80045, USA; natalia.voge@ucdenver.edu

* Correspondence: Enrique.Alvarez@ucdenver.edu;

Abstract: The global incidence of multiple sclerosis (MS) appears to be increasing. Although it may not be associated with a high mortality rate, this disease has a high morbidity rate which affects the quality of life of patients and reduces their ability to do their activities of daily living. Thankfully, the development of novel disease modifying therapies continues to increase. Monoclonal antibodies (MABs) have become a mainstay of MS treatment and they are likely to continue to be developed for the treatment of this disease. Specifically, MABs have proven to be some of the most efficacious treatments at reducing relapses and the inflammation in MS patients, including the first treatment for primary progressive MS and are being explored as reparative/remyelinating agents as well. These relatively new treatments will be reviewed here to help evaluate their efficacy, adverse events, immunogenicity, and benefit-risk ratios in the treatment of the diverse spectrum of MS. The focus will be on MABs that are currently approved or may be approved in the near future.

Keywords: monoclonal antibodies; anti-CD20; Ocrevus; Rituxan; Tysabri; multiple sclerosis; clinical trial; disease modifying therapy

---

1. Introduction

Monoclonal antibodies (MABs) are one of the preferred treatments for multiple sclerosis (MS) due to their target specificity and usually high efficacy [1]. These have usually targeted the immune system, which plays a key role in the pathogenesis of MS, especially during the early inflammatory stages. MABs bind very specifically to epitopes or parts of larger proteins (antigens) that allow them to mediate their effects on very specific pathways. In MS, MABs are able to more specifically neutralize key immune players that negatively impact the central nervous system. Because of their specificity, they tend to have few off target effects and less drug–drug interactions minimizing their side effects, which tend to arise from their downstream effects on the immune system and reactions to the drugs themselves, although this problem has been greatly reduced with the advent of humanized MABs [1,2].

Therapeutic MABs were originally developed from non-human species such as mice. The first MAB to be approved was muromonab-CD3 (Orthoclone OKT3) which targeted the CD3 surface protein of T lymphocytes to help prevent organ rejection in 1985 [3]. Reactions to murine MABs were soon associated with the development of antidrug antibodies (ADAs) against the murine-based protein with repeated exposures [4]. In order to reduce the potential immunogenicity of murine MABs, chimeric mouse-human antibodies were developed (Figure 1). This occurs by inserting the antigen-specific variable domain of a mouse antibody on the constant domains of a human antibody, producing antibodies that are up to 65% humanized [5,6]. Humanized antibodies that contain human light and heavy chains but retaining murine hypervariable regions being greater than 90% humanized will be developed. Transgenic mouse strains, which express human variable domains, have allowed the production of MABs with a reduced immunogenic potential, making them "fully humanized" and with properties similar to any human antibody [7]. These antibodies can be further modified to change their properties, for example by altering the glycosylation at amino acid N297 to increase their antigen-dependent cellular cytotoxicity (ADCC).

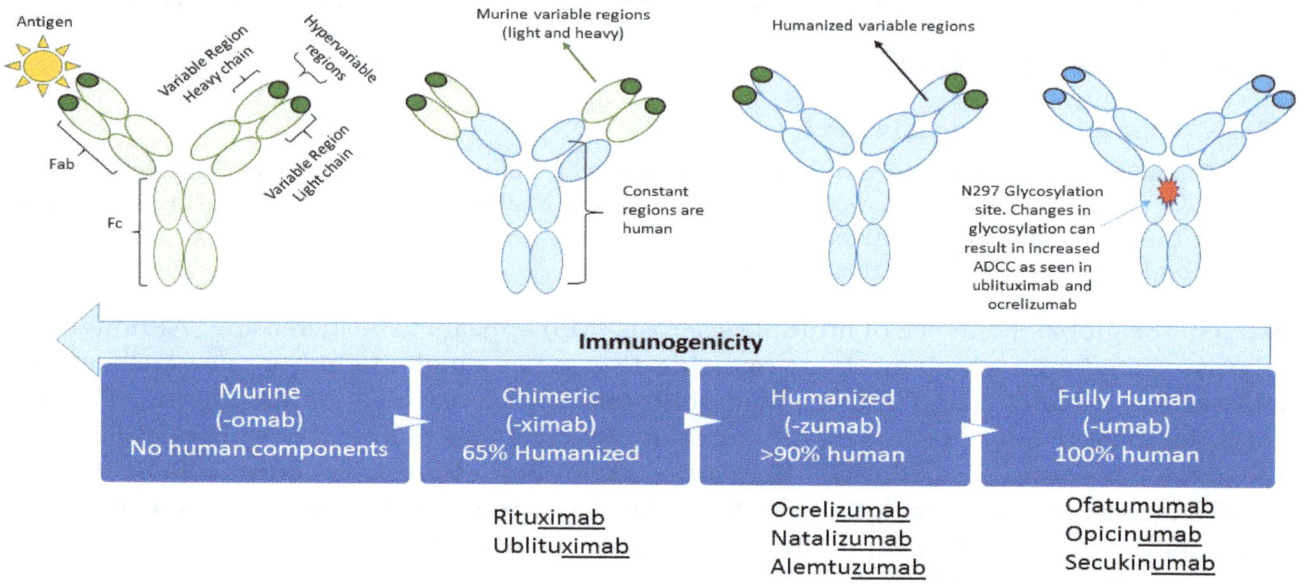

Figure 1. Bioengineering techniques have resulted in progressively more humanized antibodies. The figure shows the different fractions of the monoclonal antibodies and whether they represent mouse (green) or human (blue) sequences. As the sequences become more humanized their immunogenicity decreases. Glycosylation occurs at amino acid N297 and affects ADCC. Fragment antigen binding (Fab), Fragment crystallizable (Fc), Antigen-dependent cellular cytotoxicity (ADCC).

Natalizumab was the first MAB to be approved by the United States Food and Drug Administration (FDA) for the treatment of MS in 2004 [8], heralding the age of MABs for the treatment of MS. Other MABs have followed including alemtuzumab and ocrelizumab. Rituximab and ofatumumab have been used off label in the treatment of MS and ublituximab and ofatumumab are undergoing Phase III studies for approval in MS.

Opicinumab targets leucine-rich repeat and immunoglobulin domain-containing neurite outgrowth inhibitor receptor-interacting protein 1 (LINGO-1) [9], the remyelinating/reparative MAB that has been the most studied in MS. It has undergone phase II trials with mixed results and is currently being evaluated in another phase II study (AFFINITY). The MABs previously listed will be the focus of this review and other treatments completing phase II studies in MS can be found in Table 1; including some preliminary compounds in phase II such as Elezanumab, VAY736, and the HERV-W Env Antagonist GNbAC1.

In the past decade, several MABs were developed in an attempt to find a more efficacious and safe therapeutic option for MS patients; rigorous clinical trials have demonstrated lack of efficacy of as well as serious adverse events from some of them. For example, daclizumab (Zinbryta) [10] binds CD25, a subunit of the IL-2 receptor, was approved in 2016 for the treatment of MS, but was voluntarily withdrawn from the market due to reports of encephalitis in March 2018. Additionally, MABs that have been withdrawn or discontinued from further testing are listed in Table 2.

Table 1. Monoclonal antibodies currently on the market or being evaluated in phase II/III studies.

Therapeutic Monoclonal Antibodies					
MAB	**Composition**	**Target**	**Mechanism of Action**	**Administration**	**FDA Approval Date for MS**
Alemtuzumab	Humanized MAB IgGk	CD52	ADCC	Intravenous	November 2014
Elezanumab [11]	Fully human MAB	RGMa	Binds and neutralizes RGMa which modulates T cell responses and dendritic cells in CNS lesions	Intravenous	N/A
GNbAC1 [12]	Humanized IgG4 MAB	Envelope protein of HERV-W MSRV	Targets the envelope protein of HERV-W MSRV, which may play a critical role in multiple sclerosis	Intravenous	N/A
Natalizumab	Humanized monoclonal IgG1	Cell adhesion molecule α4-integrin	Preventing lymphocyte transport across the blood brain barrier	Intravenous	November 2004 and reapproved on June 2006
Ocrelizumab	Humanized IgG1	Phosphorylated glycoprotein CD20 on B lymphocytes	ADCC > CDC	Intravenous	March 2017
Ofatumumab	Fully humanized IgG1	CD20	CDC > ADCC	Subcutaneous	N/A
Opicinumab	Humanized MAB	Targets LINGO-1	Allows OPCs to differentiate into mature OLG for remyelination	Intravenous	N/A
Ublituximab	Chimeric IgG1 MAB	CD20	CDC and ADCC	Intravenous	N/A
Rituximab	Chimeric (murine/human) MAB	CD20	CDC and ADCC	Intravenous	N/A
VAY736 [13]	Defucosylated, human IgG1 MAB	Targets the receptor for BAFF-R	ADCC and blockade of BAFF:BAFF-R signaling that drives B cell differentiation, proliferation and survival	Intravenous	N/A

Abbreviations: monoclonal antibody (MAB), multiple sclerosis (MS), not applicable (N/A), envelope protein (Env), human endogenous multiple sclerosis-associated retrovirus (HERV-W MSRV), cluster of differentiation (CD), complement-dependent cytotoxicity (CDC), antibody-dependent cellular cytotoxicity (ADCC), T helper (Th), Leucine-rich repeat and immunoglobulin domain-containing neurite outgrowth inhibitor receptor-interacting protein 1 (LINGO-1), oligodendrocyte precursor cells (OPCs), oligodendrocytes (OLGs), repulsive guidance molecule A (RGMa), B cell activating factor of the TNF family (BAFF-R).

Table 2. Examples of MAB therapies that have been discontinued from further clinical trials due to lack of efficacy or serious adverse events in the treatment of multiple sclerosis.

MAB	Composition	Target/Mechanism	Withdrawn
Atacicept [14]	Fully humanized recombinant fusion protein containing the extracellular ligand-binding portion of the human TACI receptor	Binds to the cytokines BLyS and APRIL, involved in B-cell differentiation, maturation, and survival.	Increases relapse rates in multiple sclerosis reflected on an increase in annualized relapse rates.
Daclizumab [15]	Humanized IgG1 MAB	CD25, which is attached to the Tac epitope on the alpha chain of CD25 (IL-2 receptor) on activated lymphocytes	Post-marketing vigilance helped to detect secondary autoimmune events, including inflammatory encephalitis in 12 patients worldwide leading to at least 3 deaths where an interaction with the drug could not be ruled out.
Muromonab [16]	Chimeric MAB, first MAB to ever be approved	Inhibition of CD3 receptor	High toxicity made it unlikely to be a preferred treatment for MS.
Secukinumab [17]	Humanized IgG1kappa MAB	IL-17 receptor, inhibits proinflammatory IL-17A	Discontinued due to the development of a fully-human anti IL-17 MAB with better potential
Tabalumab [18]	Selective and fully human IgG4 MAB	Neutralization of membrane-bound and soluble B-cell activating factor (BAFF)	Results from phase 2 clinical trials in patients with RMS, showed no evidence of reduction Gd-enhancing lesions versus placebo, further analysis were discontinued.
Ustekinumab [19]	Fully humanized IgG1 MAB	Targets subunit P40 on cytokines IL-12 and IL-23 preventing them from differentiating and activating Th1 cells	Discontinued after phase 2 trials for low/lack of efficacy.
Vatelizumab [20]	Fully humanized MAB that targets VLA-2, a collagen binding integrin expressed on activated lymphocytes	Preventing the crossing of inflammatory cells into the brain, reducing inflammation and tested on RMS	Primary efficacy endpoint was not met after phase 2a and 2b studies halting further development for MS.

Abbreviations: transmembrane activator and calcium modulator and cyclophilin-ligand interactor (TACI), B-lymphocyte stimulator, also known as TNFSF20 (BLyS), a proliferation-inducing ligand, also known as TNFSF13 (APRIL), monoclonal antibody (MAB), T activation (Tac), cluster of differentiation (CD), interleukin (IL-), B-cell activating factor (BAFF), relapsing multiple sclerosis (RMS), gadolinium (Gd), T helper (Th), very late antigen-2 (VLA-2; also known as integrin $\alpha 2\beta 1$).

Although the MABs have some of the best proven efficacy in the treatment of MS, side effects remain a concern for some providers and patients alike. Figure 2 shows how these MABs affect the pathophysiology of MS and their efficacy is described below for each MAB. The incomplete understanding of the immune system and how alterations to it can lead to infections, other autoimmune conditions, and possibly neoplasms is something that we will learn with experience, especially as we look to prescribe these treatments to our patients for many years. Additionally, the relatively unpredictable events secondary to MABs leading to immune reactions, including serum sickness and anaphylaxis, can be reduced by humanizing MABs as described above. Infusion-related reactions (IRRs) can be common and are more likely related to cytokine release syndrome (CRS) than to reactions to the MABs themselves. CRS can be a serious adverse event but is more common in conditions where the target lymphocytes are in high abundance. For example, CRS is much more common and severe in the treatment of B-cell lymphomas than in the treatment of MS with anti-CD20 MABs. CRS manifestations include a wide clinical spectrum, which can vary from mild flu-like symptoms, to life-threatening manifestations including progression to uncontrolled systemic inflammatory response, vascular leakage, disseminated intravascular coagulation and multi-organ system failure [21,22]. Although CRS or milder versions of it have the highest incidence during the first infusion, they can occur with later infusions as well. These IRRs tend to occur during or soon after the infusions. Even some of the fully humanized MABs can be immunogenic, causing anaphylaxis or serum sickness in later infusions [23]. Pretreatment with steroids, acetaminophen, and/or an antihistaminic prior to infusion can reduce IRRs and CRS and are often used prior to medications that cause lymphocyte destruction.

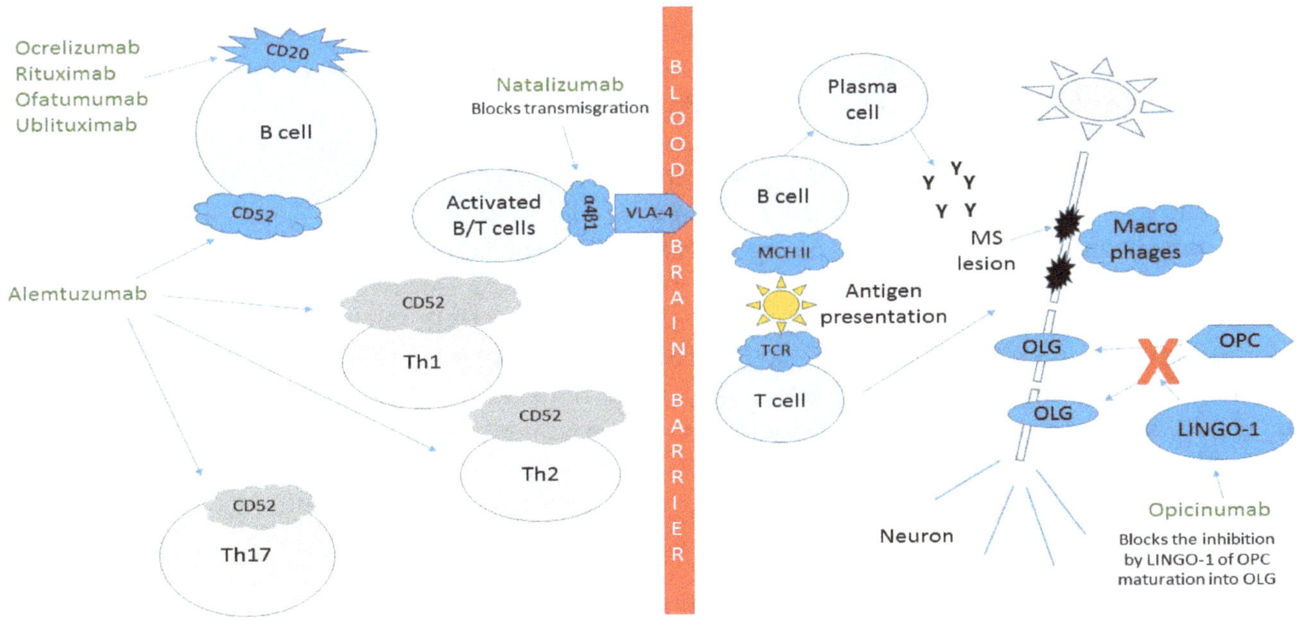

Figure 2. Mechanism of action of monoclonal antibodies in the treatment of multiple sclerosis. Ocrelizumab, rituximab, ofatumumab and ublituximab target CD20 expressing cells. Natalizumab targets transmigration of lymphocytes through the blood brain barrier. Alemtuzumab targets CD52 expressing cells. Opicinumab helps OPC differentiate into myelin producing OLGs. Cluster of differentiation (CD), T helper cells (Th), Leucine rich repeat and Immunoglobin-like domain-containing protein 1 (LINGO-1), oligodendrocyte (OLG), oligodendrocyte precursor cell (OPC).

Clinical evidence of continued disease activity, side effects, ease of administration, and costs are some of the aspects to consider when switching a patient to/from MAB therapies. Understanding the mechanism of action, how to monitor for adverse events and developing strategies for evaluating treatment failure are important tenants of personalized medicine and help to provide the safest treatment for patients with MS.

1.1. Natalizumab (Tysabri™)

Natalizumab was the first MAB approved by the FDA in 2004 for the treatment of MS (Table 1). Although it was temporarily withdrawn from the market due to cases of progressive multifocal leukoencephalopathy (PML), it was returned to the US market in 2006 after development of a risk evaluation and mitigation strategy (REMS) program to monitor the cases of PML [24] It is a recombinant humanized MAB to integrin α-4, which forms a heterodimer with β1. By binding the α4β1 integrin on the surface of activated inflammatory lymphocytes and monocytes, natalizumab blocks the interaction with VCAM-1 on endothelial cells preventing these inflammatory cells' entry into the central nervous system (Figure 2).

Natalizumab has shown great efficacy in the treatment of patients with MS. In the AFFIRM study, natalizumab reduced the annualized relapse rate (ARR) by 68% compared with placebo at one year, and with a significant reduction of 42% in the cumulative probability of sustained 3 months disability progression over two years [25]. Additionally, there was an 83% reduction in new or enlarging T2 lesions with a 92% reduction in contrast-enhancing lesions in the natalizumab group as compared to placebo.

Natalizumab is well tolerated at therapeutic doses with a very low rate of infusion reactions. It has been documented that anti-natalizumab neutralizing antibodies decrease free and cell-bound drug levels [26]. These develop and persist for at least 42 days after treatment in approximately 6% of natalizumab-treated patients [25,27]. Persistence of anti-natalizumab antibodies has been associated with reduced efficacy and increased incidence of IRRs [25,27].

The most serious adverse event consist of the brain infection PML caused by the John Cunningham virus (JCV). The risk of PML has been associated with prior chemotherapy and immunosuppressant use as well as amount of time on the drug. Additionally, a positive stratify JCV titer has been associated with higher risk of PML and this increases with higher titers. The index to assess PML risk consist in measurement of antibodies to JCV. Patients with a positive index have a higher risk of PML, which increases particularly in patients with an index >1.5 [24].

A routine monitoring strategy of the JCV titer should be part of the drug monitoring strategy for natalizumab (usually every 6 months) along with routine basic laboratories including a comprehensive metabolic panel and complete cell count with differential. In JCV seronegative patients, the benefits of natalizumab treatment still greatly outweigh the potential risks of PML [28,29] Clinical and neuroimaging follow-ups are recommended for disease activity monitoring and detection of side effects.

Other documented adverse events (AEs) with natalizumab include infections with herpes virus [27,30] and is contraindicated in patients that are severely immunocompromised. Melanoma risk may be higher in at risk-patients [31]. Liver injury can occur in patients with no previous history of liver disease, although rarely [32]. Hypereosinophilia may occur during treatment with this MAB [33].

1.2. Ocrelizumab (Ocrevus™)

Ocrelizumab is a cytotoxic recombinant humanized MAB that targets CD20 on circulating B-lymphocytes (Table 1, Figure 2). Ocrelizumab was the first anti-CD20 treatment approved for use in MS patients, although rituximab had been used off-label previously. In comparison to rituximab, ocrelizumab has a modified Fc region with enhanced ADCC [34]. As a humanized molecule, ocrelizumab is expected to be less immunogenic and might thus have fewer IRRs than rituximab [35]. Ocrelizumab reduces CD20 counts after infusion with a median time for B-cell counts to return to baseline of 72 weeks [36]. CD19 counts are often used instead of CD20 cell counts for monitoring these medications since both proteins are expressed in nearly the same cell populations and due to concerns that CD20 could be masked by a bound drug not allowing detection of cells but that did not lyse [36].

In relapsing MS, ocrelizumab showed efficacy superiority over interferon Beta-1a (IFN-β1a). The ARR was significantly reduced by 46% and 47% in the two OPERA studies [37]. Additionally, contrast enhancing lesions decreased by 94% and 95% and new or newly enlarging T2 lesions decreased by 77% and 83%. Confirmed disability progression at 12 weeks decreased by 40% in a pooled analysis of both studies.

In primary progressive MS, ocrelizumab reduced the confirmed disability progression at 12 weeks by 24% over placebo. T2-weighted lesion volume decreased by 3.4% in ocrelizumab-treated patients but increased 7.4% with a placebo. The brain volume loss in ocrelizumab-treated patients was 0.90% versus 1.09% with placebo ($p = 0.02$) [34].

Common adverse events include IRRs, which is the reason that premedication is recommended with methylprednisolone, acetaminophen and diphenhydramine. Although common, these are rarely serious. Additionally, nasopharyngitis (14.8%), upper respiratory tract infections (15.2%) [37], headache, and urinary tract infections have been seen in patients treated with ocrelizumab. An increased risk of neoplasms, particularly breast cancer were noted and will need to be studied more to understand if this was indeed related to ocrelizumab. It is recommended that vaccinations be administered at least six weeks prior to starting ocrelizumab, with avoidance of live or live attenuated vaccines during treatment [38,39]. Ocrelizumab is contraindicated in patients with active hepatitis B infections, thus patients should be screened prior to starting treatment. PML has been reported when transitioning from natalizumab or fingolimod, but should be regularly monitored for in patients on ocrelizumab long term [40]. Additionally, patients should have standardized monitoring during treatment with ocrelizumab, including immunoglobulin G levels, as these levels can decrease placing patients at increased risk of infection if their levels drop to very low levels [38].

1.3. *Rituximab (Rituxan™)*

Rituximab is a chimeric MAB that binds to CD20 and lyses B cells via complement-dependent cytotoxicity (CDC) and ADCC (Table 1) [1,41,42]. It achieves a >95% depletion of B cells, which is sustained at week 24. By 48 weeks, B cells remain at 30.7% of baseline [43]. After the initial infusion, a depletion of T cells is observed in CSF in addition to the expected decrease in B cells [41,44,45].

Rituximab, commonly prescribed off-label, is very effective in relapsing MS [43]. In the HERMES phase II study, patients in the rituximab group had a significant reduction in total number of contrast enhancing lesions over 24 weeks versus placebo (mean number 0.5 versus 5.5; relative reduction 91%). The proportion of patients in the rituximab group with relapses was decreased at week 24 (14.5% vs. 34.3%, $p = 0.02$) and week 48 (20.3% vs. 40.0%, $p = 0.04$) [43]. The OLYMPUS study in primary progressive MS failed to show a reduction in the confirmed progression of disability at 12 weeks, but did find a significant reduction of 48% in those aged <51 and of 59% in those with enhancing lesions at baseline [46].

Rituximab caused more IRRs within 24 h after the first infusion versus placebo [43]. Adverse reactions include serum sickness, PML, neutropenic fever, sinusitis, nasopharyngitis, upper respiratory infection, urinary tract infection, reactivation of hepatitis B virus, cardiac arrhythmias, cytopenias and malignancies, which have been associated with chronic B-cell depletion, among other less frequently reported [41,47]. Serious AEs were predominantly reported in patients >55 years of age [47]. The development of anti-chimeric neutralizing antibodies secondary to treatment with rituximab is reported in 26% of patients treated in progressive MS and in 37% in RRMS patients, which is partially the reason for the development of less immunogenic humanized MABs [48]. Recommended patient monitoring is similar to that with ocrelizumab.

1.4. *Ofatumumab*

Ofatumumab is currently being evaluated in phase 3 clinical trials for the treatment of relapsing MS (Table 1). Ofatumumab is a fully humanized MAB, which binds to the human CD20 antigen inducing B-cell lysis through ADCC and CDC. Its target epitope is located in a different cellular site than rituximab and ocrelizumab [49,50].

A small phase II study was completed which showed a reduction in new MRI lesions of 99% for all dose groups versus placebo by 24 weeks [50]. The MIRROR study, which compared ofatumumab to placebo in a phase IIB trial using subcutaneous dosing, showed a reduction in cumulative new gadolinium lesions of 65% for all dose groups when compared to placebo ($p < 0.001$). For all doses of >30 mg a reduction of >90% new brain lesions was seen over a 12 week period. The most common adverse event was injection related reactions at the first dose, which decreased in subsequent doses [49].

Observed adverse events included rash and urticaria, infusion reactions, pruritus, headaches, nasopharyngitis, hypersensitivity and dyspnea [50,51]. None of the patients developed human anti-human antibodies. Marginal changes in IgG, IgA, and IgM were observed [50]. Monitoring is similar to that with ocrelizumab.

1.5. *Ublituximab*

Ublituximab is a novel glycoengineered chimeric MAB antiCD20 therapy that is currently in phase III studies (ULTIMATE) (Table 1). Glycoenginering allows it to have enhanced affinity for Fc γ RIIIa receptors, eliciting increased ADCC. At week 4, a 99% B cell depletion was observed and maintained up to week 24 after treatment [52]. One particular benefit is that the infusion time duration is typically between 1 and 2 h.

Results from a phase II study with a median duration of 11 months, showed that ublituximab at week 24 has an ARR of 0.05 and a reduction in new T2 lesion volume of 7.67% compared to baseline. Additionally at week 24, 98% of participants were relapse free, no subjects had a contrast enhancing lesion, 84% did not have any new/enlarging T2 lesion, and 93% did not have confirmed disability progression at 24 weeks resulting in 76% of subjects meeting criteria for no evidence of disease activity [52].

No grade 3–4 AEs were observed, all IRRs reported were levels 1 and 2. Some adverse reactions reported include mild/moderate IRRs, fatigue, headache, numbness, common colds, dizziness, nausea/vomiting, and upper respiratory infection [52]. Monitoring is similar to that with ocrelizumab.

1.6. *Alemtuzumab (Lemtrada™)*

Alemtuzumab is a humanized anti-CD52 cytolytic MAB which targets the surface of lymphocytes and monocytes predominantly by ADCC. The repopulation of B cells occurs within 6 weeks of treatment, but T cells take longer to normalize at 9–12 months after a course of treatment [53,54]. This provides a long pharmacodynamic effect allowing the medication to be administered intravenously over two treatment courses. The first treatment consist of 12 mg/day on 5 consecutive days with the second on 3 consecutive days administered 12 months after the first treatment [53,54].

As a first line treatment, alemtuzumab in CARE-MS 1 showed an ARR of 54%, a non-significant reduction in sustained accumulation of disability, a 17% reduction in new or enlarging T2 lesion, a 63% reduction in contrast enhancing lesions, and a 42% reduction in brain parenchymal atrophy compared with IFN-β1a [53]. In CARE-MS 2, alemtuzumab showed an ARR of 50%, a non-significant reduction in sustained accumulation of disability, a 32% reduction in new or enlarging T2 lesion, a 61% reduction in contrast enhancing lesions, and a non-significant reduction in brain parenchymal atrophy compared with IFN-β1a [54]. Over 5 years, it lowered the risk of sustained accumulation of disability by 72% compared with IFN-β1a ($p < 0.0001$) and reduced the number of relapses by 69% over IFN-β1a ($p < 0.0001$) [54]. Both studies were performed in a non-blinded fashion, meaning patients knew if they were under the experimental arm of the trial and being prescribed this MAB. This approach was adopted due to the severity of the IRRs, nonetheless, blinded neurologists performed the efficacy assessments [55].

Adverse events have created the need for a REMS program. For example, recently the FDA issued a warning about elevated risk of stroke and artery damage, for this reason a black box label was added to the U.S. product label [56]. Patients can develop other autoimmune conditions such as thyroid disease (40.7%) [57], as well as immune thrombocytopenia, autoimmune hemolytic anemia, and anti-glomerular basement membrane disease [53,54]. Additionally, there has been an increased risk of malignancies such as thyroid cancer, melanoma, and lymphoproliferative disorders. IRRs are also common (>90%) [53,58], including rare cases of serum sickness and anaphylaxis. Over time, infections (>71%) can also occur including nasopharyngitis, urinary tract infections, upper respiratory tract infections, herpes viral infection, and fungal infections [59]. The monitoring labs that constitute the REMS program include complete blood count with differential, serum creatinine, urinalysis with microscopy, which should be performed monthly, and thyroid function tests, which should be done every 3 months, until 48 months after the last infusion [60].

1.7. Opicinumab

It is encouraging to see new MABs being developed for repair/remyelination of lesions in MS patients. Opicinumab is a fully humanized MAB that targets LINGO-1. By inhibiting LINGO-1, oligodendrocyte precursor cells (OPCs) can differentiate into mature oligodendrocytes (OLCs) and allow for remyelination of damaged plaques (Table 1, Figure 2) [9,38,61].

Opicinumab was evaluated in a phase II study (RENEW) as an add-on in patients with optic neuritis where it did not differ significantly in remyelination rates when compared to placebo at week 24. However, there was a small improvement of 9.1 milliseconds on full field visual evoked responses in the per protocol analysis that was not significant in the intention to treat analysis [9]. Subgroup analysis showed an improvement for baseline age $\geq$33 years of -14.17 milliseconds suggesting a greater benefit in older patients [62].

Another phase II study (SYNERGY) evaluated the efficacy of coadministration of opicinumab with IFN-β1a. The primary end point was the percentage of patients with an improvement over at least 3 months on a multicomponent endpoint comprising the expanded disability status scale, timed 25 foot walk, 9-hole peg test, and a 3-s paced auditory serial addition test. The percentage of improvement was 51.6% for placebo, 51.1% for 3 mg/kg opicinumab, 65.6% for 10 mg/kg, 68.8% for 30 mg/kg, and 41.2% for 100 mg/kg. In summary, there was an increased percentage of remyelination with opicinumab at 10 and 30 mg/kg when compared to placebo [63]. An additional study is underway (AFFINITY), which looks at patients that did better in SYNERGY, and includes those with disease activity of less than 21 years and that meet certain criteria on magnetization transfer ratio and diffusion tensor imaging on magnetic resonance scans.

Opicinumab has been well tolerated, adverse events have been similarly reported among groups treated with opicinumab and placebo [62,63]. However, some mild hypersensitivity reactions have been reported [61].

2. New Horizons and Future Trends for Therapeutic Monoclonal Antibodies

MABs have become a mainstay of MS treatment and they are likely to continue to be developed and optimized for the treatment of this disease, such as analyzing the safety of faster infusion times and administration by subcutaneous routes. MABs are some of the most effective therapies for relapsing MS without the side effects associated with chemotherapeutic agents. Additionally, new MABS are being developed to help repair the damage/disability that has already occurred, which is promising. New advancements in bioengineering are being incorporated to antibodies that are more humanized to help optimize their effectiveness and improve their tolerability and safety. The newer MABs that are being developed (Table 1) are based on lessons learned from past studies and drug development programs of drugs that have already been approved (Table 1) or stopped (Table 2). Overall, it is expected that MABs will continue to be a preferred therapy for MS in the foreseeable future.

Author Contributions: N.V.V. and E.A. designed and wrote this paper.

References

1. Wootla, B.; Watzlawik, J.O.; Stavropoulos, N.; Wittenberg, N.J.; Dasari, H.; Abdelrahim, M.A.; Henley, J.R.; Oh, S.H.; Warrington, A.E.; Rodriguez, M. Recent Advances in Monoclonal Antibody Therapies for Multiple Sclerosis. *Expert Opin. Biol. Ther.* **2016**, *16*, 827–839. [CrossRef] [PubMed]

2. Steinman, L.; Carlson, C.M. Monoclonal Antibody Therapy in Multiple Sclerosis. *Pract. Neurol.* **2018**, 28–31.
3. Smith, S.L. Ten years of Orthoclone OKT3 (muromonab-CD3): A review. *J. Transpl. Coord.* **1996**, *6*, 109–121. [CrossRef] [PubMed]
4. Ober, R.J.; Radu, C.G.; Ghetie, V.; Ward, E.S. Differences in promiscuity for antibody-FcRn interactions across species: Implications for therapeutic antibodies. *Int. Immunol.* **2001**, *13*, 1551–1559. [CrossRef] [PubMed]
5. Buss, N.A.; Henderson, S.J.; McFarlane, M.; Shenton, J.M.; de Haan, L. Monoclonal antibody therapeutics: History and future. *Curr. Opin. Pharmacol.* **2012**, *12*, 615–622. [CrossRef] [PubMed]
6. Morrison, S.L.; Johnson, M.J.; Herzenberg, L.A.; Oi, V.T. Chimeric human antibody molecules: Mouse antigen-binding domains with human constant region domains. *Proc. Natl. Acad. Sci. USA* **1984**, *81*, 6851–6855. [CrossRef]
7. Lonberg, N. Fully human antibodies from transgenic mouse and phage display platforms. *Curr. Opin. Immunol.* **2008**, *20*, 450–459. [CrossRef]
8. Yaldizli, O.; Putzki, N. Natalizumab in the treatment of multiple sclerosis. *Ther. Adv. Neurol. Disord.* **2009**, *2*, 115–128. [CrossRef]
9. Cadavid, D.; Balcer, L.; Galetta, S.; Aktas, O.; Ziemssen, T.; Vanopdenbosch, L.; Frederiksen, J.; Skeen, M.; Jaffe, G.J.; Butzkueven, H.; et al. Safety and efficacy of opicinumab in acute optic neuritis (RENEW): A randomised, placebo-controlled, phase 2 trial. *Lancet Neurol.* **2017**, *16*, 189–199. [CrossRef]
10. Giovannoni, G.; Gold, R.; Selmaj, K.; Havrdova, E.; Montalban, X.; Radue, E.W.; Stefoski, D.; McNeill, M.; Amaravadi, L.; Sweetser, M.; et al. Daclizumab high-yield process in relapsing-remitting multiple sclerosis (selection): A multicentre, randomised, double-blind extension trial. *Lancet Neurol.* **2014**, *13*, 472–481. [CrossRef]
11. Cree, B.; Rosebraugh, M.; Barger, B.; Ziemann, A. A Phase 1, Multiple-Dose Study of Elezanumab (ABT-555) in Patients with Relapsing Forms of Multiple Sclerosis. In Proceedings of the European Committee for Treatment and Research in Multiple Sclerosis Conference, Berlin, Germay, 11 October 2018.
12. Curtin, F.; Perron, H.; Kromminga, A.; Porchet, H.; Lang, A.B. Preclinical and early clinical development of gnbac1, a humanized igg4 monoclonal antibody targeting endogenous retroviral msrv-env protein. *MAbs* **2015**, *7*, 265–275. [CrossRef] [PubMed]
13. Dörner, T.; Posch, M.; Wagner, F.; Hüser, A.; Fischer, T.; Mooney, L.; Petricoul, O.; Maguire, P.; Pal, P.; Doucet, J.; et al. THU0313 Double-Blind, Randomized Study of VAY736 Single Dose Treatment in Patients with Primary Sjögren's Syndrome (PSS). *Ann. Rheum. Dis.* **2016**, *75*, 300–301. [CrossRef]
14. Bible, E. Multiple sclerosis: Atacicept increases relapse rates in multiple sclerosis. *Nat. Rev. Neurol.* **2014**, *10*, 182. [CrossRef]
15. EMA Recommends Immediate Suspension and Recall of Multiple Sclerosis Medicine Zinbryta. Available online: https://www.ema.europa.eu/en/news/ema-recommends-immediate-suspension-recall-multiple-sclerosis-medicine-zinbryta (accessed on 12 March 2019).
16. Weinshenker, B.G.; Bass, B.; Karlik, S.; Ebers, G.C.; Rice, G.P. An open trial of OKT3 in patients with multiple sclerosis. *Neurology* **1991**, *41*, 1047–1052. [CrossRef]
17. Havrdová, E.; Belova, A.; Goloborodko, A.; Tisserant, A.; Wright, A.; Wallstroem, E.; Garren, H.; Maguire, R.P.; Johns, D.R. Activity of secukinumab, an anti-IL-17A antibody, on brain lesions in RRMS: Results from a randomized, proof-of-concept study. *J. Neurol.* **2016**, *263*, 1287–1295. [CrossRef]
18. Silk, M.; Nantz, E. Efficacy and Safety of Tabalumab in Patients with Relapsing-Remitting Multiple Sclerosis: A Randomized, Double-Blind, Placebo-Controlled Study (P3.397). *Neurology* **2018**, *90*.
19. Segal, B.M.; Constantinescu, C.S.; Raychaudhuri, A.; Kim, L.; Fidelus-Gort, R.; Kasper, L.H.; Ustekinumab, M.S.I. Repeated subcutaneous injections of IL12/23 p40 neutralising antibody, ustekinumab, in patients with relapsing-remitting multiple sclerosis: A phase II, double-blind, placebo-controlled, randomised, dose-ranging study. *Lancet Neurol.* **2008**, *7*, 796–804. [CrossRef]
20. Vatelizumab. Available online: https://multiplesclerosisnewstoday.com/vatelizumab-gbr-500 (accessed on 1 February 2019).
21. Wing, M.G.; Moreau, T.; Greenwood, J.; Smith, R.M.; Hale, G.; Isaacs, J.; Waldmann, H.; Lachmann, P.J.; Compston, A. Mechanism of first-dose cytokine-release syndrome by CAMPATH 1-H: Involvement of CD16 (FcgammaRIII) and CD11a/CD18 (LFA-1) on NK cells. *J. Clin. Investig.* **1996**, *98*, 2819–2826. [CrossRef]

21. Wing, M.G.; Moreau, T.; Greenwood, J.; Smith, R.M.; Hale, G.; Isaacs, J.; Waldmann, H.; Lachmann, P.J.; Compston, A. Mechanism of first-dose cytokine-release syndrome by CAMPATH 1-H: Involvement of CD16 (FcgammaRIII) and CD11a/CD18 (LFA-1) on NK cells. *J. Clin. Investig.* **1996**, *98*, 2819–2826. [CrossRef]
22. Klinger, M.; Brandl, C.; Zugmaier, G.; Hijazi, Y.; Bargou, R.C.; Topp, M.S.; Gokbuget, N.; Neumann, S.; Goebeler, M.; Viardot, A.; et al. Immunopharmacologic response of patients with B-lineage acute lymphoblastic leukemia to continuous infusion of T cell-engaging CD19/CD3-bispecific BiTE antibody blinatumomab. *Blood* **2012**, *119*, 6226–6233. [CrossRef]
23. Del Boccio, P.; Rossi, C.; di Ioia, M.; Cicalini, I.; Sacchetta, P.; Pieragostino, D. Integration of metabolomics and proteomics in multiple sclerosis: From biomarkers discovery to personalized medicine. *Proteom. Clin. Appl.* **2016**, *10*, 470–484. [CrossRef]
24. McGuigan, C.; Craner, M.; Guadagno, J.; Kapoor, R.; Mazibrada, G.; Molyneux, P.; Nicholas, R.; Palace, J.; Pearson, O.R.; Rog, D.; et al. Stratification and monitoring of natalizumab-associated progressive multifocal leukoencephalopathy risk: Recommendations from an expert group. *J. Neurol. Neurosurg. Psychiatry* **2016**, *87*, 117–125. [CrossRef] [PubMed]
25. Polman, C.H.; O'Connor, P.W.; Havrdova, E.; Hutchinson, M.; Kappos, L.; Miller, D.H.; Phillips, J.T.; Lublin, F.D.; Giovannoni, G.; Wajgt, A.; et al. A randomized, placebo-controlled trial of natalizumab for relapsing multiple sclerosis. *N. Engl. J. Med.* **2006**, *354*, 899–910. [CrossRef] [PubMed]
26. Sehr, T.; Proschmann, U.; Thomas, K.; Marggraf, M.; Straube, E.; Reichmann, H.; Chan, A.; Ziemssen, T. New insights into the pharmacokinetics and pharmacodynamics of natalizumab treatment for patients with multiple sclerosis, obtained from clinical and in vitro studies. *J. Neuroinflamm.* **2016**, *13*, 164. [CrossRef]
27. Rudick, R.A.; Stuart, W.H.; Calabresi, P.A.; Confavreux, C.; Galetta, S.L.; Radue, E.W.; Lublin, F.D.; Weinstock-Guttman, B.; Wynn, D.R.; Lynn, F.; et al. Natalizumab plus interferon beta-1a for relapsing multiple sclerosis. *N. Engl. J. Med.* **2006**, *354*, 911–923. [CrossRef]
28. Walker, A.; Watson, C.; Alexopoulos, S.T.; Deniz, B.; Arnold, R.; Bates, D. A benefit–risk analysis of natalizumab in the treatment of patients with multiple sclerosis when considering the risk of progressive multifocal leukoencephalopathy. *Curr. Med. Res. Opin.* **2014**, *30*, 629–635. [CrossRef]
29. Thompson, J.P.; Noyes, K.; Dorsey, E.R.; Schwid, S.R.; Holloway, R.G. Quantitative risk-benefit analysis of natalizumab. *Neurology* **2008**, *71*, 357–364. [CrossRef]
30. Bloomgren, G.; Richman, S.; Hotermans, C.; Subramanyam, M.; Goelz, S.; Natarajan, A.; Lee, S.; Plavina, T.; Scanlon, J.V.; Sandrock, A.; et al. Risk of natalizumab-associated progressive multifocal leukoencephalopathy. *N. Engl. J. Med.* **2012**, *366*, 1870–1880. [CrossRef] [PubMed]
31. Mullen, J.T.; Vartanian, T.K.; Atkins, M.B. Melanoma Complicating Treatment with Natalizumab for Multiple Sclerosis. *N. Engl. J. Med.* **2008**, *358*, 647–648. [CrossRef] [PubMed]
32. Bezabeh, S.; Flowers, C.M.; Kortepeter, C.; Avigan, M. Clinically significant liver injury in patients treated with natalizumab. *Aliment. Pharmacol. Ther.* **2010**, *31*, 1028–1035. [CrossRef] [PubMed]
33. Abbas, M.; Lalive, P.H.; Chofflon, M.; Simon, H.-U.; Chizzolini, C.; Ribi, C. Hypereosinophilia in patients with multiple sclerosis treated with natalizumab. *Neurology* **2011**, *77*, 1561–1564. [CrossRef]
34. Montalban, X.; Hauser, S.L.; Kappos, L.; Arnold, D.L.; Bar-Or, A.; Comi, G.; de Seze, J.; Giovannoni, G.; Hartung, H.P.; Hemmer, B.; et al. Ocrelizumab versus Placebo in Primary Progressive Multiple Sclerosis. *N. Engl. J. Med.* **2017**, *376*, 209–220. [CrossRef] [PubMed]
35. Sorensen, P.S.; Blinkenberg, M. The potential role for ocrelizumab in the treatment of multiple sclerosis: Current evidence and future prospects. *Ther. Adv. Neurol. Disord.* **2016**, *9*, 44–52. [CrossRef] [PubMed]
36. Pasic, I.; Lipton, J.H. Current approach to the treatment of chronic myeloid leukaemia. *Leuk. Res.* **2017**, *55*, 65–78. [CrossRef] [PubMed]
37. Hauser, S.L.; Bar-Or, A.; Comi, G.; Giovannoni, G.; Hartung, H.-P.; Hemmer, B.; Lublin, F.; Montalban, X.; Rammohan, K.W.; Selmaj, K.; et al. Ocrelizumab versus Interferon Beta-1a in Relapsing Multiple Sclerosis. *N. Engl. J. Med.* **2017**, *376*, 221–234. [CrossRef] [PubMed]
38. Calabresi, P.A. B-Cell Depletion—A Frontier in Monoclonal Antibodies for Multiple Sclerosis. *N. Engl. J. Med.* **2017**, *376*, 280–282. [CrossRef] [PubMed]
39. Kappos, L.; Li, D.; Calabresi, P.A.; O'Connor, P.; Bar-Or, A.; Barkhof, F.; Yin, M.; Leppert, D.; Glanzman, R.; Tinbergen, J.; et al. Ocrelizumab in relapsing-remitting multiple sclerosis: A phase 2, randomised, placebo-controlled, multicentre trial. *Lancet* **2011**, *378*, 1779–1787. [CrossRef]

40. Diem, L.; Nedeltchev, K.; Kahles, T.; Achtnichts, L.; Findling, O. Long-term evaluation of NEDA-3 status in relapsing-remitting multiple sclerosis patients after switching from natalizumab to fingolimod. *Ther. Adv. Neurol. Disord.* **2018**, *11*. [CrossRef] [PubMed]
41. He, D.; Guo, R.; Zhang, F.; Zhang, C.; Dong, S.; Zhou, H. Rituximab for relapsing-remitting multiple sclerosis. *Cochrane Database Syst. Rev.* **2013**. [CrossRef] [PubMed]
42. Di Gaetano, N.; Cittera, E.; Nota, R.; Vecchi, A.; Grieco, V.; Scanziani, E.; Botto, M.; Introna, M.; Golay, J. Complement Activation Determines the Therapeutic Activity of Rituximab In Vivo. *J. Immunol.* **2003**, *171*, 1581–1587. [CrossRef]
43. Hauser, S.L.; Waubant, E.; Arnold, D.L.; Vollmer, T.; Antel, J.; Fox, R.J.; Bar-Or, A.; Panzara, M.; Sarkar, N.; Agarwal, S.; et al. B-cell depletion with rituximab in relapsing-remitting multiple sclerosis. *N. Engl. J. Med.* **2008**, *358*, 676–688. [CrossRef]
44. Bar-Or, A.; Calabresi, P.A.; Arnold, D.; Markowitz, C.; Shafer, S.; Kasper, L.H.; Waubant, E.; Gazda, S.; Fox, R.J.; Panzara, M.; et al. Rituximab in relapsing-remitting multiple sclerosis: A 72-week, open-label, phase I trial. *Ann. Neurol.* **2008**, *63*, 395–400. [CrossRef] [PubMed]
45. Cross, A.H.; Stark, J.L.; Lauber, J.; Ramsbottom, M.J.; Lyons, J.A. Rituximab reduces B cells and T cells in cerebrospinal fluid of multiple sclerosis patients. *J. Neuroimmunol.* **2006**, *180*, 63–70. [CrossRef] [PubMed]
46. Hawker, K.; O'Connor, P.; Freedman, M.S.; Calabresi, P.A.; Antel, J.; Simon, J.; Hauser, S.; Waubant, E.; Vollmer, T.; Panitch, H.; et al. Rituximab in patients with primary progressive multiple sclerosis: Results of a randomized double-blind placebo-controlled multicenter trial. *Ann. Neurol.* **2009**, *66*, 460–471. [CrossRef]
47. Memon, A.B.; Javed, A.; Caon, C.; Srivastawa, S.; Bao, F.; Bernitsas, E.; Chorostecki, J.; Tselis, A.; Seraji-Bozorgzad, N.; Khan, O. Long-term safety of rituximab induced peripheral B-cell depletion in autoimmune neurological diseases. *PLoS ONE* **2018**, *13*, e0190425. [CrossRef] [PubMed]
48. Dunn, N.; Juto, A.; Ryner, M.; Manouchehrinia, A.; Piccoli, L.; Fink, K.; Piehl, F.; Fogdell-Hahn, A. Rituximab in multiple sclerosis: Frequency and clinical relevance of anti-drug antibodies. *Mult. Scler. J.* **2018**, *24*, 1224–1233. [CrossRef]
49. Bar-Or, A.; Grove, R.A.; Austin, D.J.; Tolson, J.M.; VanMeter, S.A.; Lewis, E.W.; Derosier, F.J.; Lopez, M.C.; Kavanagh, S.T.; Miller, A.E.; et al. Subcutaneous ofatumumab in patients with relapsing-remitting multiple sclerosis: The MIRROR study. *Neurology* **2018**, *90*, e1805–e1814. [CrossRef] [PubMed]
50. Sorensen, P.S.; Lisby, S.; Grove, R.; Derosier, F.; Shackelford, S.; Havrdova, E.; Drulovic, J.; Filippi, M. Safety and efficacy of ofatumumab in relapsing-remitting multiple sclerosis: A phase 2 study. *Neurology* **2014**, *82*, 573–581. [CrossRef]
51. Kurrasch, R.; Brown, J.C.; Chu, M.; Craigen, J.; Overend, P.; Patel, B.; Wolfe, S.; Chang, D.J. Subcutaneously administered ofatumumab in rheumatoid arthritis: A phase I/II study of safety, tolerability, pharmacokinetics, and pharmacodynamics. *J. Rheumatol.* **2013**, *40*, 1089–1096. [CrossRef] [PubMed]
52. Inglese, M.; Petracca, M.; Cocozza, S.; Wray, S.; Racke, M.; Shubin, R.; Twyman, C.; Eubanks, J.L.; Mok, K.; Weiss, M.; Fox, E. Final MRI results at 6 months from a Phase 2 Multicenter Study of Ublituximab, A Novel Glycoengineered Anti-CD20 Monoclonal Antibody, In Patients With Relapsing Forms of Multiple Sclerosis (RMS), Demonstrates Complete Elimination of Gd-Enhancing Lesions. In Proceedings of the AAN Enterprises, Los Angeles, CA, USA, 21–27 April 2018.
53. Cohen, J.A.; Coles, A.J.; Arnold, D.L.; Confavreux, C.; Fox, E.J.; Hartung, H.P.; Havrdova, E.; Selmaj, K.W.; Weiner, H.L.; Fisher, E.; et al. Alemtuzumab versus interferon beta 1a as first-line treatment for patients with relapsing-remitting multiple sclerosis: A randomised controlled phase 3 trial. *Lancet* **2012**, *380*, 1819–1828. [CrossRef]
54. Coles, A.J.; Twyman, C.L.; Arnold, D.L.; Cohen, J.A.; Confavreux, C.; Fox, E.J.; Hartung, H.P.; Havrdova, E.; Selmaj, K.W.; Weiner, H.L.; et al. Alemtuzumab for patients with relapsing multiple sclerosis after disease-modifying therapy: A randomised controlled phase 3 trial. *Lancet* **2012**, *380*, 1829–1839. [CrossRef]
55. Coles, A.J.; Compston, A. Product licences for alemtuzumab and multiple sclerosis. *Lancet* **2014**, *383*, 867–868. [CrossRef]
56. FDA. FDA Warns about Rare but Serious Risks of Stroke and Blood Vessel Wall Tears with Multiple Sclerosis Drug Lemtrada (Alemtuzumab). Available online: https://www.fda.gov/Drugs/DrugSafety/ucm624247.htm (accessed on 3 July 2019).

57. Decallonne, B.; Bartholome, E.; Delvaux, V.; D'Haeseleer, M.; El Sankari, S.; Seeldrayers, P.; Van Wijmeersch, B.; Daumerie, C. Thyroid disorders in alemtuzumab-treated multiple sclerosis patients: A Belgian consensus on diagnosis and management. *Acta Neurol. Belg.* **2018**, *118*, 153–159. [CrossRef] [PubMed]
58. LaCasce, A.S.; Castells, M.C.; Burstein, H.J.; Meyerhardt, J.A. Infusion-Related Reactions to Therapeutic Monoclonal Antibodies Used for Cancer Therapy. Available online: https://www.uptodate.com/contents/infusion-related-reactions-to-therapeutic-monoclonal-antibodies-used-for-cancer-therapy (accessed on 6 February 2019).
59. Daniels, G.H.; Vladic, A.; Brinar, V.; Zavalishin, I.; Valente, W.; Oyuela, P.; Palmer, J.; Margolin, D.H.; Hollenstein, J. Alemtuzumab-related thyroid dysfunction in a phase 2 trial of patients with relapsing-remitting multiple sclerosis. *J. Clin. Endocrinol. Metab.* **2014**, *99*, 80–89. [CrossRef] [PubMed]
60. Van Den Neste, E.; Cazin, B.; Janssens, A.; Gonzalez-Barca, E.; Terol, M.J.; Levy, V.; Perez de Oteyza, J.; Zachee, P.; Saunders, A.; de Frias, M.; et al. Acadesine for patients with relapsed/refractory chronic lymphocytic leukemia (cll): A multicenter phase i/ii study. *Cancer Chemother. Pharmacol.* **2013**, *71*, 581–591. [CrossRef]
61. McCroskery, P.; Selmaj, K.; Fernandez, O.; Grimaldi, L.M.E.; Silber, E.; Pardo, G.; Freedman, S.M.; Zhang, Y.; Xu, L.; Cadavid, D.; et al. Safety and Tolerability of Opicinumab in Relapsing Multiple Sclerosis: The Phase 2b SYNERGY Trial (P5.369). *Neurology* **2017**, *88*.
62. Cadavid, D.; Balcer, L.; Galetta, S.; Aktas, O.; Ziemssen, T.; Vanopdenbosch, L.J.; Leocani, L.; Freedman, M.S.; Plant, G.T.; Preiningerova, J.L.; et al. Predictors of response to opicinumab in acute optic neuritis. *Ann. Clin. Transl. Neurol.* **2018**, *5*, 1154–1162. [CrossRef] [PubMed]
63. Mellion, M.; Edwards, K.R.; Hupperts, R.; Drulović, J.; Montalban, X.; Hartung, H.-P.; Brochet, B.; Calabresi, P.A.; Rudick, R.; Ibrahim, A.; et al. Efficacy Results from the Phase 2b SYNERGY Study: Treatment of Disabling Multiple Sclerosis with the Anti-LINGO-1 Monoclonal Antibody Opicinumab (S33.004). *Neurology* **2017**, *88*, S33.004.

5

No Immediate Effects of Transcranial Direct Current Stimulation at Various Intensities on Cerebral Blood Flow in People with Multiple Sclerosis

Craig D. Workman [1], Laura L. Boles Ponto [2], John Kamholz [3] and Thorsten Rudroff [1,3,*]

1 Department of Health and Human Physiology, University of Iowa, Iowa City, IA 52242, USA; craig-workman@uiowa.edu
2 Department of Radiology, University of Iowa Hospitals and Clinics, Iowa City, IA 52242, USA; laura-ponto@uiowa.edu
3 Department of Neurology, University of Iowa Hospitals and Clinics, Iowa City, IA 52242, USA; john-kamholz@uiowa.edu
* Correspondence: thorsten-rudroff@uiowa.edu;

Abstract: Animal and transcranial magnetic stimulation motors have evoked potential studies suggesting that the currently used transcranial direct current stimulation (tDCS) intensities produce measurable physiological changes. However, the validity, mechanisms, and general efficacy of this stimulation modality are currently being scrutinized. The purpose of this pilot study was to investigate the effects of dorsolateral prefrontal cortex tDCS on cerebral blood flow. A sample of three people with multiple sclerosis underwent two blocks of five randomly assigned tDCS intensities (1, 2, 3, 4 mA, and sham; 5 min each) and [^{15}O]water positron emission tomography imaging. The relative regional (i.e., areas under the electrodes) and global cerebral blood flow were calculated. The results revealed no notable differences in regional or global cerebral blood flow from the different tDCS intensities. Thus, 5 min of tDCS at 1, 2, 3, and 4 mA did not result in immediate changes in cerebral blood flow. To achieve sufficient magnitudes of intracranial electrical fields without direct peripheral side effects, novel methods may be required.

Keywords: tDCS; neuroimaging; positron emission tomography; cerebral blood flow; multiple sclerosis

---

1. Introduction

Multiple sclerosis (MS) is a chronic central nervous system disease that affects approximately 2.3 million people worldwide [1]. Because some MS symptoms (e.g., neuropathic pain) are treatment-resistant [2], practical and inexpensive adjunctive therapies, like transcranial direct current stimulation (tDCS), are of high interest. Despite promising findings in tDCS studies in people with multiple sclerosis (PwMS) [3–5] (see [6] for a review), the validity and utility of tDCS is under scrutiny. For example, a critical review [7] did not support the idea that tDCS has a reliable neurophysiological effect beyond motor evoked potential (MEP) amplitude modulation. Though MEP amplitude appears to be sensitive to tDCS modulation, other reliable transcranial magnetic stimulation (TMS) measures that rely on similar neural mechanisms (e.g., short interval intracortical inhibition (SICI), intracortical facilitation (ICF), and cortical silent period (cSP)) have all shown no tDCS effect. Questions concerning the mechanistic foundations and general efficacy of this stimulation modality are on the rise.

Animal studies have suggested that the intensities that are typically employed in human research are sufficient to produce measurable physiological changes [8]. Unfortunately, findings from animal models, especially in vitro approaches, may have poor applicability to human studies. Thus, a vital concern is that tDCS may not induce a sufficient current in the cortex to have a measurable effect on neural function—at least not for the commonly used stimulation intensities (≤2 mA). Therefore, it is necessary to combine tDCS with human neuroimaging to complement animal studies and to further clarify whether tDCS can affect neural function.

Cerebral activity in PwMS has been investigated with [^{15}O]water [9]. A close coupling of perfusion and metabolism was assumed, as this reflects the oxidative phosphorylation of glucose as the predominant energy source. Consequently, cerebral blood flow (CBF) is often considered an indirect measure of neuronal function and integrity [10]. This is supported by the significant association of glucose metabolism with regional CBF (rCBF) across different brain regions and global CBF (gCBF) across varying states of consciousness.

2. Materials and Methods

We conducted a pilot investigation on the effects of tDCS on CBF with semi-quantitative [^{15}O]water Positron Emission Tomography (PET), the gold standard for CBF measurements [11–15], in a sample of three people with relapsing–remitting MS (Table 1). Scans were completed in two blocks, one at baseline and five immediately after randomized tDCS stimulation intensities (1, 2, 3, 4 mA, and sham; six scans per block). The second block (intensity re-randomized) helped verify the reliability of the first. Therefore, each subject experienced 12 total scans in one session (Figure 1). The subjects performed a simple counting task for the duration of each scan (100 sec). This study was approved by the University of Iowa's Institutional Review Board (IRB-01: IRB#201905826; clinicaltrials.gov NCT04033133). All subjects provided written informed consent before participating.

Table 1. Subject demographic information (n = 3). Data are mean ± SD.

Sex (M/F)	2/1
Age (years)	45.3 ± 19.0
Height (cm)	171.9 ± 18.7
Weight (kg)	83.5 ± 19.9
Time since diagnosis (years)	8.0 ± 5.3
Patient-Determined Disease Steps [1]	2.3 ± 2.1

[1] Provides an indication of disease severity. A score of 2–4 out of 8 indicates moderate disability.

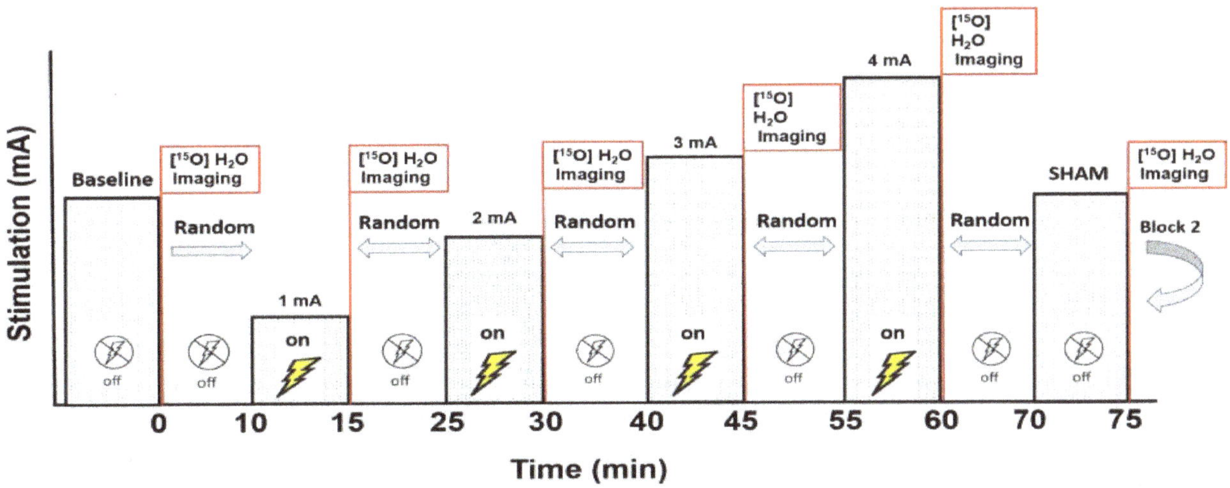

Figure 1. The stimulation and scan protocol. After the baseline scan, the five stimulation intensities (1, 2, 3, 4 mA, and sham) were delivered for 5 min each in a random order (six total scans per block). Ten minutes after the final scan of Block 1, Block 2 began with a new baseline scan and a different intensity randomization. Each subject experienced 12 total scans.

A battery-operated tDCS device (Soterix Medical Inc., New York, NY, USA) administered the stimulation. A previous study indicated that 5 min of tDCS over the primary motor cortex (M1) was sufficient to induce significant increases in MEP amplitude and that the effects of the stimulation returned to baseline after 10 min [16], and another study indicated significant blood flow changes from 4 min of motor cortex stimulation [17]. Thus, the tDCS parameters in this study included 5 min of stimulation at each intensity, each separated by ≥10 min, to avoid stimulation carry-over effects; this also allowed for sufficient time for the [^{15}O]water tracer to decay before the next injection. The stimulation was ramped up to the target intensity (1, 2, 3, or 4 mA) over 30 s, after which time the intensity was maintained for 5 min before ramping down to 0 mA over 30 s. The anode was over the left dorsolateral prefrontal cortex (dlPFC), and the cathode was over the contralateral supraorbital area. A dlPFC target helped to avoid potentially confounding M1 activity from counting or spontaneous movement during scanning.

Because significant excitability increases from 5 min of tDCS have been found at 1 min post-tDCS [16], imaging commenced 1 min after the ramp-down process was completed. A summed image of the 40 seconds immediate post-bolus transit was generated for each scan. The summed images were co-registered with the subject's T1-weighted magnetic resonance imaging (MRI). Individual, anatomically-based regions were defined by using the PNEURO tool of the PMOD Biomedical Image Quantification software package (PMOD Technologies, Ltd. Zürich, Switzerland. The mean global activity (gCBF) was calculated based on the volume-weighted average of all intracerebral regions. The CBF relative to the global activity was calculated for each region (rCBF = regional activity/gCBF; e.g., ratio 1.2 = rCBF 20% higher than gCBF) for each condition. Changes in gCBF and rCBF, focusing on regions under the electrodes, at the different tDCS intensities were investigated.

3. Results

The results revealed no notable differences in the gCBF or rCBF for the areas under the electrodes from the different tDCS intensities (Figure 2). We did not find any immediate effects (i.e., ~1–2 min post-stimulation) of tDCS on CBF in this functional [^{15}O]water PET study. None of the stimulation intensities (1, 2, 3, and 4 mA) over dlPFC were associated with changes in gCBF (not shown) or rCBF under the electrodes.

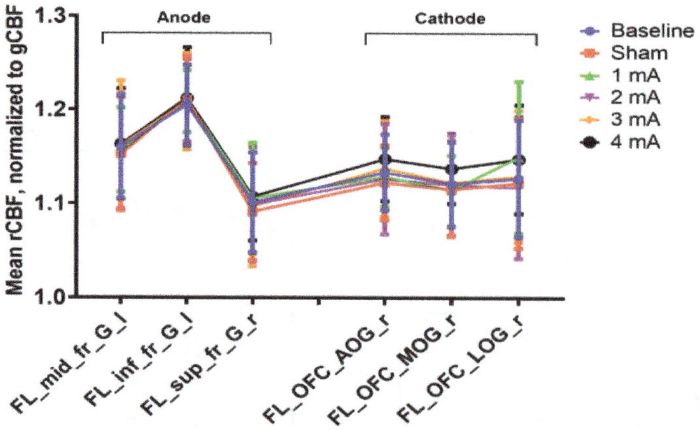

Figure 2. Mean tracer uptake (regional cerebral blood flow (rCBF)) relative to global tracer uptake (global CBF (gCBF)) by region and condition. Data are mean ± SEM. FL_mid_fr_G_l = left middle frontal gyrus, FL_inf_fr_G_l = left inferior frontal gyrus, FL_sup_fr_G_l = left superior frontal gyrus, FL_OFC_AOG_r = right anterior orbital gyrus, FL_OFC_MOG_r = right medial orbital gyrus, and FL_OFC_LOG_r = right lateral orbital gyrus.

4. Discussion

There are several possible explanations for this finding: (1) tDCS may not induce a sufficient current in the cortex to have a measurable effect on neural function. Vöröslakos et al. [18] suggested that a 1 V/m minimum voltage gradient was required for measurable online stimulation effects on neuronal spiking or membrane potentials in a rat model. To achieve 1 V/m at the cortex, the current applied at the scalp may need to be as high as 4–6 mA; however, the 4 mA that was used in this study did not elicit any CBF changes. (2) Only a small fraction of the transcranial current may reach the brain. One study [18] in rodents and human cadavers demonstrated that >75% of applied current is lost at the scalp, subcutaneous tissue, and muscle. These tissues serve as an effective shunt, resulting in at least a 50% reduction of current intensity. In addition, the serial resistance of the skull further reduces the current flow by 10%–25%, depending on skull thickness [18]. (3) Inter-individual variability in tDCS, with approximately 50% of people having poor or absent responses [19], may have biased our results. (4) Previous neuroimaging studies on the neurophysiological effects of tDCS detected immediate effects of tDCS on CBF by using [^{15}O]water PET [17,20]. However, these studies targeted M1 during a motor task, and diverse tDCS effects on different brain regions cannot be excluded. (5) Stimulating nerves on the scalp could also send signals to the brain or influence circulation, and/or other non-neuronal cells may react to the induced electrical fields and gradually alter brain function. Lastly, (6) the significant findings reported in the tDCS literature have assumed to have reflected one or more of a number of factors including placebo effects, influences from peripheral nerve stimulation, poor experimental designs, low statistical power, or inappropriate control conditions or analyses.

The sample size of this pilot study was small, and more subjects are recommended to confirm or refute these results. However, the study design, which included 12 injections that encompassed all conditions in duplicate, provided robust and remarkably consistent information, both between conditions and between subjects. Additionally, given that PET studies are costly and exposing the fewest subjects as possible to radiation is a major consideration [21], collecting images from additional subjects when there were no evident effects in these three PwMS was not justified. Furthermore, one of the purposes of reports like the present study is to encourage discussion and highlight the need to confirm the mechanistic effects of tDCS with neuroimaging (e.g., [^{15}O]water PET, [^{18}F]-fluorodeoxyglucose PET, functional magnetic resonance imaging (fMRI), and arterial spin labelling (ASL)). It should also be mentioned that multiple interventions over short periods might have complex and non-linear effects on the brain. Thus, any effect (or lack of effect) should to be interpreted with caution. Additionally, the absence of immediate tDCS effects on the cortex does not preclude longer-term effects. Furthermore, these findings were in a sample of PwMS, and different effects in healthy or patient populations cannot be excluded. Finally, this is a growing field for research, and a comprehensive understanding of how tDCS modulates the cortex is necessary. In humans, physiological changes associated with tDCS at different intensities and durations can be assessed with a variety of different neuroimaging methods (e.g., PET, fMRI, and ASL). All of these techniques have their limitations, but [^{15}O]water PET is considered to be the most "direct" measurement of cerebral blood flow. Thus, routinely combining neuroimaging with tDCS will help provide the necessary evidence that tDCS can affect neural function in humans.

5. Conclusions

In conclusion, we have demonstrated that 5 min of dlPFC tDCS at 1, 2, 3, or 4 mA did not result in immediate changes in CBF in PwMS. Thus, to achieve sufficient magnitudes of intracranial electrical fields without direct peripheral side effects, novel methods may be required.

Author Contributions: Conceptualization, C.D.W., T.R., and L.L.B.P.; methodology, C.D.W., T.R., and L.L.B.P.; data analysis, C.D.W. and L.L.B.P.; investigation, C.D.W. and L.L.B.P.; resources: T.R.; writing—original draft preparation: C.D.W. and T.R.; writing—review and editing; C.D.W., L.L.B.P., J.K., and T.R.; All authors approved the final version. All authors have read and agreed to the published version of the manuscript.

Acknowledgments: The authors would like to thank all of the study participants for their time and effort during participation. In addition, the authors thank Lisa Dunnwald and Shannon Lehman for their assistance in data collection and study coordination.

References

1. Bishop, M.; Rumrill, P.D. Multiple sclerosis: Etiology, symptoms, incidence and prevalence, and implications for community living and employment. *Work* **2015**, *52*, 725–734. [CrossRef]
2. Solaro, C.; Tanganelli, P.; Messmer Uccelli, M. Pharmacological treatment of pain in multiple sclerosis. *Exp. Rev. Neurotherap.* **2007**, *7*, 1165–1174. [CrossRef]
3. Berra, E.; Bergamaschi, R.; De Icco, R.; Dagna, C.; Perrotta, A.; Rovaris, M.; Grasso, M.G.; Anastasio, M.G.; Pinardi, G.; Martello, F.; et al. The Effects of Transcutaneous Spinal Direct Current Stimulation on Neuropathic Pain in Multiple Sclerosis: Clinical and Neurophysiological Assessment. *Front. Hum. Neurosci.* **2019**, *13*, 31. [CrossRef]
4. Oveisgharan, S.; Karimi, Z.; Abdi, S.; Sikaroodi, H. The use of brain stimulation in the rehabilitation of walking disability in patients with multiple sclerosis: A randomized double-blind clinical trial study. *Iran J. Neurol.* **2019**, *18*, 57–63. [CrossRef]
5. Workman, C.D.; Kamholz, J.; Rudroff, T. Transcranial direct current stimulation (tDCS) for the treatment of a Multiple Sclerosis symptom cluster. *Brain Stimul.* **2020**, *13*, 263–264. [CrossRef]
6. Sanchez-Kuhn, A.; Perez-Fernandez, C.; Canovas, R.; Flores, P.; Sanchez-Santed, F. Transcranial direct current stimulation as a motor neurorehabilitation tool: An empirical review. *Biomed. Eng. Online* **2017**, *16*, 76. [CrossRef]
7. Horvath, J.C.; Forte, J.D.; Carter, O. Evidence that transcranial direct current stimulation (tDCS) generates little-to-no reliable neurophysiologic effect beyond MEP amplitude modulation in healthy human subjects: A systematic review. *Neuropsychologia* **2015**, *66*, 213–236. [CrossRef]
8. Krause, M.R.; Vieira, P.G.; Csorba, B.A.; Pilly, P.K.; Pack, C.C. Transcranial alternating current stimulation entrains single-neuron activity in the primate brain. *Proc. National Acad. Sci. USA* **2019**, *116*, 5747–5755. [CrossRef]
9. Sun, X.; Tanaka, M.; Kondo, S.; Okamoto, K.; Hirai, S. Clinical significance of reduced cerebral metabolism in multiple sclerosis: A combined PET and MRI study. *Ann. Nucl. Med.* **1998**, *12*, 89–94. [CrossRef]
10. Iadecola, C. Neurovascular regulation in the normal brain and in Alzheimer's disease. *Nat. Rev. Neurosci.* **2004**, *5*, 347–360. [CrossRef]
11. Herscovitch, P.; Markham, J.; Raichle, M.E. Brain blood flow measured with intravenous $H_2{}^{(15)}O$. I. Theory and error analysis. *J. Nucl. Med.* **1983**, *24*, 782–789.
12. Raichle, M.E.; Martin, W.R.; Herscovitch, P.; Mintun, M.A.; Markham, J. Brain blood flow measured with intravenous H2(15)O. II. Implementation and validation. *J. Nucl. Med.* **1983**, *24*, 790–798.
13. Giovannella, M.; Andresen, B.; Andersen, J.B.; El-Mahdaoui, S.; Contini, D.; Spinelli, L.; Torricelli, A.; Greisen, G.; Durduran, T.; Weigel, U.M.; et al. Validation of diffuse correlation spectroscopy against (15)O-water PET for regional cerebral blood flow measurement in neonatal piglets. *J. Cereb. Blood Flow Metab.* **2019**. [CrossRef]
14. Guo, J.; Gong, E.; Fan, A.P.; Goubran, M.; Khalighi, M.M.; Zaharchuk, G. Predicting (15)O-Water PET cerebral blood flow maps from multi-contrast MRI using a deep convolutional neural network with evaluation of training cohort bias. *J. Cereb. Blood Flow Metab.* **2019**. [CrossRef]
15. Puig, O.; Henriksen, O.M.; Vestergaard, M.B.; Hansen, A.E.; Andersen, F.L.; Ladefoged, C.N.; Rostrup, E.; Larsson, H.B.; Lindberg, U.; Law, I. Comparison of simultaneous arterial spin labeling MRI and (15)O-H2O PET measurements of regional cerebral blood flow in rest and altered perfusion states. *J. Cereb. Blood Flow Metab.* **2019**. [CrossRef]
16. Nitsche, M.A.; Paulus, W. Sustained excitability elevations induced by transcranial DC motor cortex stimulation in humans. *Neurology* **2001**, *57*, 1899–1901. [CrossRef]
17. Paquette, C.; Sidel, M.; Radinska, B.A.; Soucy, J.P.; Thiel, A. Bilateral transcranial direct current stimulation modulates activation-induced regional blood flow changes during voluntary movement. *J. Cereb. Blood Flow Metab.* **2011**, *31*, 2086–2095. [CrossRef]
18. Vöröslakos, M.; Takeuchi, Y.; Brinyiczki, K.; Zombori, T.; Oliva, A.; Fernández-Ruiz, A.; Kozák, G.; Kincses, Z.T.; Iványi, B.; Buzsáki, G.; et al. Direct effects of transcranial electric stimulation on brain circuits in rats and humans. *Nat. Commun.* **2018**, *9*, 483. [CrossRef]

19. Wiethoff, S.; Hamada, M.; Rothwell, J.C. Variability in response to transcranial direct current stimulation of the motor cortex. *Brain Stimul.* **2014**, *7*, 468–475. [CrossRef]
20. Lang, N.; Siebner, H.R.; Ward, N.S.; Lee, L.; Nitsche, M.A.; Paulus, W.; Rothwell, J.C.; Lemon, R.N.; Frackowiak, R.S. How does transcranial DC stimulation of the primary motor cortex alter regional neuronal activity in the human brain? *Eur. J. Neurosci.* **2005**, *22*, 495–504. [CrossRef]
21. Andreasen, N.C.; Arndt, S.; Cizadlo, T.; O'Leary, D.S.; Watkins, G.L.; Ponto, L.L.; Hichwa, R.D. Sample size and statistical power in [^{15}O]H_2O studies of human cognition. *J. Cereb. Blood Flow Metab.* **1996**, *16*, 804–816. [CrossRef]

6

Sphingosine-1-Phosphate: Its Pharmacological Regulation and the Treatment of Multiple Sclerosis

Stanley Cohan, Elisabeth Lucassen, Kyle Smoot, Justine Brink and Chiayi Chen *

Providence Multiple Sclerosis Center, Providence Brain and Spine Institute, Providence St, Vincent Medical Center, Portland, OR 97225, USA; Stanley.Cohan@providence.org (S.C.); elisabeth.lucassen@providence.org (E.L.); Kyle.smoot@providence.org (K.S.); Justine.Brink@providence.org (J.B.)

* Correspondence: Chiayi.Chen@providence.org;

Abstract: Sphingosine-1-phosphate (S1P), via its G-protein-coupled receptors, is a signaling molecule with important regulatory properties on numerous, widely varied cell types. Five S1P receptors (S1PR1-5) have been identified, each with effects determined by their unique G-protein-driven downstream pathways. The discovery that lymphocyte egress from peripheral lymphoid organs is promoted by S1P via S1PR-1 stimulation led to the development of pharmacological agents which are S1PR antagonists. These agents promote lymphocyte sequestration and reduce lymphocyte-driven inflammatory damage of the central nervous system (CNS) in animal models, encouraging their examination of efficacy in the treatment of multiple sclerosis (MS). Preclinical research has also demonstrated direct protective effects of S1PR antagonists within the CNS, by modulation of S1PRs, particularly S1PR-1 and S1PR-5, and possibly S1PR-2, independent of effects upon lymphocytes. Three of these agents, fingolimod, siponimod and ozanimod have been approved, and ponesimod has been submitted for regulatory approval. In patients with MS, these agents reduce relapse risk, sustained disability progression, magnetic resonance imaging markers of disease activity, and whole brain and/or cortical and deep gray matter atrophy. Future opportunities in the development of more selective and intracellular S1PR-driven downstream pathway modulators may expand the breadth of agents to treat MS.

Keywords: multiple sclerosis; sphingosine-1-phosphate modulators

---

1. Introduction

Although it was long thought that sphingosine, largely generated from hydrolysis of ceramides within lysosomes [1,2], served primarily as a component of the structural sphingolipid family of molecules, it is now recognized for its importance as a component of sphingosine-1-phosphate (S1P), a crucial messenger molecule. S1P is generated by sphingosine kinase 1 or 2 (sk1, sk2), primarily in red blood cells, platelets and endothelial cells [3,4] (Figure 1). Their G-protein-coupled receptors are widely distributed in many organs and tissues, on cell surface plasma membranes, and on the endoplasmic reticulum and cell nuclei, but it is cytoplasmic membrane-bound receptor sites that have attracted the greatest attention [4]. Five S1P receptor (S1PR-1-5) subtypes have been identified [5,6] (Figure 2a). The translational intracellular pathways activated by S1P-receptor (S1PR) interaction are highly varied because of the multiplicity of receptor subtypes, the varied G-proteins to which they are coupled, the multiple downstream pathways linked to G proteins, and the wide variety cells which express S1PRs (Figure 2b; Table 1). Investigations into the physiological impact of S1P and its receptors, as well as its potential contribution to disease pathogenesis, have revealed important opportunities for therapeutic interventions. This is particularly the case in the treatment of multiple sclerosis (MS). In the past 10 years, three disease modifying therapies (DMT)s which modulate S1PRs, fingolimod (FGM), siponimod (SPM), and ozanimod (OZM), have been approved for treatment of MS, and a fourth agent, ponesimod (PNM) is under regulatory review.

The first part of this article describes the results of preclinical research, which has expanded the knowledge of the physiological roles of S1P and its receptors, and a discussion of the specific mechanisms of action of the S1PR modulators. This work did not only reveal important insights into S1PR-based DMT mechanisms of action, but also widened the perspective on future therapeutic opportunities for this class of molecules. The second part of this chapter summarizes the results of the pivotal clinical trials of FGM, SPM, OZM, and the phase II and phase III trials of PNM upon clinical efficacy, as well as the reported adverse events (AE) of these S1PR modulators.

Fingolimod (FGM) was the first S1PR modulator to be approved for the treatment of relapsing forms of MS (RMS). Preclinical and clinical studies demonstrated that its use results in the sequestration of lymphocytes, particularly central memory and naïve T and B cell lymphocytes in peripheral lymphoid organs [7–11]. Pathological studies also demonstrated reduced pro-inflammatory cells within the CNS following treatment with this class of agents, and it had been widely believed that the sequestration of these potentially pro-inflammatory cells within lymphoid organs accounted for their therapeutic efficacy in MS [7–10]. However, preclinical investigations, further detailed below, strongly suggest that these agents may also act directly within the CNS, where there is an abundance of S1PR expression, to ameliorate the impact of inflammatory disease.

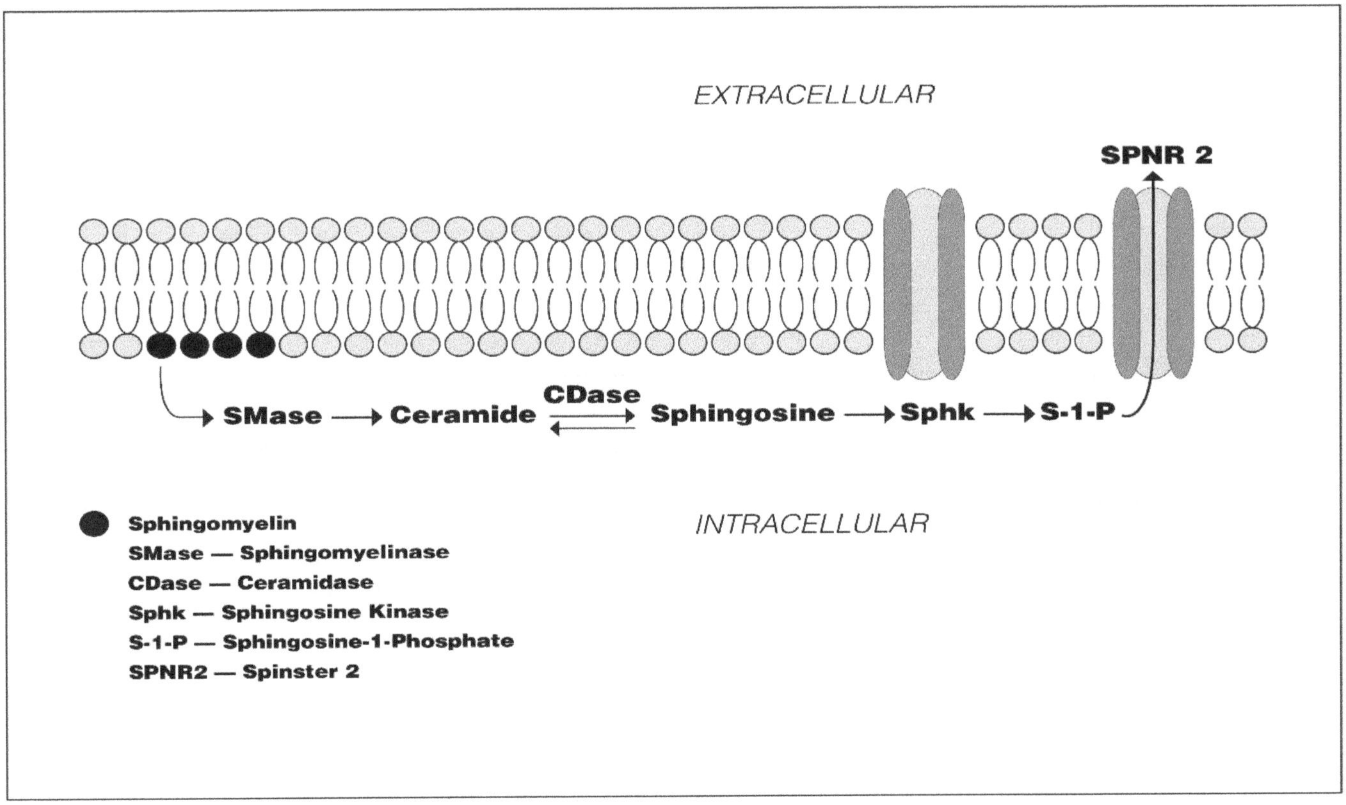

Figure 1. Metabolic Pathway to Sphingosine-1-phosphate Synthesis and Migration from the Intracellular to Extracellular Space via Sphingosine-1-phosphate Transmembrane Transporters.

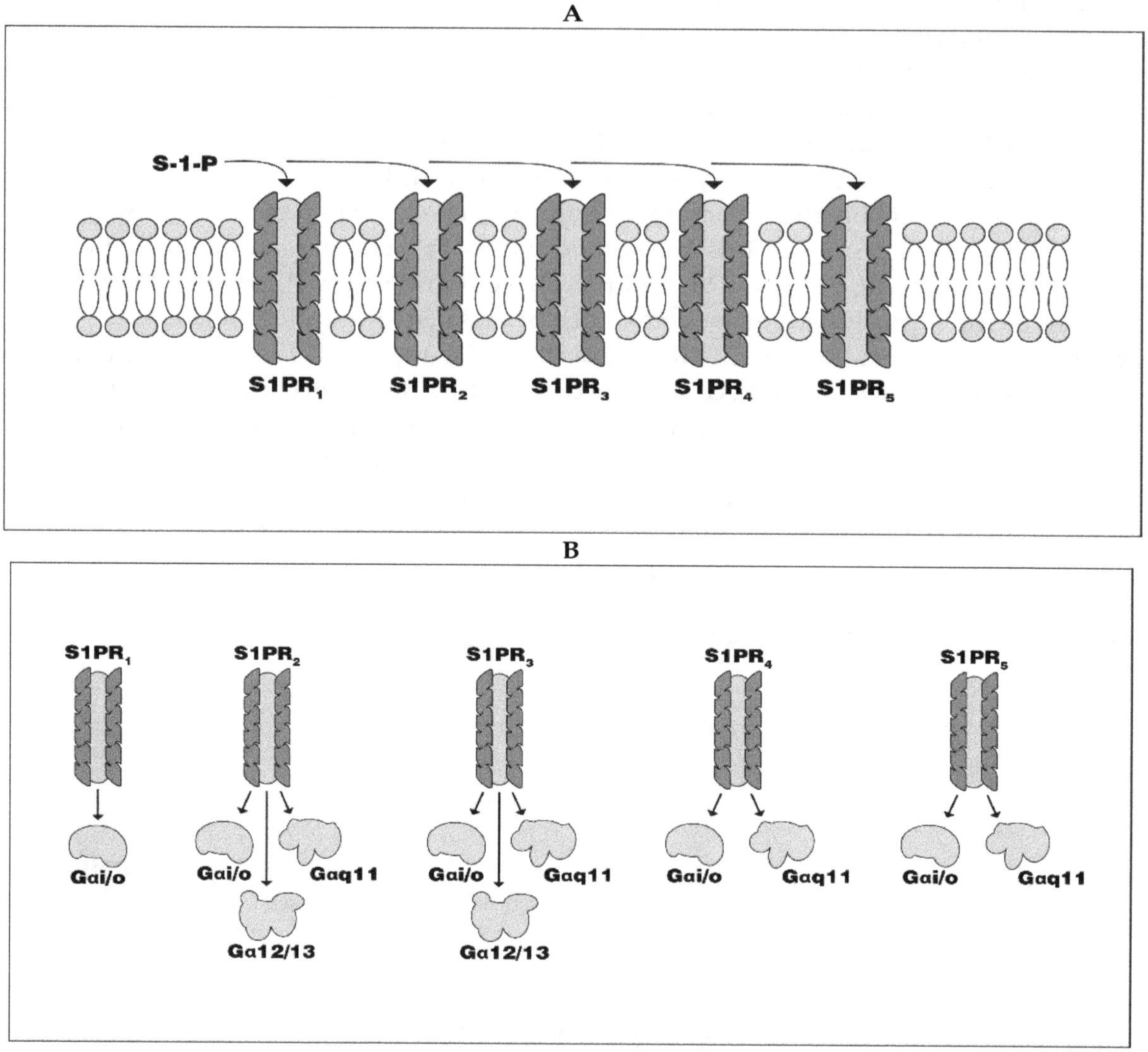

Figure 2. (**A**) Five G protein-coupled Sphingosine-1-phosphate receptors have been identified. (**B**) Each of the S1PRs is coupled to one or more G proteins, resulting in multiple different downstream messaging targets (See Table 1). S-1-P = Sphingosne-1-phosphate (S-1-P), S1PR = Sphingosine-1-phosphate Receptor.

Table 1. G protein-coupled Sphingosine-1-phosphate receptor subset modulation of downstream signaling pathways.

S1PR	G Protein	Downstream Signaling Pathways
S1PR 1–5	Gαi/o→	Akt→Ras→MAPK→Rac
S1PR 2–5	Gαq11→	DAG→PKC→Ca2+
S1PR 2 and 3	Gα12/13→	Rho→ROCK

S1PR = Sphingosine-1-phosphate Receptor, Akt = serine/threonine kinase (protein kinase B), Ras = small GTPase, MAPK = mitogen-activated protein kinase, Rac = member of Rho family of small GTPases, DAG = Diacyl Glycerol, PKC = protein kinase C, Rho = ras homolog gene family, ROCK = Rho kinase.

2. Preclinical Studies

As noted above, S1P is a major intracellular signaling molecule via its G-protein-coupled membrane bound receptors [12–15]. Because the S1PR subsets are coupled to different G-proteins, they can modulate multiple downstream intracellular pathways (Table 1).

Although S1P is critically essential for normal CNS development and maturation [3,4,16,17] and may regulate synaptic function [18], it may also be cytotoxic at elevated concentrations, such as when there is a genetic deficiency in its degradative enzymes, producing neuronal apoptosis [19–24]. S1P also regulates calcium signaling [25], and may promote presynaptic calcium overload and cell death [26].

It is now known that S1P, through its interaction with S1PR-1, expressed on the surface of CCR7+ naïve, central memory B, and T cell lymphocytes, regulates the trafficking of these cells from peripheral lymphoid organs [27–30]. The S1PR-1-expressing lymphocytes egress in response to the S1P gradient (Figure 3). This effect of S1P makes its metabolic and translational pathways attractive potential therapeutic targets for the treatment of cell-mediated immunologic disorders such as MS.

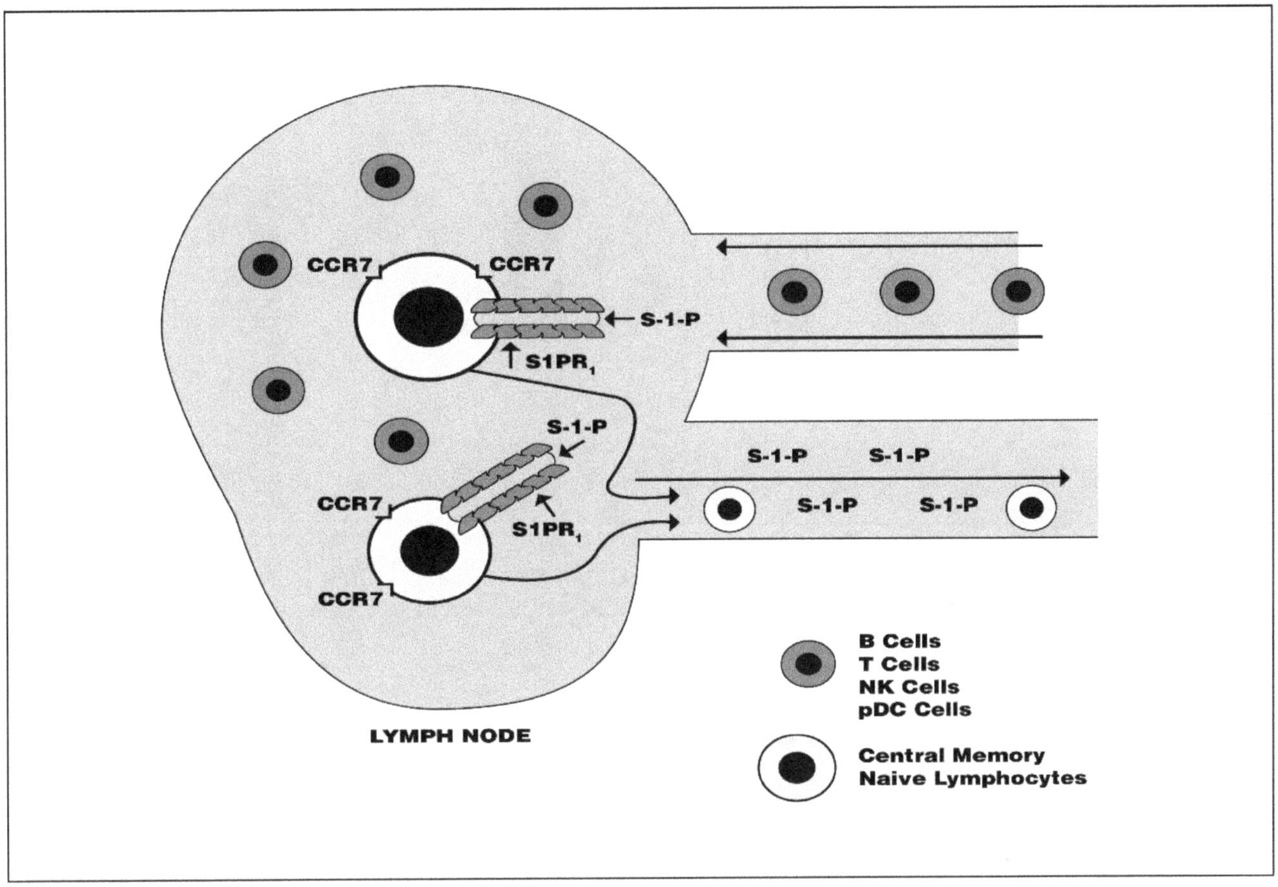

Figure 3. The effect of Sphingosine-1-phosphate on lymphocyte mobilization from peripheral lymphoid organs. Sphingosine-1-phosphate interaction with S1PR1-expressing lymphocytes over-rides CCR7-induced retention signaling, which results in mobilization and egress of naïve and central memory lymphocytes into circulation in response to the S-1-P gradient. Non-CCR7-expressing lymphocytes, such as effector memory cells, are not S-1-P dependent for their entry into the peripheral circulation. B Cells = B cell lymphocytes, T Cells = T cell lymphocyte, NK cells = natural killer cells, pDC Cells = plasmacytoid dendritic cell, S-1-P = Sphingosine-1-phosphate, S1PR1 = Sphingosine-1-Phosphate Receptor, CCR7 = Chemokine Receptor 7.

2.1. S1P Receptors

Fingolimod, approved for the treatment of relapsing forms of MS, is a non-selective S1PR modulator, which once phosphorylated (FGM-P) by sk2 [31], has affinity for S1PRs 1, 3, 4, and 5 [7,31]. The interaction of FGM-P with the S1PR-1 on the surface of CCR7+ lymphocytes results in the internalization and degradation of S1PR-1 [32,33] (Figure 4), promoting the sequestration of naïve, central memory T, and central memory B cell lymphocytes in peripheral lymphoid organs [34]. The circulation of central effector B and T cells, which do not express CCR7, are unaffected by FGM-P. When used in patients with relapsing forms of MS, FGM results in robust clinical and MRI evidence of efficacy, in parallel with marked reduction in circulating B and T cell numbers.

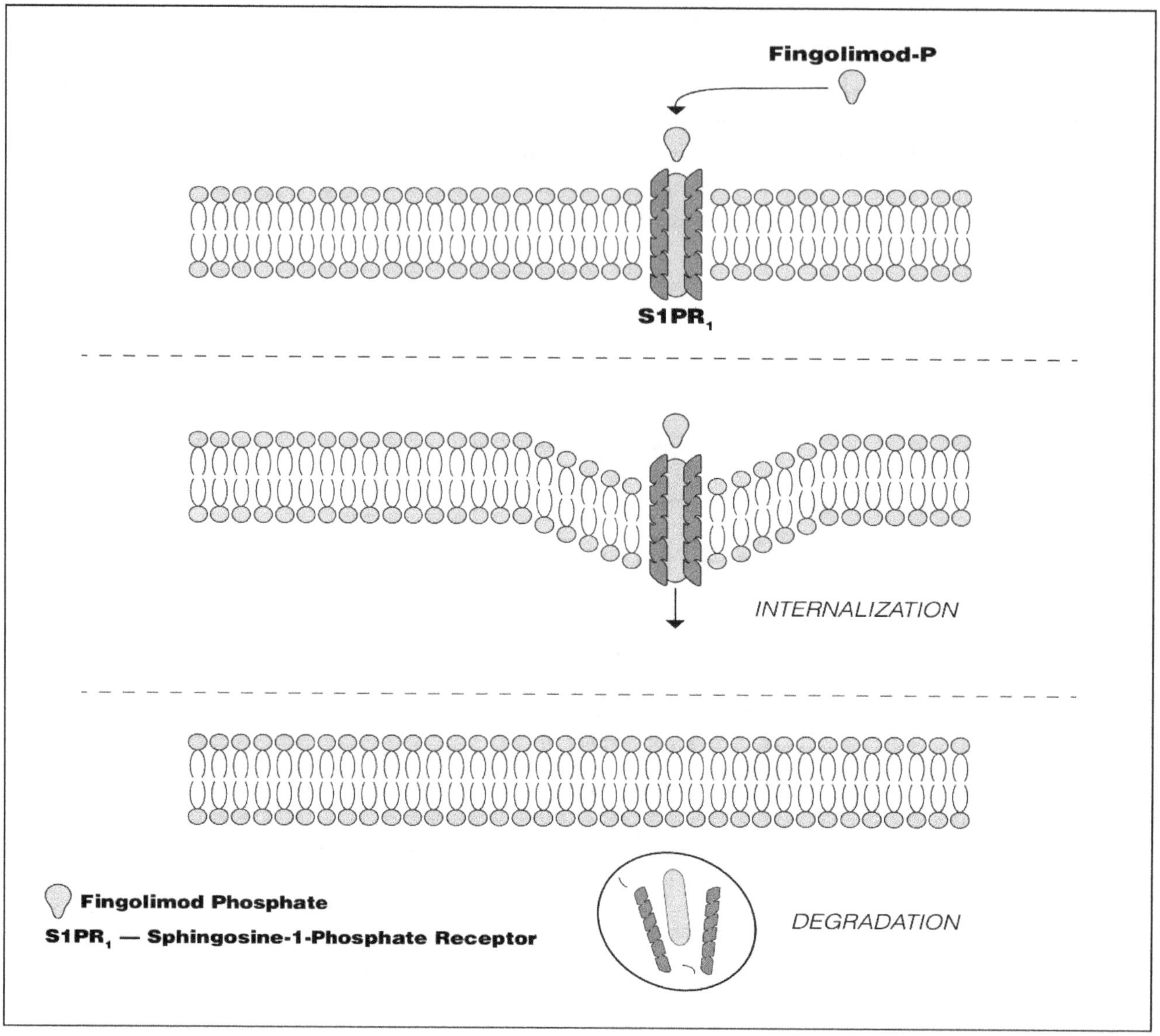

Figure 4. The effect of fingolimod-phosphate upon lymphocyte Sphinogosine-1-phosphate receptor-1. Although initially acting as an agonist, sustained exposure of sphingosine-1-phosphate receptor to fingolimod-phosphate results in receptor internalization and intracellular degradation. As a consequence of sphingosine-phosphate receptor-1 internalization, CCR7-expressing lymphocytes are no longer capable of responding to the sphingosine-1-phhosphate gradient. This results in naïve and central memory cell retention in peripheral lymphoid organs. S1PR$_1$ = Sphingosine-1-phosphate receptor-1.

It has been well-established that the CNS also expresses S1PRs, on neurons, astrocytes, microglia, and oligodendroglia (OLG) during development, maturation, and adult cell states [35–37]. Furthermore, FGM-P, and the newer S1PR modulators SPM, OZM, and PNM, readily cross the blood brain barrier (BBB), and are selectively accumulated within the CNS. Unlike FGM, these latter 3 agents do not require prior phosphorylation to be pharmacologically active. It is possible that some of the therapeutic benefits of S1PR modulators result directly from their effects upon CNS receptors, and in the discussion that follows, we present evidence that supports such a role for these agents. Furthermore, there is evidence to suggest that the therapeutic effects of these agents depends, at least in part, upon their interaction with CNS S1PRs [38].

The use of whole animal inflammatory CNS models, such as experimental allergic encephalitis (EAE), non-inflammatory models of CNS demyelination using in situ cuprizone or lyolecithin, in whole animal, brain tissue slice, and CNS cell culture models [39–42] have all provided important insights into fundamental S1P and S1PR physiology. They have also expanded knowledge of the mechanisms by which S1PR modulation regulates CNS development [4,17], and may protect the CNS during inflammatory insult [38]. What follows is a description of preclinical research which has provided important insights into the role of selective S1PR subtypes, the effects of their modulation/inhibition, and also the use of selective S1PR agonists and antagonists to further clarify the physiological roles of these receptors, and their impact on inflammatory CNS insults.

Although multiple S1PRs are expressed in the mammalian CNS, S1PR-1, 2 and 5 have attracted the most interest because of the pivotal roles they play in the development and myelinating function of OLGs, the regulation of astrocytes and microglia, and in maintaining the integrity of the BBB.

2.1.1. S1PR-1

During CNS inflammation, both S1PR-1 and S1PR-3 are up-regulated by astrocytes and are associated with astrocyte activation and increased production of glial acidic fibrillary protein (GFAP) [3]. The up-regulation of S1PR-1 is seen on activated GFAP-expressing astrocytes in or near active MS lesions [43–45]. During active inflammation there is also S1PR-1-dependent up-regulation of microglia (MGL) that is enhanced in the presence of S1P to further increase inflammation [46]. By contrast, in EAE produced in astrocyte S1PR-1 knockdown mice, there is an inhibition of astrocyte activation [38]. Furthermore, selective S1PR-1 blockade enhances maturation of OLGs [40]. Thus S1PR-1 blockade is a potentially important pharmacological target to reduce astrogliosis and promote remyelination in MS. Although S1PR3 up-regulation occurs in activated astrocytes, the role of S1PR-3 in producing significant cardiovascular effects, via its regulation of the KACh potassium channel [47–50], has diminished interest in it as a target for modulation in MS.

2.1.2. S1PR-2

S1PR-2 is expressed on oligodendroglial progenitor cells (OPC) and macrophages (MPG) [51,52]. In mice with EAE, S1PR-2 activation promotes breakdown of BBB, which is prevented by the use of selective endothelial cell S1PR-2 blocking agents [53], and in endothelial S1PR-2 knockout EAE mice. In these latter models there is also an inhibition of fibrinogen extravasation into the CNS, as well as the inhibition of MPG and MGL recruitment into CNS lesions [41]. To eliminate the potentially confounding effects of systemic inflammation in EAE, models employing in situ injection of lyolecithin-induced demyelination, have produced the same results: S1PR-2 knockout or pharmacologic S1PR-2 inhibition reduced MCP and MGL infiltration of the lesions [41]. S1PR-2 is also a negative regulator of oligodendroglial progenitor cell (OPC) maturation into OLGs. Following demyelination, the inhibition of S1PR-2 promoted maturation of OPCs, increased re-myelination and increased the number of mature myelinated axons [41]. In addition to being a receptor for S1P, S1PR-2 has a high affinity for NOGO A, which also inhibits remyelination [54], providing a second S1PR-2 pathway for the inhibition of re-myelination [55–57]. Consistent with these observations, the pharmacological inhibition of S1PR-2, or use of S1PR-2 knockout mice, results in improved EAE scores, reduced BBB leakage, less fibrinogen extravasation, reduced macrophage (MPG) and MGL recruitment, as well as increased OLG accumulation and re-myelination [53]. Although not a target of any current clinically employed S1PR modulators, S1PR-2 activation, because of its effects on BBB integrity, macrophage/MGL activation, and myelination, could be an important potential therapeutic target of future drug development.

2.1.3. S1P Neurotropism and S1PR-1/S1PR-2 Synergy

Sphingosine-1-P, by stimulating both S1PR-1 and S1PR-2, may induce gene expression encoding for the production of protective astrocyte neurotrophic factors, not achieved by S1PR-1 modulation alone [58]. Bi-receptor S1PR-1 and S1PR-2 stimulation [59] appears to be necessary to up-regulate neurotrophic mRNA expression, which only takes place in astrocytes [60,61]. To date there are no pharmacological agents of which we are aware that operate jointly or exclusively at both S1PR-1 and S1PR-2 under investigation as potential medications for MS, yet the importance of regulating astrocyte proliferation and astrogliosis would be reasons enough to examine agents that can synergistically modulate both receptor subsets.

2.1.4. S1PR-5

The S1PR-5 is mainly expressed on OLGs in white matter tracts, and on brain endothelial cells [51,62]. S1P5 receptor mRNA has been found primarily in the white matter of the CNS, but has not been detected in neurons, microglia, or astrocytes [63,64]. S1PR-5 is expressed throughout the development timeline of OLGs, from immature stages to the mature myelin-forming cell [62,65,66]. In mature OLGs, S1P5 receptors co-localize with myelin basic protein exclusively on myelinated axons and not on OLG cell bodies [64].

Although S1P5 appears to mediate S1P-induced survival of mature OLGs, it may also induce cell process retraction on immature OLGs [51,62], thus regulating a dual-signaling developmental pathway. It appears that activation of S1PR-5 may be important in the maturation and survival of OLGs by playing a role in their modulation, formation, and myelin repair [62].

As has been shown for S1PR-2, S1PR-5 influences BBB integrity and is highly expressed on human brain endothelial cells. Studies have demonstrated that S1PR-5 plays a key role in BBB maintenance and modulation of endothelial cell inflammatory state. S1PR-5 knockdown endothelial cells have reduced barrier integrity [67]. Activation of S1PR-5 reduces the expression of inflammatory cell adhesion molecules on their surface, and enhances the capacity of brain endothelial cells to prevent monocyte penetration. It has been suggested [67] that the role of S1PR-5 may include induction of specific BBB properties such as low paracellular permeability and increased expression of key brain endothelial proteins such as tight junction, ATP binding cassette and glucose transporter molecules. These results point out the potential importance of investigating pharmacological agents which have high affinity and selectivity to promote S1PR-5 preservation in maintaining BBB integrity and protecting OLG maturation and myelination.

2.2. Direct Pharmacological Actions of the S1PR Modulators in the CNS

Established and approved S1P agonists include fingolimod (FGM), siponimod (SPM), and ozanimod (OZM). Ponesimod (PNM) has recently been submitted for regulatory approval based upon Phase III clinical study outcomes. Because it has been available the longest, most data on modulation of S1P receptors by these agents come from studies utilizing FGM. At low doses, FGM has been shown to cause process extension of human OPCs via interaction with S1PR-1, but at high doses, causes process retraction via S1PR-3 and S1PR-5 [42]. Furthermore, short-term FGM treatment causes retraction and prevention of migration of OPCs via an S1PR-3 and S1PR-5-mediated pathway, whereas long-term exposure led to increased cell survival via an S1PR-1-driven pathway [42,51]. Fingolimod also enhances BBB integrity, probably by modulation of S1PR-5, reducing transendothelial migration of monocytes in vitro, the latter being an initial step in the formation of new MS lesions [67].

2.2.1. Fingolimod

As noted above, the therapeutic effects of FGM appear to result at least in part from control of lymphocyte trafficking via down-regulation of lymphocyte S1PR-1 (Figure 4) [68,69]. There is also growing evidence from preclinical studies, that some of FGM's therapeutic effects may be independent of lymphocyte sequestration in peripheral lymphoid organs [38,69]. FGM readily crosses the BBB, potentially enabling its subsequent modulation of S1PRs [35,69,70].

There is up-regulation of S1PR-1- and S1PR-3-expressing astrocytes [71] during active inflammation, and there is growing evidence that astrocytes expressing S1PR-1 may be a primary FGM therapeutic target in the CNS [72]. Consistent with this view has been the demonstration of diminished therapeutic benefit of FGM in EAE in the absence of S1PR-1 expression on astrocytes in genetic knock down mice [38].

Fingolimod, which causes the internalization and destruction of astrocytic S1PR-1 [38] also enhances remyelination in a number of different in vitro models and in EAE mice [40,45,73–75], prevents OLG death, reduces the number of reactive astrocytes and reduces the number of reactive MGL. These beneficial effects are mimicked by the selective S1PR-1 antagonist CYM5442, which also prevents the up-regulation of S1PR-1 on astrocytes [45]. As further evidence of the importance of the astrocyte S1PR-1 receptor, the S1PR-1 gene is primarily expressed in astrocytes, its coupled-G-protein-regulated pathway promotes astrocyte proliferation, and its selective blockade inhibits astrogliosis, potentially reducing OLG death and demyelination. These results are supporting evidence that at least some of the protective effects of FGM are mediated via S1PR-1 negative modulation in the CNS [45]. As further support, deletion of the astrocyte S1PR-1 gene reduces production of the pro-inflammatory cytokines IL-1β, IL-6 and IL-17, reduces demyelination, and eliminates any additive benefit of CNS protection by FGM treatment [38].

2.2.2. Siponimod

Siponimod is a selective modulator of S1PR-1 and S1PR-5 [76,77], and was originally synthesized to reduce cardiovascular effects by eliminating S1PR-3 affinity [78,79]. Its structure favors avid penetration of the BBB. It has a short T1/2 elimination, and lymphocyte counts may return to baseline within 48 h of the last dose (see Table 2) [78]. Recent studies in both human and rodent astrocytes have demonstrated that SPM modulates cellular pro-survival pathways [80–82], primarily via S1PR-1 [82]. SPM also demonstrates anti-inflammatory effects, reducing phosphatidyl choline, TNFα and IL-17-induced IL-6 production by via S1PR-1 modulation. In an in-situ injected curpizone mouse model, SPM treatment reduces myelin breakdown-associated proteins, decreases the number of damaged axons, decreases OLG loss, increases the number of myelinated axons, and reduces MPG and MGL infiltration [83]. In studies of EAE-induced excitotoxic synaptic degeneration, SPM treatment preserves gabaergic neurons in the striatum, and reduces microgliosis, even in the absence of pro-inflammatory lymphocyte affects. These results have been replicated in brain slices, further supporting a direct SPM affect upon the CNS. It has been hypothesized that SPM, via its actions on S1PR-1, reduces MGL activation, which in turn reduces pro-inflammatory lymphocyte recruitment into the CNS [83]. Lastly, since SPM is also a modulator of S1PR-5, preservation of OLGs and myelinated axons in demyelination models following its use is not unexpected. Although, to our knowledge, not yet reported, SPM may also preserve BBB function via S1PR-5 modulation.

Table 2. Pharmacokinetics and pharmacodynamics of the S1PR antagonists.

S1PR Antagonist	T $\frac{1}{2}$ Elimination	Time to Max Concentration	Median Decrease in Maximum Lymphocyte Count	Maximum Decrease in Steady State Lymphocyte Count	Median recovery Time to Normal Lymphocyte Count
fingolimod	6–9 days *	12–26 h	60% of baseline in 4–6 h	18–30% of baseline	1–2 months
siponimod	30 h	4 h	20–30% of baseline	20–30% of baseline	10 days, but up to 3–4 weeks for some patients
ozanimod CC112273 **	21 h 11 days	6–8 h	30% of baseline	45%	30 days ***
ponesimod	21–33 h	2.5–5 h	Not available	70%	4 days

* Increased by 50% in patients with moderate to severe heart disease, ** CC112273 the major ozanimod active metabolite, *** 90% recovery to baseline lymphocyte count with 3 months.

2.2.3. Ozanimod

Ozanimod has a high affinity for S1PR-1 and to a lesser extent for S1PR-5. It selectively crosses the BBB with brain to blood ratio of 10-16:1 [30] and its affinity for the S1PR-1 is comparable to FGM-P and SPM [30]. Like FGM-P and SPM, it induces rapid internalization and degradation of S1PR-1 in rodents and produces reduction in circulating B and T cell lymphocytes [30,84]. Compared to FGM and SPM, there is more rapid lymphocyte reconstitution after it is discontinued. The t1/2 elimination of its major active metabolites, cc112273 and cc1084037, is only 11 days (see Table 2) [85]. Of note, OZM treatment significantly improves EAE scores in mice, even in the presence of restored blood lymphocyte counts [30], supporting a direct CNS therapeutic role. We are unaware of extensive preclinical studies of OZM modulation of S1PR-5, its effects on OPCs, OLGs or myelination, or BBB integrity.

2.2.4. Ponesimod

Ponesimod is a selective S1PR-1 modulator [86,87], with a t1/2 elimination of 21-33 h [87], which like FGM, SPM and OZM, reduces circulating B and T cell lymphocytes by up to 70%, with return to baseline values within 4 days of cessation (see Table 2) [84,88–90], PNM readily crosses the BBB and reduces EAE scores in mice [84].

3. Clinical Trial Results

3.1. *Fingolimod*

Fingolimod was the first oral medication, approved in patients with relapsing forms of MS. The therapeutic efficacy of FGM for RMS was initially established in two pivotal, phase III, double-blind, randomized clinical trials of adults, comparing FGM to placebo (FREEDOMS) and comparing FGM to IFN-β-1a (TRANSFORMS). This was followed by the phase III extension studies FREEDOMS II and extended TRANSFORMS. The regulatory approval for use of FGM in the treatment of RRMS in children ages 10–17 years of age in 2018 [91] followed the results of the pivotal trial, PARADIGM [92].

3.1.1. FREEDOMS

FREEDOMS was a phase III double-blind, placebo-controlled trial with 1272 patients that demonstrated superior efficacy of FGM in RMS when compared to placebo [93]. Inclusion criteria included a diagnosis of RMS, Expanded Disability Status Scale (EDSS) score ≤5.5, and evidence of active disease over the previous 2 years. The median disease duration was 6.7 years, and median EDSS at baseline was 2.0. Patients were randomized in a 1:1:1 ratio to receive placebo, FGM 0.5 mg, or 1.25 mg once daily. The primary endpoint was annualized relapse rate (ARR) and the main secondary endpoint was time to three-month confirmed disability progression (CDP). Other secondary endpoints included: time to first relapse, change in EDSS score and the MS Functional Composite (MSFC) z-score at baseline compared to 24-months, conventional MRI measurements, drug tolerability, and safety. Because the 1.25 mg dose of FGM did not demonstrate therapeutic superiority to the 0.5 mg dose, it was the latter that received regulatory approval, and for that reason only the data for the 0.5 mg dose are presented.

The ARR was 0.18 for 0.5 mg FGM, and 0.40 for placebo-treated patients ($p < 0.0001$), a relative reduction of 54% in favor of FGM. Time to first relapse was significantly longer in FGM than in placebo-treated patients and more FGM patients remained relapse free over 24-months. Cumulative probability of three months of CDP was 17.7% for FGM and 24.1% for placebo (Hazard ratio 0.70). During the 24-month study period, EDSS score and MSFC z-scores remained stable in the FGM-treated group and minimally worsened in the placebo group. FGM treatment was associated with a significant relative decrease in the number of new or enlarging T2 lesions (74%), gadolinium-enhancing (Gd+) lesions (79%) and a relative reduction in brain volume loss (36%), all MRI comparisons being significant at 24 months ($p < 0.001$).

3.1.2. TRANSFORMS

TRANSFORMS was a Phase III clinical trial, enrolling 1292 patients, comparing efficacy of FGM to intramuscular IFNβ-1a in a 12-month, randomized, double-dummy, parallel group study in patients with active RMS over the previous 24 months [94]. The inclusion criteria included a diagnosis of RMS, EDSS ≤ 5.5. Patients were randomized 1:1:1 to oral FGM 0.5 mg or 1.25 mg once daily, or IFNβ-1a 30 μg IM once weekly, and we only report on the FGM 0.5 mg vs. IFNβ-1a results. The primary endpoint was ARR and major secondary endpoints included number of new or enlarging T2 MRI lesions at one year and 3-month CDP during the 12-month duration of the study. At 12 months, ARR was 0.16 for FGM, and 0.33 for IFNβ-1a patients ($p < 0.001$), a relative reduction in ARR of 52%. In the FGM arm time to first relapse was longer and more patients remained relapse free than the IFNβ-1a treated patients. FGM treatment was associated with a relative reduction in the mean number of new and enlarged T2 lesions (FGM 1.7 and IFNβ-1a 2.6; $p < 0.004$), a 54% relative reduction in Gd+ lesions ($p < 0.001$), a 31% relative reduction in percent brain volume loss from baseline ($p < 0.001$). In contrast, there was no significant difference observed between the treatment arms with respect to 3 month CDP.

3.1.3. FREEDOMS II

FREEDOMS II, a phase III trial to evaluate the efficacy and safety of FGM [95] was a 24-month, randomized, double-blind, placebo-controlled, evaluating the efficacy of FGM compared to placebo in 1083 patients. Inclusion criteria included: a diagnosis of RMS, evidence of active disease over the previous 24 months, and an EDSS ≤ 5.5. Patients were randomized in a 1:1:1 ratio to receive FGM 0.5 mg, or 1.25 mg, or placebo once daily but only the FGM 0.5 mg and placebo data are reported; patients randomized to the FGM 1.25 mg arm were switched to 0.5 mg a day at the recommendation of the data and safety committee. The primary endpoint of the trial was ARR. Secondary endpoints included the effect of FGM upon time to 3-month CDP, change in MSFC score, and effect on MRI measurements in comparison to placebo.

The ARR over 24 months was 0.21 for FGM and 0.40 for placebo ($p < 0.0001$), a relative reduction of 48%. The percent change in brain volume from baseline to 24 months, was 0.9% for FGM and 1.3% for placebo, a relative reduction of 31% ($p < 0.001$). The mean number of new and enlarged T2 lesions at 24 months was 2.3 for FGM, and 8.9 for placebo, a relative reduction of 74%; there was a 70% relative reduction in number of Gd+ lesions. There was no significant difference between FGM and placebo in 3- or 6-month CDP. The time to first confirmed relapse was longer, and more patients remained relapse-free in the FGM treated arm compared to placebo-treated patients at 24-months. MSFC scores were also improved at month 24 in the FGM versus the placebo-treated arm.

3.1.4. Extended TRANSFORMS

Extended TRANSFORMS reported long-term results (up to 4.5 years) for the core TRANSFORMS patients [96]. A total of 92% ($n = 1027$) of patients completing TRANSFORMS entered and 75.2% completed the extension phase. Patients randomized to FGM 0.5 mg or FGM 1.25 mg in the core study continued at the same dose in the extension study, whereas patients receiving IFNβ-1a were re-randomized 1:1 to either FGM 0.5 mg or FGM 1.25 mg daily. Following the sponsor's decision to discontinue FGM 1.25 mg in 2009, all patients subsequently received FGM 0.5 mg until completion of the extension phase. It is only the 0.5 mg FGM results vs. IFNβ-1a which are reported below.

The primary endpoint, ARR at 4.5 years, was significantly reduced in patients who initiated FGM treatment in TRANSFORMS compared to those patients switching from IFNβ-1a to FGM during Extended TRANSFORMS: (0.17 versus 0.27), a 35% relative reduction in risk of relapse ($p < 0.001$). Patients initially treated with IFNβ-1a who switched to FGM, experienced a subsequent 50% reduction in ARR, 0.4 to 0.2, by the end of the extension study. MRI outcomes in the extended TRANSFORMS revealed a 63% reduction in new or newly-enlarged T2 lesion count in the group switching from IFNβ-1a to FGM. The proportion of patients with no evidence of disease activity (NEDA: no relapses, no MRI worsening, and no sustained disability progression) increased by 50% in the first year after switching to FGM (43% to 66%). During the extension phase, there was no statistical difference in the number of patients in either group who remained without Gd+ lesions. The relative reduction in brain volume loss observed during the core study in patients continuously treated with FGM was maintained through the extension study, whereas the patients switched from IFNβ to FGM experienced a reduction in the rate of brain volume loss during the extension phase.

3.1.5. PARADIGM

PARADIGM [92] was a 24 month randomized double-blind, active-controlled, parallel group phase III study of 215 patients with RRMS between the ages of 10 and 17 years of age randomized to either daily oral FGM (107) 0.5 mg (0.25 mg for those weighing 40 kg or less), vs. IFNβ-1a 30 μg IM weekly. All patients had evidence of disease activity in the previous 2 years. The primary outcome, ARR, was 0.12 in FGM versus 0.67 in the IFNβ-1a treated patients, a relative decrease of 82% ($p < 0.001$). The mean percentage of relapse-free patients was 85.7 versus 38.8 favoring the FGM treatment arm. Secondary outcomes included the total number of new and enlarged T2 lesions, which was 4.39 in FGM versus 9.27 in IFNβ-1a treated patients, a 53% relative decrease ($p < 0.001$). The mean number of Gd+ lesions/scan was 0.44 in FGM versus 1.28 in IFNβ-1a treated patients. The mean rate in brain volume change was -0.48% in FGM versus −0.8% in IFNβ-1a treated patients.

3.2. Siponimod

As previously indicated, SPM is a selective S1P1R and S1P5R modulator that readily crosses the BBB [78]. Preclinical studies indicate that it may preserve neurons by preventing excitotoxic synaptic degeneration [83], enhancing cell survival pathways [80,82], and promoting remyelination in the CNS [83]. Given the results of these preclinical studies, and because of the need to develop DMTs that might slow disability worsening in patients with secondary progressive multiple sclerosis (SPMS), it was decided to evaluate SPM efficacy in this patient population.

EXPAND

EXPAND [97] was a double-blind, randomized phase III study of 1645 adults, age 18–60, with SPMS and an EDSS score of 3.0–6.5. Patients were assigned (2:1) to once daily oral SPM 2 mg or placebo for up to three years, or until the occurrence of a pre-specified number of CDP events. The primary endpoint was time to three-month CDP. At baseline, the mean time since first MS symptoms was 16.8 years and time since conversion to SPMS was 3.8 years. Sixty-four percent of patients (n = 1055) had not had a relapse in the previous two years; 56% (n = 918) needed walking assistance. Twenty-six percent (288/1096) of patients receiving SPM and 32% (173/545) receiving placebo had three-month CDP (hazard ratio 0.79, 95% CI 0.65–0.95), a relative risk reduction of 21% (p = 0.013). Of the secondary endpoints, there was no significant difference between SPM and placebo-treated patients in the time to three-month confirmed worsening of at least 20% in Timed 25 Foot Walk (T25FW). The increase in T2 lesion volume from baseline was significantly lower in SPM-treated versus placebo-treated patients, with a between group difference of −695.3 mm^3 (95% CI –877.3 to –513.3; $p < 0.0001$). Numerically more patients receiving SPM were free of Gd+ lesions (89% vs. 67%) and of new or enlarging T2 lesions (57% vs. 37%) than their placebo-treated counterparts. Siponimod was approved for the treatment of "active forms" of SPMS, defined as patients having had a relapse in the previous 2 years, because this was the only subgroup in which the primary end-point was achieved. Following completion of the core EXPAND trial, an open label extension was initiated which is expected to conclude in 2024.

3.3. Ozanimod

Ozanimod, a S1PR1 and S1PR5 modulator, that has been studied in two phase III clinical trials, RADIANCE Part B and SUNBEAM, the most recent agent in this class to receive regulatory approval. Each of these trials was a randomized, double-blind, double-dummy, parallel group, active-controlled study, evaluating the efficacy and safety of daily oral OZM 0.5 mg or 1 mg versus weekly IFNβ-1a 30 μg IM in patients with RRMS. Following its ingestion, OZM is partly transformed into 2 primary metabolites, CC112273 and CC1084037, which account for the bulk of OZM pharmacological effects, each with a t1/2 elimination of approximately 11 days, compared to 19–22 h for OZM itself [85].

3.3.1. RADIANCE Part B

RADIANCE Part B [98], a 24 month trial, included 1,313 patients with RRMS randomized to daily oral OZM 0.5 mg ($n = 439$), OZM 1 mg ($n = 433$) or weekly IFN β-1a 30 μg IM ($n = 441$). Inclusion criteria were ages 18–55 years, EDSS 0.0–5.0, diagnosis of RRMS, and evidence of active disease over the prior 24 months. Exclusion criteria included recent myocardial infarction, TIA, stroke, prolonged QTc interval, resting heart rate < 55 bpm, Type I diabetes, or uncontrolled Type II diabetes.

The primary endpoint in RADIANCE Part B was ARR at each OZM dose versus interferon β-1a over 24 months of treatment. Key secondary endpoints included number of new or enlarging T2 brain lesions, number of Gd+ brain lesions, and time to three-month CDP. Other secondary endpoints included relative rate of whole brain volume loss. Exploratory outcomes included relative changes in cortical grey matter and thalamic volumes over the 2 years of observation. Because of its superior efficacy, regulatory approval was only given the 1.0 mg dose. The 0.5 mg data are not presented. ARR at two years was 0.172 for OZM and 0.276 for IFN β-1a, a relative reduction of 38% favoring OZM ($p < 0.0001$). There was a 42% relative reduction in new and enlarging T2 lesions with OZM treatment compared to IFNβ-1a ($p < 0.001$). The relative reduction in number of Gd+ enhancing brain lesions at two years was 53% in OZM-treated patients ($p = 0.0006$) compared to patients treated with IFNβ-1a. There were no statistically significant differences between OZM and IFNβ-1a treatment in time to three-month CDP. Relative reduction in brain volume loss at 2 years was 27% less in OZM ($p < 0.0001$) than in IFNβ-1a treated patients. Relative cortical gray volume loss was reduced by 58% in patients treated with OZM ($p < 0.0001$) and relative thalamic volume loss at 2 years was reduced by 32% ($p < 0.0001$) in patients receiving OZM.

3.3.2. SUNBEAM

The SUNBEAM phase III study [99] included 1,346 patients with RRMS, randomized to daily oral OZM 0.5 mg ($n = 451$) or 1 mg ($n = 447$) versus weekly intramuscular 30 μg IFNβ-1a IM ($n = 448$). Inclusion criteria included ages 18–55 years, EDSS 0.0–5.0, diagnosis of RRMS, with the same remaining inclusion and exclusion criteria as RADIANCE Part B. Only the data for 1 mg OZM is presented.

The primary endpoint in SUNBEAM was ARR with OZM treatment versus IFNβ-1a over 12 months of observation. Key secondary endpoints included number of new or enlarging T2 brain lesions, number of Gd+ brain lesions at one year, and time to three-month CDP. Other secondary endpoints included whole brain volume loss. Exploratory endpoints included cortical grey matter and thalamic volume changes at one year. ARR at one year was 0.181 for OZM and 0.35 for IFNβ -1a treated patients, a relative risk reduction of 48% ($p < 0.0001$) favoring OZM treated patients. There was a 48% relative reduction in the number of new or enlarging T2 brain lesions favoring OZM-treated patients ($p < 0.001$) and total number of Gd+-brain lesions reduced by 63% in the OZM treatment arm ($p < 0.0001$) compared to IFNβ-1a. There was no statistically significant difference between OZM and IFNβ-1a for time to three-month CDP. There was a 33% relative reduction ($p < 0.0001$) in percentage whole brain volume decrease for OZM treated patients, as well as an 84% ($p < 0.0001$) relative reduction in cortical grey matter loss and a 39% ($p < 0.0001$) relative reduction in thalamic volume loss in OZM treated patients. It is of particular interest to learn the results of on-going studies which are focused on cognitive functioning and patient reported outcome status [100] in light of the demonstrated relative reduction in cortical gray matter and thalamic volume loss in OZM treated patients.

The regulatory approval for the higher OZM dose is a 92 mg capsule, as opposed to the 1.0 mg OZM hydrochloride tablets used in the clinical trials [85].

3.4. *Ponesimod*

Ponesimod (PNM), a selective S1PR-1 modulator without known effect on the remaining four S1PRs, has been studied in one phase III clinical trial.

OPTIMUM

OPTIMUM [101], was a 108 week multicenter, randomized, double-blind, parallel group, and active controlled study, evaluating the efficacy, safety, and tolerability of daily oral PNM 20 mg versus daily oral teriflunomide (TFM) 14 mg in adults with RRMS. OPTIMUM enrolled 1,133 patients, randomized to receive PNM ($n = 567$) or TFM ($n = 566$). Inclusion criteria included ages 18 to 55 years, EDSS 0.0-5.0, diagnosis of RRMS, and active disease in the 24 months prior to screening. The primary end-point was ARR over 108 weeks. Key secondary end-points included change from baseline to week 108 in fatigue-related symptoms, as measured by the symptoms domain of the FSIQ-RMS. Other secondary endpoints included the mean number of combined unique active lesions (CUAL) per year, defined as new Gd+1 lesions and any new or enlarging T2 lesions. In addition, time to 12-week and 24-week CDP was also determined.

There was a 30.5% relative reduction ($p = 0.0003$) in ARR in PNM treated patients (0.202 versus 0.290) compared to TFM treated patients. Ponesimod demonstrated superior improvement in fatigue scores at week 108 compared to TFM as measured by the FSIQ-RMS weekly symptom score (mean difference −3.57, $p = 0.0019$). There was a 56% relative reduction in CUALs per year (1.405 versus 3.164) in patients treated with PNM. No significant differences between PNM and TFM seen for 12-week or 24-week CDP.

4. Safety

4.1. Fingolimod

In FREEDOMS, 94% of patients receiving FGM compared to 93% of patients receiving placebo had an AE. The majority of these events were mild to moderate with 7.5% of patients on FGM stopping due to side effects compared to 7.7% on placebo. In TRANSFORMS, 86% of FGM 0.5 mg patients compared to 92% of patients on IFNβ-1a had an AE. However, 6% of patients on FGM versus 4% or patients on IFNβ-1a discontinued due to an AE [93,94].

In FREEDOMS, overall, incidence of infections was the same in all treatment groups; however, lower respiratory infections were more common in patients receiving FGM. There were two deaths in the 1.25 mg FGM group, one each of disseminated primary varicella zoster and herpes simplex encephalitis. The overall rate of herpes infections receiving FGM was 0.01 (10/854) and 0.01 (4/418) in placebo treated patients. As of this writing, there have been 36 confirmed cases of PML in greater than 746,700 patient years since FGM approval. In an analysis of 21 PML cases, age at treatment initiation was not a risk factor for the development of PML; however, longer duration of exposure to FGM increased the risk of developing PML [102]. As of February 2019, 46 cases of cryptococcal infections have been reported. (Novartis data on file), the majority of whom were treated for 2 or more years

Macular edema was slightly more common in patients on 0.5 mg of FGM compared to placebo, 0.5 verses 0.4%, and typically occurred within the first 3 to 4 months of therapy. Because patients with diabetes and uveitis are at higher risk of developing macular edema, they were excluded from the clinical trials. Given the risk of macular edema, a baseline eye exam is recommended within 6 months of starting and then 3 to 4 months after beginning FGM [91].

Fingolimod, on average, lowered the heart rate by eight beats per minute. Following the first dose, 0.6% of patients receiving FGM developed symptomatic bradycardia compared to 0.1% in the placebo group, with rare cases of second degree AV block reported. Nonetheless, patients are required to undergo an ECG prior to the first dose observation (FDO), and then at least a 6 h FDO, during which time hourly pulse and blood pressure are obtained, followed by an additional ECG at the end of monitoring. Medications which can cause bradycardia or prolong the QT interval, such as beta blockers. Selective serotonin and norepinephrine reuptake inhibitors are to be used with caution and may prompt, overnight or more prolonged ambulatory cardiac rhythm monitoring. Fingolimod is contraindicated in patients with recent myocardial infarction, unstable angina, stroke, transient ischemic attack, or heart failure within the last 6 months [91]. There was also an average 3 mm Hg increase in systolic blood pressure and 2 mm Hg increase in diastolic pressure in patients on FGM. Elevation in liver enzymes was more commonly seen in the patients receiving FGM, with elevations of three times the upper limit of normal (ULN) or greater were seen in 14% of patients treated with FGM and in 3% of patients on placebo, typically occurring within 6 to 9 months of starting FGM. Peripheral lymphocyte counts dropped by 73% on average in patients receiving FGM, and typically return to baseline values 1–2 after stopping FGM (Novartis data on file). To date, there has been no evidence that lower lymphocyte counts are predictive of increased infection risk [103].

Skin cancer, particularly basal cell carcinoma, may be more common in patients on FGM [91]. Post-marketing studies have also reported rare cases of cutaneous melanoma and squamous cell carcinoma [104,105].

In the pediatric population (PARADIGM), the incidence of AEs was 88.8% in FGM and 95.3% in IFNβ-1a treated patients. The most common side effects in the FGM treated patients were headache (31.8%), viral upper respiratory infections (21.5%), Upper respiratory infections (15.9%), leukopenia (14%), influenza (1.2%), cough (9%), and pyrexia (7.5%). Serious AEs occurred in the FGM treated cohort and 4.7 % of FGM treated patients discontinued the trial because of SAEs. These AEs included convulsions (5.6%), and 3.7% of patients had serious infections, including one case each of appendicitis, cellulitis, oral abscess, and viral pharyngitis. Single SAE cases also included agranulocytosis, arthralgia, auto-immune uveitis, gastrointestinal necrosis, vasculitis, second degree AV conduction block, and small bowel obstruction.

Fingolimod is not recommended during pregnancy and lactation, based upon its teratogenicity, increased fetal loss and its presence in the milk of lactating animals. Prescribing information currently recommends stopping FGM 3-months prior to planning conception; however this recommendation may require revision in light of recent reports of increased MS breakthrough activity, occurring in 10–25% of patients within 12 weeks of discontinuing FGM [106,107]. Patients with a higher annualized risk of relapse or higher EDSS prior to starting FGM may be at greater risk of rebound disease once stopping FGM [108].

4.2. *Siponimod*

The SPM safety profile is similar to that of FGM. In EXPAND [97], 89% of patients receiving SPM and 82% of patients receiving placebo had an AE. Non-serious adverse events leading to discontinuation in the study was 4% versus 3% respectively. Serious adverse events occurred in 18% of the SPM group compared to 15% in the placebo group.

Rate of infections were also similar in both groups, but upper and lower respiratory infections, as well as herpes zoster reactivation, were more common in the SPM treated group. The risk of herpes infection was 2.5% in SPM versus 0.7% in placebo treated patients. No cases of PML or cryptococcal infections were reported, although these opportunistic infections may emerge as larger populations are treated for longer durations, given the similar mechanism of action compared to FNM. The reduction in the peripheral lymphocyte count was between 20 to 30% which is less than that observed in patients treated with FGM [93,94], but whether this impacts the comparative rate of infection is yet to be determined.

Liver function abnormalities were observed in 10.7% of SPM treated patients and 3.7% in the placebo group.

Rate of macular edema was 1.8% in patients on SPM and 0.2% of patients treated with placebo. This is higher than 0.4% reported in the phase III clinical trials with FGM [93,94].

Seizures occurred in 1.7% of SPM treated patients and was 0.4% in the placebo group.

The reduction in heart rate was a mean of six beats per minute in the SPM treated group, with the maximum reduction occurring on average 4 h after the first dose. Bradycardia was reported as an AE in 6% of patients receiving SPM compared to 3% receiving placebo. Cases of Mobitz type II or higher degree atrio-ventricular (AV) block were not observed. As a result, first dose observation is not required except for patients with recent history of myocardial infarction, unstable angina, recent stroke, TIA or baseline heart rate of less than 55 beats per minute [109]. Clinicians may also recommend first dose observation for patients on medication which may lower heart rate, particularly those medication that slow AV conduction.

Elevation in liver enzymes was 10.1% in patients on SPM, versus 3.7% of patients on placebo. Overall, rate of malignancies was the same in each group.

Medications which inhibit the hepatic enzymes CYP2C9 and CYP3A4 can result in elevated concentration of SPM, and the opposite is true for hepatic enzyme inducers. Furthermore, in patients with the CYP2C9 genotype variants CYP2C9 1*/3* or 2*/3* should receive only 1.0 mg a day maintenance dosing and those with the 3*/3* genotype should not receive SPM at all due to their inhibition of SPM degradation in the liver [109].

4.3. Ozanimod

In RADIANCE and SUNBEAM, overall AEs and AEs leading to discontinuation were lower in both groups of patients taking OZM compared to interferon beta-1a. Nasopharyngitis, elevated liver enzymes, hypertension, and urinary tract infections were commonly seen in the OZM groups in both clinic trials. No serious opportunistic infections were reported, and the rate of herpes infections were the same across the three treatment groups.

There was one case of posterior reversible encephalopathy syndrome (PRES) in a patient receiving 1.0 mg OZM, occurring 10 months after starting the medication. Of note, post-approval cases have also been reported in patients treated with FGM [110,111]. Mean absolute lymphocyte count in patients on OZM 1.0 mg were reduced by approximately 45% by 3 months, and maintained at that level thereafter. The rate of macular edema was 0.3% in each OZM and the IFNβ-1a group. Maximum mean reduction in heart rate on day 1 was 0.6 bpm at 5 h in RADIANCE. Four patients treated with OZM had a heart rate less than 45, but had baseline heart rates of 55-64 bpm, and no symptoms were reported. In SUNBEAM, the maximum mean reduction was 1.8 bpm at 5 h, with no rate below 45 bpm reported. No second- or third-degree heart block was observed in either study. Given the minimal reduction in heart rate, FDO is not required for most patients.

As with the other S1PR-1 modulators, mild elevations in liver function enzymes were observed. In RADIANCE, 6.7% of patients on 1.0 mg of OZM had an ALT of 3 X ULN normal, as did 3.9% of patients on IFNβ-1a. In SUNBEAM, the rate was 4.3% for OZM and 2.2% for IFNβ-1a treated patients.

4.4. Contraindications and Cautions

The use of FGM, SPM, and OZM is contraindicated in patients with recent (within the past 6 months) myocardial infarction or stroke, unstable angina, class III/IV heart failure4.4, recent transient ischemic attack and in patients receiving class I and Class III anti-arrhythmics, patients with Mobitz type 2 s or third degree heart block, sino-atrial block, or sick sinus syndrome without a functioning pacemaker. In addition, specifically for OZM there is a contraindication for the concomitant use of monoamine oxidase inhibitors and in patients with untreated severe sleep apnea. The concomitant use of SSRIs, SNRIs and narcotics is not recommended for any of the S1PR modulators [85,91,109].

4.5. Ponesimod

The proportion of patients experiencing at least one treatment emergent AE (TEAE) in OPTIMUM was similar for both PNM and TFM, although discontinuation due to TEAE was higher in the PMN than the TFM group, 8.7% vs. 6.0% respectively. Premature discontinuations due to elevated liver enzymes and respiratory events were relatively higher in the PNM than TFM groups. The most common AEs of special interest were elevated liver function tests in the PNM group, (22.7% vs. 12.2%), hypertension (10.1% vs. 9.0%), and pulmonary events (8.0% vs. 2.7%). Most ALT increases ≥3X ULN were single transient asymptomatic events that spontaneously resolved on treatment or resulted in protocol mandated discontinuation. Eight seizures were reported in patients treated with PMN compared to one patient on TFM.

Skin malignancies occurred in five patients treated with PMN and in one patient in the TFM group. Four cases of bradycardia (0.7%) occurred in the PMN 20 mg group and an additional three patients experienced first degree atrioventricular block. None of the events were serious or led to treatment discontinuation.

5. Potential Therapeutic Opportunities

As is evident from the data presented, the S1PR modulators are an important addition to the list of DMTs for the treatment of MS. In addition to their oral route of administration, an important addition to patient quality of life, with a higher likelihood of compliance and persistence, they offer significant improvement in clinical efficacy at acceptable levels of risk in studies in which they have been compared to "platform" injectable or oral therapies. Important questions and research opportunities remain. Will agents with more potent S1PR-5 modulation improve remyelination, as a result of improved maturation of OPCs and enhanced myelin formation by OLGs? Will their use reduce inflammatory impact of MS by the enhancement of BBB integrity? Will selective S1PR-2 inhibition stimulate remyelination by blocking the NOGO/LOGO membrane complex, and will simultaneous S1PR-1 and S1PR-2 provide greater synergistic regulation of astrocytes than either agent alone? Since S1PR-3 is up-regulated on astrocytes during CNS inflammation [112] can CNS selective S1PR-3 modulators be developed which do not also increase cardiovascular side effects? Lastly, as more is learned about the intracellular pathways activated or inhibited by S1P and its receptors, the development of pharmacological agents which can manipulate these pathways, and the development of agents that can interact with intracellular S1PRs, offer highly specific, potentially fruitful therapeutic opportunities for MS and numerous other diseases, including rheumatoid arthritis [113–115], systemic lupus [116,117], polymyotisis [118], ulcerative colitis [119], psoriasis [120], colon cancer [121–123], breast cancer [124–126], lung cancer [127,128] and atherosclerosis [129,130].

Author Contributions: Conceptualization, S.C., E.L., K.S., and J.B.; writing—original draft preparation, S.C., E.L., K.S., J.B., and C.C.; writing—review and editing, S.C. and C.C. All authors have read and agreed to the published version of the manuscript.

Acknowledgments: The authors acknowledge and thank Jessica Garten for producing Figures 1–4.

References

1. Spiegel, S.; Milstien, S. Sphingosine-1-phosphate: An enigmatic signalling lipid. *Nat. Rev. Mol. Cell Boil.* **2003**, *4*, 397–407. [CrossRef] [PubMed]
2. Merrill, A.H. Sphingolipid and Glycosphingolipid Metabolic Pathways in the Era of Sphingolipidomics. *Chem. Rev.* **2011**, *111*, 6387–6422. [CrossRef] [PubMed]
3. Grassi, S.; Mauri, L.; Prioni, S.; Cabitta, L.; Sonnino, S.; Prinetti, A.; Giussani, P. Sphingosine 1-Phosphate Receptors and Metabolic Enzymes as Druggable Targets for Brain Diseases. *Front. Pharmacol.* **2019**, *10*, 807. [CrossRef] [PubMed]
4. Proia, R.L.; Hla, T. Emerging biology of sphingosine-1-phosphate: Its role in pathogenesis and therapy. *J. Clin. Investig.* **2015**, *125*, 1379–1387. [CrossRef]
5. Brunkhorst, R.; Vutukuri, R.; Pfeilschifter, W. Fingolimod for the treatment of neurological diseases-state of play and future perspectives. *Front. Cell. Neurosci.* **2014**, *8*. [CrossRef]
6. Blaho, V.A.; Hla, T. An update on the biology of sphingosine 1-phosphate receptors. *J. Lipid Res.* **2014**, *55*, 1596–1608. [CrossRef]
7. Brinkmann, V.; Davis, M.D.; Heise, C.E.; Albert, R.; Cottens, S.; Hof, R.; Bruns, C.; Prieschl, E.; Baumruker, T.; Hiestand, P.; et al. The Immune Modulator FTY720 Targets Sphingosine 1-Phosphate Receptors. *J. Boil. Chem.* **2002**, *277*, 21453–21457. [CrossRef]
8. Webb, M.; Tham, C.-S.; Lin, F.-F.; Lariosa-Willingham, K.; Yu, N.; Hale, J.; Mandala, S.; Chun, J.; Rao, T.S. Sphingosine 1-phosphate receptor agonists attenuate relapsing–remitting experimental autoimmune encephalitis in SJL mice. *J. Neuroimmunol.* **2004**, *153*, 108–121. [CrossRef]

9. Matloubian, M.; Lo, C.G.; Cinamon, G.; Lesneski, M.J.; Xu, Y.; Brinkmann, V.; Allende, M.L.; Proia, R.L.; Cyster, J.G. Lymphocyte egress from thymus and peripheral lymphoid organs is dependent on S1P receptor 1. *Nature* **2004**, *427*, 355–360. [CrossRef]
10. Pappu, R.; Schwab, S.R.; Cornelissen, I.; Pereira, J.P.; Regard, J.B.; Xu, Y.; Camerer, E.; Zheng, Y.-W.; Huang, Y.; Cyster, J.G.; et al. Promotion of Lymphocyte Egress into Blood and Lymph by Distinct Sources of Sphingosine-1-Phosphate. *Science* **2007**, *316*, 295–298. [CrossRef]
11. Cyster, J.G.; Schwab, S.R. Sphingosine-1-Phosphate and Lymphocyte Egress from Lymphoid Organs. *Annu. Rev. Immunol.* **2012**, *30*, 69–94. [CrossRef] [PubMed]
12. Harrison, S.M.; Reavill, C.; Brown, G.; Brown, J.T.; Cluderay, J.E.; Crook, B.; Davies, C.H.; Dawson, L.A.; Grau, E.; Heidbreder, C.; et al. LPA1 receptor-deficient mice have phenotypic changes observed in psychiatric disease. *Mol. Cell Neurosci.* **2003**, *24*, 1170–1179. [CrossRef] [PubMed]
13. Chun, J.; Brinkmann, V. Faculty Opinions recommendation of A mechanistically novel, first oral therapy for multiple sclerosis: The development of fingolimod (FTY720, Gilenya). *Fac. Opin. Post-Pub. Peer Rev. Biomed. Lit.* **2014**, *12*, 213–228. [CrossRef]
14. Choi, J.W.; Chun, J. Lysophospholipids and their receptors in the central nervous system. *Biochim. Biophys. Acta (BBA)-Mol. Cell Boil. Lipids* **2013**, *1831*, 20–32. [CrossRef]
15. Giussani, P.C.; Tringali, C.A.; Riboni, L.; Viani, P.; Venerando, B. Sphingolipids: Key Regulators of Apoptosis and Pivotal Players in Cancer Drug Resistance. *Int. J. Mol. Sci.* **2014**, *15*, 4356–4392. [CrossRef] [PubMed]
16. Bassi, R.; Anelli, V.V.; Giussani, P.C.; Tettamanti, G.; Viani, P.; Riboni, L. Sphingosine-1-phosphate is released by cerebellar astrocytes in response to bFGF and induces astrocyte proliferation through Gi-protein-coupled receptors. *Glia* **2006**, *53*, 621–630. [CrossRef]
17. Mizugishi, K.; Yamashita, T.; Olivera, A.; Miller, G.F.; Spiegel, S.; Proia, R.L. Essential Role for Sphingosine Kinases in Neural and Vascular Development. *Mol. Cell. Boil.* **2005**, *25*, 11113–11121. [CrossRef]
18. Riganti, L.; Antonucci, F.; Gabrielli, M.; Prada, I.; Giussani, P.C.; Viani, P.; Valtorta, F.; Menna, E.; Matteoli, M.; Verderio, C. Sphingosine-1-Phosphate (S1P) Impacts Presynaptic Functions by Regulating Synapsin I Localization in the Presynaptic Compartment. *J. Neurosci.* **2016**, *36*, 4624–4634. [CrossRef]
19. Moore, A.N.; Kampfl, A.W.; Zhao, X.; Hayes, R.L.; Dash, P.K. Sphingosine-1-phosphate induces apoptosis of cultured hippocampal neurons that requires protein phosphatases and activator protein-1 complexes. *Neuroscience* **1999**, *94*, 405–415. [CrossRef]
20. Hagen, N.; Van Veldhoven, P.P.; Proia, R.L.; Park, H.; Merrill, A.H.; Van Echten-Deckert, G. Subcellular Origin of Sphingosine 1-Phosphate Is Essential for Its Toxic Effect in Lyase-deficient Neurons. *J. Boil. Chem.* **2009**, *284*, 11346–11353. [CrossRef]
21. Hagen, N.; Hans, M.; Hartmann, D.; Swandulla, D.; Van Echten-Deckert, G. Sphingosine-1-phosphate links glycosphingolipid metabolism to neurodegeneration via a calpain-mediated mechanism. *Cell Death Differ.* **2011**, *18*, 1356–1365. [CrossRef] [PubMed]
22. Mitroi, D.N.; Karunakaran, I.; Gräler, M.; Saba, J.D.; Ehninger, D.; Ledesma, M.D.; Van Echten-Deckert, G. SGPL1 (sphingosine phosphate lyase 1) modulates neuronal autophagy via phosphatidylethanolamine production. *Autophagy* **2017**, *13*, 885–899. [CrossRef]
23. Karunakaran, I.; Alam, S.; Jayagopi, S.; Frohberger, S.J.; Hansen, J.N.; Kuehlwein, J.; Hölbling, B.V.; Schumak, B.; Hübner, M.P.; Gräler, M.H.; et al. Neural sphingosine 1-phosphate accumulation activates microglia and links impaired autophagy and inflammation. *Glia* **2019**, *67*, 1859–1872. [CrossRef] [PubMed]
24. Choi, Y.-J.; Saba, J.D. Sphingosine phosphate lyase insufficiency syndrome (SPLIS): A novel inborn error of sphingolipid metabolism. *Adv. Boil. Regul.* **2019**, *71*, 128–140. [CrossRef] [PubMed]
25. Giussani, P.C.; Ferraretto, A.; Gravaghi, C.; Bassi, R.; Tettamanti, G.; Riboni, L.; Viani, P. Sphingosine-1-Phosphate and Calcium Signaling in Cerebellar Astrocytes and Differentiated Granule Cells. *Neurochem. Res.* **2006**, *32*, 27–37. [CrossRef] [PubMed]
26. Mitroi, D.N.; Deutschmann, A.U.; Raucamp, M.; Karunakaran, I.; Glebov, K.; Hans, M.; Walter, J.; Saba, J.; Gräler, M.; Ehninger, D.; et al. Sphingosine 1-phosphate lyase ablation disrupts presynaptic architecture and function via an ubiquitin- proteasome mediated mechanism. *Sci. Rep.* **2016**, *6*, 37064. [CrossRef] [PubMed]
27. Brinkmann, V.; Cyster, J.G.; Hla, T. FTY720: Sphingosine 1-Phosphate Receptor-1 in the Control of Lymphocyte Egress and Endothelial Barrier Function. *Arab. Archaeol. Epigr.* **2004**, *4*, 1019–1025. [CrossRef]
28. Chiba, K. FTY720, a new class of immunomodulator, inhibits lymphocyte egress from secondary lymphoid tissues and thymus by agonistic activity at sphingosine 1-phosphate receptors. *Pharmacol. Ther.* **2005**, *108*, 308–319. [CrossRef]

29. Thangada, S.; Khanna, K.M.; Blaho, V.A.; Oo, M.L.; Im, D.-S.; Guo, C.; Lefrancois, L.; Hla, T. Cell-surface residence of sphingosine 1-phosphate receptor 1 on lymphocytes determines lymphocyte egress kinetics. *J. Exp. Med.* **2010**, *207*, 1475–1483. [CrossRef]
30. Scott, F.L.; Clemons, B.; Brooks, J.; Brahmachary, E.; Powell, R.; Dedman, H.; Desale, H.G.A.; Timony, G.; Martinborough, E.; Rosen, H.; et al. Ozanimod (RPC1063) is a potent sphingosine-1-phosphate receptor-1 (S1P1) and receptor-5 (S1P5) agonist with autoimmune disease-modifying activity. *Br. J. Pharmacol.* **2016**, *173*, 1778–1792. [CrossRef]
31. Mandala, S. Alteration of Lymphocyte Trafficking by Sphingosine-1-Phosphate Receptor Agonists. *Science* **2002**, *296*, 346–349. [CrossRef] [PubMed]
32. Oo, M.L.; Thangada, S.; Wu, M.T.; Liu, C.H.; Macdonald, T.L.; Lynch, K.R.; Lin, C.Y.; Hla, T. Immunosuppressive and anti-angiogenic sphingosine 1-phosphate receptor-1 agonists induce ubiquitinylation and proteasomal degradation of the receptor. *J. Biol. Chem.* **2007**, *282*, 9082–9089. [CrossRef]
33. Gräler, M.H.; Goetzl, E.J. The immunosuppressant FTY720 down-regulates sphingosine 1-phosphate G protein-coupled receptors. *FASEB J.* **2004**, *18*, 551–553. [CrossRef]
34. Mullershausen, F.; Zecri, F.; Çetin, C.; Billich, A.; Guerini, D.; Seuwen, K. Persistent signaling induced by FTY720-phosphate is mediated by internalized S1P1 receptors. *Nat. Methods* **2009**, *5*, 428–434. [CrossRef] [PubMed]
35. Groves, A.; Kihara, Y.; Chun, J. Fingolimod: Direct CNS effects of sphingosine 1-phosphate (S1P) receptor modulation and implications in multiple sclerosis therapy. *J. Neurol. Sci.* **2013**, *328*, 9–18. [CrossRef] [PubMed]
36. Subei, A.M.; Cohen, J.A. Sphingosine 1-phosphate receptor modulators in multiple sclerosis. *CNS Drugs* **2015**, *29*, 565–575. [CrossRef] [PubMed]
37. Mao-Draayer, Y.; Sarazin, J.; Fox, D.; Schiopu, E. The sphingosine-1-phosphate receptor: A novel therapeutic target for multiple sclerosis and other autoimmune diseases. *Clin. Immunol.* **2016**, *175*, 10–15. [CrossRef]
38. Choi, J.W.; Gardell, S.E.; Herr, D.R.; Rivera, R.; Lee, C.-W.; Noguchi, K.; Teo, S.T.; Yung, Y.C.; Lu, M.; Kennedy, G.; et al. FTY720 (fingolimod) efficacy in an animal model of multiple sclerosis requires astrocyte sphingosine 1-phosphate receptor 1 (S1P1) modulation. *Proc. Natl. Acad. Sci. USA* **2010**, *108*, 751–756. [CrossRef]
39. Kim, H.J.; Miron, V.E.; Dukala, D.; Proia, R.L.; Ludwin, S.K.; Traka, M.; Antel, J.P.; Soliven, B. Neurobiological effects of sphingosine 1-phosphate receptor modulation in the cuprizone model. *FASEB J.* **2011**, *25*, 1509–1518. [CrossRef]
40. Nystad, A.E.; Lereim, R.R.; Wergeland, S.; Oveland, E.; Myhr, K.-M.; Bø, L.; Torkildsen, Ø. Fingolimod downregulates brain sphingosine-1-phosphate receptor 1 levels but does not promote remyelination or neuroprotection in the cuprizone model. *J. Neuroimmunol.* **2020**, *339*, 577091. [CrossRef]
41. Seyedsadr, M.S.; Weinmann, O.; Amorim, A.; Ineichen, B.V.; Egger, M.; Mirnajafi-Zadeh, J.; Becher, B.; Javan, M.; Schwab, M.E. Inactivation of sphingosine-1-phosphate receptor 2 (S1PR2) decreases demyelination and enhances remyelination in animal models of multiple sclerosis. *Neurobiol. Dis.* **2019**, *124*, 189–201. [CrossRef]
42. Miron, V.E.; Jung, C.-G.; Kim, H.J.; Kennedy, T.E.; Soliven, B.; Antel, J.P. FTY720 modulates human oligodendrocyte progenitor process extension and survival. *Ann. Neurol.* **2008**, *63*, 61–71. [CrossRef]
43. Brana, C.; Frossard, M.J.; Gobert, R.P.; Martinier, N.; Boschert, U.; Seabrook, T.J. Immunohistochemical detection of sphingosine-1-phosphate receptor 1 and 5 in human multiple sclerosis lesions. *Neuropathol. Appl. Neurobiol.* **2014**, *40*, 564–578. [CrossRef]
44. Van Doorn, R.; Van Horssen, J.; Verzijl, D.; Witte, M.; Ronken, E.; Hof, B.V.H.; Lakeman, K.; Dijkstra, C.D.; Van Der Valk, P.; Reijerkerk, A.; et al. Sphingosine 1-phosphate receptor 1 and 3 are upregulated in multiple sclerosis lesions. *Glia* **2010**, *58*, 1465–1476. [CrossRef] [PubMed]
45. Kim, S.; Bielawski, J.; Yang, H.; Kong, Y.; Zhou, B.; Li, J. Functional antagonism of sphingosine-1-phosphate receptor 1 prevents cuprizone-induced demyelination. *Glia* **2017**, *66*, 654–669. [CrossRef] [PubMed]
46. Assi, E.; Cazzato, D.; De Palma, C.; Perrotta, C.; Clementi, E.; Cervia, D. Sphingolipids and Brain Resident Macrophages in Neuroinflammation: An Emerging Aspect of Nervous System Pathology. *Clin. Dev. Immunol.* **2013**, *2013*, 1–8. [CrossRef]

47. Koyrakh, L.; Roman, M.I.; Brinkmann, V.; Wickman, K. The Heart Rate Decrease Caused by Acute FTY720 Administration Is Mediated by the G Protein-Gated Potassium Channel I KACh. *Arab. Archaeol. Epigr.* **2005**, *5*, 529–536. [CrossRef] [PubMed]
48. Bünemann, M.; Brandts, B.; Zu Heringdorf, D.M.; Van Koppen, C.J.; Jakobs, K.H.; Pott, L. Activation of muscarinic K+ current in guinea-pig atrial myocytes by sphingosine-1-phosphate. *J. Physiol.* **1995**, *489*, 701–707. [CrossRef] [PubMed]
49. Sanna, M.G.; Liao, J.; Jo, E.; Alfonso, C.; Ahn, M.-Y.; Peterson, M.S.; Webb, B.; Lefebvre, S.; Chun, J.; Gray, N.; et al. Sphingosine 1-Phosphate (S1P) Receptor Subtypes S1P1and S1P3, Respectively, Regulate Lymphocyte Recirculation and Heart Rate. *J. Boil. Chem.* **2004**, *279*, 13839–13848. [CrossRef] [PubMed]
50. Li, N.; Zhang, F. Implication of sphingosin-1-phosphate in cardiovascular regulation. *Front. Biosci.* **2016**, *21*, 1296–1313. [CrossRef] [PubMed]
51. Novgorodov, A.S.; El-Alwani, M.; Bielawski, J.; Obeid, L.M.; Gudz, T.I. Activation of sphingosine-1-phosphate receptor S1P5 inhibits oligodendrocyte progenitor migration. *FASEB J.* **2007**, *21*, 1503–1514. [CrossRef] [PubMed]
52. Adada, M.; Canals, D.; Hannun, Y.A.; Obeid, L.M. Sphingosine-1-phosphate receptor 2. *FEBS J.* **2013**, *280*, 6354–6366. [CrossRef] [PubMed]
53. Cruz-Orengo, L.; Daniels, B.P.; Dorsey, D.; Basak, S.A.; Grajales-Reyes, J.G.; McCandless, E.E.; Piccio, L.; Schmidt, R.E.; Cross, A.H.; Crosby, S.D.; et al. Enhanced sphingosine-1-phosphate receptor 2 expression underlies female CNS autoimmunity susceptibility. *J. Clin. Investig.* **2014**, *124*, 2571–2584. [CrossRef]
54. Kempf, A.; Tews, B.; Arzt, M.; Weinmann, O.; Obermair, F.J.; Pernet, V.; Zagrebelsky, M.; Delekate, A.; Iobbi, C.; Zemmar, A.; et al. The Sphingolipid Receptor S1PR2 Is a Receptor for Nogo-A Repressing Synaptic Plasticity. *PLoS Boil.* **2014**, *12*, e1001763. [CrossRef] [PubMed]
55. Chong, S.Y.C.; Rosenberg, S.S.; Fancy, S.P.J.; Zhao, C.; Shen, Y.-A.A.; Hahn, A.T.; McGee, A.W.; Xu, X.; Zheng, B.; Zhang, L.I.; et al. Neurite outgrowth inhibitor Nogo-A establishes spatial segregation and extent of oligodendrocyte myelination. *Proc. Natl. Acad. Sci. USA* **2011**, *109*, 1299–1304. [CrossRef]
56. Ishii, M.; Kikuta, J.; Shimazu, Y.; Meier-Schellersheim, M.; Germain, R.N. Chemorepulsion by blood S1P regulates osteoclast precursor mobilization and bone remodeling in vivo. *J. Exp. Med.* **2010**, *207*, 2793–2798. [CrossRef]
57. Thurnherr, T.; Benninger, Y.; Wu, X.; Chrostek, A.; Krause, S.M.; Nave, K.-A.; Franklin, R.; Brakebusch, C.; Suter, U.; Relvas, J.B. Cdc42 and Rac1 Signaling Are Both Required for and Act Synergistically in the Correct Formation of Myelin Sheaths in the CNS. *J. Neurosci.* **2006**, *26*, 10110–10119. [CrossRef]
58. Hoffmann, F.S.; Hofereiter, J.; Rübsamen, H.; Melms, J.; Schwarz, S.; Faber, H.; Weber, P.; Pütz, B.; Loleit, V.; Weber, F.; et al. Fingolimod induces neuroprotective factors in human astrocytes. *J. Neuroinflamm.* **2015**, *12*, 184. [CrossRef] [PubMed]
59. Tran, C.; Heng, B.; Teo, J.D.; Humphrey, S.J.; Qi, Y.; Couttas, T.A.; Stefen, H.; Brettle, M.; Fath, T.; Guillemin, G.J.; et al. Sphingosine 1-phosphate but not Fingolimod protects neurons against excitotoxic cell death by inducing neurotrophic gene expression in astrocytes. *J. Neurochem.* **2019**, *153*, 173–188. [CrossRef]
60. Zhang, Y.; Chen, K.; Sloan, S.A.; Bennett, M.L.; Scholze, A.R.; O'Keeffe, S.; Phatnani, H.P.; Guarnieri, P.; Caneda, C.; Ruderisch, N.; et al. An RNA-Sequencing Transcriptome and Splicing Database of Glia, Neurons, and Vascular Cells of the Cerebral Cortex. *J. Neurosci.* **2014**, *34*, 11929–11947. [CrossRef] [PubMed]
61. Zhang, Y.; Sloan, S.A.; Clarke, L.E.; Caneda, C.; Plaza, C.A.; Blumenthal, P.D.; Vogel, H.; Steinberg, G.K.; Edwards, M.S.B.; Li, G.; et al. Purification and Characterization of Progenitor and Mature Human Astrocytes Reveals Transcriptional and Functional Differences with Mouse. *Neuron* **2016**, *89*, 37–53. [CrossRef] [PubMed]
62. Jaillard, C.; Harrison, S.; Stankoff, B.; Aigrot, M.S.; Calver, A.R.; Duddy, G.; Walsh, F.S.; Pangalos, M.N.; Arimura, N.; Kaibuchi, K.; et al. Edg8/S1P5: An oligodendroglial receptor with dual function on process retraction and cell survival. *J. Neurosci.* **2005**, *25*, 1459–1469. [CrossRef] [PubMed]
63. Allard, J.; Barron, S.; Diaz, J.; Lubetzki, C.; Zalc, B.; Schwartz, J.C.; Sokoloff, P. A rat G protein-coupled receptor selectively expressed in myelin-forming cells. *J. Neurosci.* **1998**, *10*, 1045–1053. [CrossRef] [PubMed]
64. Im, N.-S.; Clemens, J.; Macdonald, T.L.; Lynch, K.R. Characterization of the Human and Mouse Sphingosine 1-Phosphate Receptor, S1P5(Edg-8): Structure−Activity Relationship of Sphingosine1-Phosphate Receptors. *Biochemistry* **2001**, *40*, 14053–14060. [CrossRef]

65. Terai, K.; Soga, T.; Takahashi, M.; Kamohara, M.; Ohno, K.; Yatsugi, S.; Okada, M.; Yamaguchi, T. Edg-8 receptors are preferentially expressed in oligodendrocyte lineage cells of the rat CNS. *Neuroscice* **2003**, *116*, 1053–1062. [CrossRef]
66. Yu, N.; Lariosa-Willingham, K.D.; Lin, F.-F.; Webb, M.; Rao, T.S. Characterization of lysophosphatidic acid and sphingosine-1-phosphate-mediated signal transduction in rat cortical oligodendrocytes. *Glia* **2003**, *45*, 17–27. [CrossRef]
67. Van Doorn, R.; Pinheiro, M.A.L.; Kooij, G.; Lakeman, K.; Hof, B.V.H.; Van Der Pol, S.M.A.; Geerts, D.; Van Horssen, J.; Van Der Valk, P.; Van Der Kam, E.; et al. Sphingosine 1-phosphate receptor 5 mediates the immune quiescence of the human brain endothelial barrier. *J. Neuroinflamm.* **2012**, *9*, 133. [CrossRef] [PubMed]
68. Brinkmann, V.; Pinschewer, D.; Chiba, K.; Feng, L. FTY720: A novel transplantation drug that modulates lymphocyte traffic rather than activation. *Trends Pharmacol. Sci.* **2000**, *21*, 49–52. [CrossRef]
69. Chun, J.; Hartung, H.-P. Mechanism of Action of Oral Fingolimod (FTY720) in Multiple Sclerosis. *Clin. Neuropharmacol.* **2010**, *33*, 91–101. [CrossRef] [PubMed]
70. Brinkmann, V. Sphingosine 1-phosphate receptors in health and disease: Mechanistic insights from gene deletion studies and reverse pharmacology. *Pharmacol. Ther.* **2007**, *115*, 84–105. [CrossRef] [PubMed]
71. Farez, M.F.; Correale, J.; Information, P.E.K.F.C. Sphingosine 1-phosphate signaling in astrocytes: Implications for progressive multiple sclerosis. *J. Neurol. Sci.* **2016**, *361*, 60–65. [CrossRef] [PubMed]
72. Rothhammer, V.; Kenison, J.E.; Tjon, E.; Takenaka, M.C.; De Lima, K.A.; Borucki, D.M.; Chao, C.-C.; Wilz, A.; Blain, M.; Healy, L.; et al. Sphingosine 1-phosphate receptor modulation suppresses pathogenic astrocyte activation and chronic progressive CNS inflammation. *Proc. Natl. Acad. Sci. USA* **2017**, *114*, 2012–2017. [CrossRef]
73. Miron, V.E.; Ludwin, S.K.; Darlington, P.J.; Jarjour, A.A.; Soliven, B.; Kennedy, T.E.; Antel, J.P. Fingolimod (FTY720) Enhances Remyelination Following Demyelination of Organotypic Cerebellar Slices. *Am. J. Pathol.* **2010**, *176*, 2682–2694. [CrossRef] [PubMed]
74. Yazdi, A.; Baharvand, H.; Javan, M. Enhanced remyelination following lysolecithin-induced demyelination in mice under treatment with fingolimod (FTY720). *Neuroscience* **2015**, *311*, 34–44. [CrossRef] [PubMed]
75. Zhang, J.; Zhang, Z.; Li, Y.; Ding, X.; Shang, X.; Lü, M.; Elias, S.B.; Chopp, M. Fingolimod treatment promotes proliferation and differentiation of oligodendrocyte progenitor cells in mice with experimental autoimmune encephalomyelitis. *Neurobiol. Dis.* **2015**, *76*, 57–66. [CrossRef] [PubMed]
76. Fryer, R.M.; Muthukumarana, A.; Harrison, P.C.; Nodop, M.S.; Chen, R.R.; Harrington, K.E.; Dinallo, R.M.; Horan, J.C.; Patnaude, L.; Modis, L.K.; et al. The clinically-tested S1P receptor agonists, FTY720 and BAF312, demonstrate subtype-specific bradycardia (S1P(1)) and hypertension (S1P(3)) in rat. *PLoS ONE* **2012**, *7*, e52985. [CrossRef]
77. Gergely, P.; Nuesslein-Hildesheim, B.; Guerini, D.; Brinkmann, V.; Traebert, M.; Bruns, C.; Pan, S.; Gray, N.; Hinterding, K.; Cooke, N.; et al. The selective sphingosine 1-phosphate receptor modulator BAF312 redirects lymphocyte distribution and has species-specific effects on heart rate. *Br. J. Pharmacol.* **2012**, *167*, 1035–1047. [CrossRef]
78. Pan, S.; Gray, N.S.; Gao, W.; Mi, Y.; Fan, Y.; Wang, X.; Tuntland, T.; Che, J.; Lefebvre, S.; Chen, Y.; et al. Discovery of BAF312 (Siponimod), a Potent and Selective S1P Receptor Modulator. *ACS Med. Chem. Lett.* **2013**, *4*, 333–337. [CrossRef]
79. Forrest, M.; Sun, S.-Y.; Hajdu, R.; Bergstrom, J.; Card, D.; Doherty, G.; Hale, J.; Keohane, C.; Meyers, C.; Milligan, J.; et al. Immune Cell Regulation and Cardiovascular Effects of Sphingosine 1-Phosphate Receptor Agonists in Rodents Are Mediated via Distinct Receptor Subtypes. *J. Pharmacol. Exp. Ther.* **2004**, *309*, 758–768. [CrossRef]
80. Coelho, R.P.; Payne, S.G.; Bittman, R.; Spiegel, S.; Sato-Bigbee, C. The Immunomodulator FTY720 Has a Direct Cytoprotective Effect in Oligodendrocyte Progenitors. *J. Pharmacol. Exp. Ther.* **2007**, *323*, 626–635. [CrossRef]
81. Jung, C.G.; Kim, H.J.; Miron, V.E.; Cook, S.; Kennedy, T.E.; Foster, C.A.; Antel, J.P.; Soliven, B. Functional consequences of S1P receptor modulation in rat oligodendroglial lineage cells. *Glia* **2007**, *55*, 1656–1667. [CrossRef] [PubMed]
82. O'Sullivan, C.; Schubart, A.; Mir, A.K.; Dev, K.K. The dual S1PR1/S1PR5 drug BAF312 (Siponimod) attenuates demyelination in organotypic slice cultures. *J. Neuroinflamm.* **2016**, *13*, 31.

83. Gentile, A.; Musella, A.; Bullitta, S.; Fresegna, D.; De Vito, F.; Fantozzi, R.; Piras, E.; Gargano, F.; Borsellino, G.; Battistini, L.; et al. Siponimod (BAF312) prevents synaptic neurodegeneration in experimental multiple sclerosis. *J. Neuroinflamm.* **2016**, *13*, 207. [CrossRef]
84. Cohen, J.A.; Comi, G.; Arnold, D.L. Efficacy and safety of ozanimod in multiple sclerosis: Dose-blinded extension of a randomized phase II study. *Mult. Scler.* **2019**, *25*, 1255–1262. [CrossRef]
85. ZEPOSIA (Ozanimod) (Package Insert). Celgene Corporation: Summit, NJ, USA. 2020. Available online: https://www.accessdata.fda.gov/drugsatfda_docs/label/2020/209899s000lbl.pdf (accessed on 18 July 2020).
86. Bolli, M.H.; Abele, S.; Binkert, C.; Bravo, R.; Buchmann, S.; Bur, D.; Gatfield, J.; Hess, P.; Kohl, C.; Mangold, C.; et al. 2-Imino-thiazolidin-4-one Derivatives as Potent, Orally Active S1P1Receptor Agonists. *J. Med. Chem.* **2010**, *53*, 4198–4211. [CrossRef] [PubMed]
87. D'Ambrosio, D.; Freedman, M.S.; Prinz, J. Ponesimod, a selective S1P1 receptor modulator: A potential treatment for multiple sclerosis and other immune-mediated diseases. *Ther. Adv. Chronic Dis.* **2016**, *7*, 18–33. [CrossRef]
88. You, S.; Piali, L.; Kuhn, C.; Steiner, B.; Sauvaget, V.; Valette, F.; Clozel, M.; Bach, J.-F.; Chatenoud, L. Therapeutic Use of a Selective S1P1 Receptor Modulator Ponesimod in Autoimmune Diabetes. *PLoS ONE* **2013**, *8*, e77296. [CrossRef]
89. Piali, L.; Froidevaux, S.; Hess, P.; Nayler, O.; Bolli, M.H.; Schlosser, E.; Kohl, C.; Steiner, B.; Clozel, M. The Selective Sphingosine 1-Phosphate Receptor 1 Agonist Ponesimod Protects against Lymphocyte-Mediated Tissue Inflammation. *J. Pharmacol. Exp. Ther.* **2011**, *337*, 547–556. [CrossRef]
90. Brossard, P.; Derendorf, H.; Xu, J.; Maatouk, H.; Halabi, A.; Dingemanse, J. Pharmacokinetics and pharmacodynamics of ponesimod, a selective S1P1 receptor modulator, in the first-in-human study. *Br. J. Clin. Pharmacol.* **2013**, *76*, 888–896. [CrossRef]
91. GILENYA (Fingolimod) (Package Insert). Novartis Pharmaceuticals Coporation: East Hanover, NJ, USA. 2019. Available online: https://www.novartis.us/sites/www.novartis.us/files/gilenya.pdf (accessed on 18 July 2020).
92. Chitnis, T.; Arnold, U.L.; Banwell, B.; Brück, W.; Ghezzi, A.; Giovannoni, G.; Greenberg, B.M.; Krupp, L.; Rostásy, K.; Tardieu, M.; et al. Trial of Fingolimod versus Interferon Beta-1a in Pediatric Multiple Sclerosis. *N. Engl. J. Med.* **2018**, *379*, 1017–1027. [CrossRef]
93. Kappos, L.; Radue, E.-W.; O'Connor, P.; Polman, C.; Hohlfeld, R.; Calabresi, P.; Selmaj, K.; Agoropoulou, C.; Leyk, M.; Zhang-Auberson, L.; et al. A Placebo-Controlled Trial of Oral Fingolimod in Relapsing Multiple Sclerosis. *N. Engl. J. Med.* **2010**, *362*, 387–401. [CrossRef] [PubMed]
94. Cohen, J.; Barkhof, F.; Comi, G.; Hartung, H.-P.; Khatri, B.O.; Montalban, X.; Pelletier, J.; Capra, R.; Gallo, P.; Izquierdo, G.; et al. Oral Fingolimod or Intramuscular Interferon for Relapsing Multiple Sclerosis. *N. Engl. J. Med.* **2010**, *362*, 402–415. [CrossRef] [PubMed]
95. Kappos, L.; Li, D.K.B.; Stuve, O.; Hartung, H.-P.; Freedman, M.S.; Hemmer, B.; Rieckmann, P.; Montalban, X.; Ziemssen, F.; Hunter, B.; et al. Safety and Efficacy of Siponimod (BAF312) in Patients with Relapsing-Remitting Multiple Sclerosis. *JAMA Neurol.* **2016**, *73*, 1089–1098. [CrossRef] [PubMed]
96. Cohen, J.; Khatri, B.; Barkhof, F.; Comi, G.; Hartung, H.-P.; Montalban, X.; Pelletier, J.; Stites, T.; Ritter, S.; Von Rosenstiel, P.; et al. Long-term (up to 4.5 years) treatment with fingolimod in multiple sclerosis: Results from the extension of the randomised TRANSFORMS study. *J. Neurol. Neurosurg. Psychiatry* **2015**, *87*, 468–475. [CrossRef]
97. Kappos, L.; Bar-Or, A.; Cree, B.A.C.; Fox, R.J.; Giovannoni, G.; Gold, R.; Vermersch, P.; Arnold, D.L.; Arnould, S.; Scherz, T.; et al. Siponimod versus placebo in secondary progressive multiple sclerosis (EXPAND): A double-blind, randomised, phase 3 study. *Lancet* **2018**, *391*, 1263–1273. [CrossRef]
98. Cohen, J.; Comi, G.; Selmaj, K.W.; Bar-Or, A.; Arnold, D.L.; Steinman, L.; Hartung, H.-P.; Montalban, X.; Havrdová, E.K.; Cree, B.A.C.; et al. Safety and efficacy of ozanimod versus interferon beta-1a in relapsing multiple sclerosis (RADIANCE): A multicentre, randomised, 24-month, phase 3 trial. *Lancet Neurol.* **2019**, *18*, 1021–1033. [CrossRef]
99. Comi, G.; Kappos, L.; Selmaj, K.W.; Bar-Or, A.; Arnold, D.L.; Steinman, L.; Hartung, H.-P.; Montalban, X.; Havrdová, E.K.; Cree, B.A.C.; et al. Safety and efficacy of ozanimod versus interferon beta-1a in relapsing multiple sclerosis (SUNBEAM): A multicentre, randomised, minimum 12-month, phase 3 trial. *Lancet Neurol.* **2019**, *18*, 1009–1020. [CrossRef]

100. Deluca, J.; Huang, D.; Cohen, J.A.; Cree, B.A.C.; Chen, Y.; Campanolo, D.; Sheffield, J.K.; Comi, G.; Kappos, L. *Ozanimod-Treated Patients Exhibited Improvements in Cognitive Processing Speed in the Phase 3 SUNBEAM Trial of Relapsing Multiple Sclerosis (RMS)*; ECTRIMS: Berlin, Germany, 2018.
101. Kappos, L.; Burcklen, M.; Freedman, M.S.; Fox, R.; Havrdová, E.K.; Hennessy, B.; Hohlfeld, R.; Lublin, F.; Montalban, X.; Pozzilli, C.; et al. *Efficacy and Safety of Ponesimod Compared to Teriflunomide in Patients with Relapsing Multiple Sclerosis: Results of the Randomized, Active-Controlled, Double-Blind, Parallel-Group Phase 3 OPTIMUM Study*; ECTRIMS: Stockholm, Sweden, 2019.
102. Ontaneda, D.; Moore, A.; Bakshi, R.; Zajicheck, A.; Kattan, M.; Fox, R. *Risk Estimates of Progressive Multifocal Leukoencephalopathy Related to Fingolimod*; ECTRIMS: Berlin, Germany, 2018.
103. Boffa, G.; Bruschi, N.; Cellerino, M.; Lapucci, C.; Novi, G.; Sbragia, E.; Capello, E.; Uccelli, A.; Inglese, M. Fingolimod and Dimethyl-Fumarate-Derived Lymphopenia is not Associated with Short-Term Treatment Response and Risk of Infections in a Real-Life MS Population. *CNS Drugs* **2020**, *34*, 425–432. [CrossRef]
104. Conzett, K.B.; Kolm, I.; Jelčić, I.; Kamarachev, J.; Dummer, R.; Braun, R.; French, L.; Linnebank, M.; Hofbauer, G.F.L. Melanoma Occurring During Treatment with Fingolimod for Multiple Sclerosis: A Case Report. *Arch. Dermatol.* **2011**, *147*, 991–992. [CrossRef]
105. Robinson, C.L.; Guo, M. Fingolimod (Gilenya) and melanoma. *BMJ Case Rep.* **2016**, *2016*. [CrossRef]
106. Hatcher, S.E.; Waubant, E.; Nourbakhsh, B.; Crabtree-Hartman, E.; Graves, J.S. Rebound Syndrome in Patients with Multiple Sclerosis After Cessation of Fingolimod Treatment. *JAMA Neurol.* **2016**, *73*, 790. [CrossRef]
107. Frau, J.; Sormani, M.P.; Signori, A.; Realmuto, S.; Baroncini, D.; Annovazzi, P.; Signoriello, E.; Maniscalco, G.T.; La Gioia, S.; Cordioli, C.; et al. Clinical activity after fingolimod cessation: Disease reactivation or rebound? *Eur. J. Neurol.* **2018**, *25*, 1270–1275. [CrossRef] [PubMed]
108. Uygunoğlu, U.; Tütüncü, M.; Altintas, A.; Saip, S.; Siva, A. Factors Predictive of Severe Multiple Sclerosis Disease Reactivation After Fingolimod Cessation. *Neurology* **2018**, *23*, 12–16. [CrossRef]
109. Bobes, N.S. Package inserts. *N. Engl. J. Med.* **1968**, *278*, 282.
110. Linda, H.; von Heijne, A. A case of posterior reversible encephalopathy syndrome associated with gilenya((R)) (fingolimod) treatment for multiple sclerosis. *Front. Neurol.* **2015**, *6*, 39. [CrossRef] [PubMed]
111. Downey, C.; Robertson, D.; Casady, L.; Maldonado, J. A Rare Complication of Fingolimod: Case Report of Posterior Reversible Encephalopathy Syndrome. *Neurology* **2019**, *92*, 2–16.
112. Fischer, A.; Prüfer, K.; Good, J.M.; Halbwax, M.; Wiebe, V.; Andre, C.; Atencia, R.; Mugisha, L.; Ptak, S.E.; Pääbo, S. Bonobos Fall within the Genomic Variation of Chimpanzees. *PLoS ONE* **2011**, *6*, e21605. [CrossRef] [PubMed]
113. Zhao, C.; Fernandes, M.J.; Turgeon, M.; Tancrède, S.; Di Battista, J.; Poubelle, P.E.; Bourgoin, S.G. Specific and overlapping sphingosine-1-phosphate receptor functions in human synoviocytes: Impact of TNF-α. *J. Lipid Res.* **2008**, *49*, 2323–2337. [CrossRef] [PubMed]
114. Tsunemi, S.; Iwasaki, T.; Kitano, S.; Imado, T.; Miyazawa, K.; Sano, H. Effects of the novel immunosuppressant FTY720 in a murine rheumatoid arthritis model. *Clin. Immunol.* **2010**, *136*, 197–204. [CrossRef]
115. Militsakh, O.; Day, T.; Hornig, J.; Lentsch, E.; Skoner, J.; Gillespie, M.B.; Sharma, A.; Neville, B.; Rumboldt, Z.; James, R.; et al. Sphingosine-1-Phosphate. *Encyclopedia Cancer* **2011**, *38*, 3485. [CrossRef]
116. Clark, D.N.; Markham, J.L.; Sloan, C.S.; Poole, B. Cytokine inhibition as a strategy for treating systemic lupus erythematosus. *Clin. Immunol.* **2013**, *148*, 335–343. [CrossRef]
117. Gottschalk, T.; Tsantikos, E.; Hibbs, M.L. Pathogenic Inflammation and Its Therapeutic Targeting in Systemic Lupus Erythematosus. *Front. Immunol.* **2015**, *6*, 1. [CrossRef] [PubMed]
118. Danko, K.; Vencovsky, J.; Lundberg, I.; Amato, A.; Oddis, C.; Malnar, M.; Moher, A.; Colin, L. *The Selective Sphingosine-1-Phosphate Receptor 1/5 Modulator Siponimod (BAF312) Shows Beneficial Effects in Patients with Active, Treatment Refractory Polymyositis and Dermatomyositis: A Phase IIa Proof-of-Concept, Double-Blind, Randomized Trial*; American College of Rheumatology: Boston, MA, USA, 2014.
119. Sandborn, W.J.; Feagan, B.G.; Mutneja, H.; Arora, S.; Vij, A. Ozanimod Treatment for Ulcerative Colitis. *N. Engl. J. Med.* **2016**, *375*, e17. [CrossRef] [PubMed]
120. Vaclavkova, A.; Chimenti, S.; Arenberger, P.; Hollo, P.; Sator, P.G.; Burcklen, M.; Stefani, M.; D'Ambrosio, D. Oral ponesimod in patients with chronic plaque psoriasis: A randomised, double-blind, placebo-controlled phase 2 trial. *Lancet* **2014**, *384*, 2036–2045. [CrossRef]

121. Oskouian, B.; Sooriyakumaran, P.; Borowsky, A.D.; Crans, A.; Dillard-Telm, L.; Tam, Y.Y.; Bandhuvula, P.; Saba, J.D. Sphingosine-1-phosphate lyase potentiates apoptosis via p53- and p38-dependent pathways and is down-regulated in colon cancer. *Proc. Nat. Acad. Sci. USA* **2006**, *103*, 17384–17389. [CrossRef] [PubMed]
122. Degagne, E.; Pandurangan, A.; Bandhuvula, P.; Kumar, A.; Eltanawy, A.; Zhang, M.; Yoshinaga, Y.; Nefedov, M.; de Jong, P.J.; Fong, L.G.; et al. Sphingosine-1-phosphate lyase downregulation promotes colon carcinogenesis through STAT3-activated microRNAs. *J. Clin. Investig.* **2014**, *124*, 5368–5384. [CrossRef]
123. Bao, Y.; Guo, Y.; Zhang, C.; Fan, F.; Yang, W. Sphingosine Kinase 1 and Sphingosine-1-Phosphate Signaling in Colorectal Cancer. *Int. J. Mol. Sci.* **2017**, *18*, 2109. [CrossRef]
124. Wang, S.; Liang, Y.; Chang, W.; Hu, B.; Zhang, Y. Triple Negative Breast Cancer Depends on Sphingosine Kinase 1 (SphK1)/Sphingosine-1-Phosphate (S1P)/Sphingosine 1-Phosphate Receptor 3 (S1PR3)/Notch Signaling for Metastasis. *Med. Sci. Monit.* **2018**, *24*, 1912–1923. [CrossRef]
125. Watson, C.; Long, J.S.; Orange, C.; Tannahill, C.L.; Mallon, E.; McGlynn, L.M.; Pyne, S.; Pyne, N.J.; Edwards, J. High expression of sphingosine 1-phosphate receptors, S1P1 and S1P3, sphingosine kinase 1, and extracellular signal-regulated kinase-1/2 is associated with development of tamoxifen resistance in estrogen receptor-positive breast cancer patients. *Am. J. Pathol.* **2010**, *177*, 2205–2215. [CrossRef]
126. Ohotski, J.; Long, J.S.; Orange, C.; Elsberger, B.; Mallon, E.; Doughty, J.; Pyne, S.; Pyne, N.J.; Edwards, J. Expression of sphingosine 1-phosphate receptor 4 and sphingosine kinase 1 is associated with outcome in oestrogen receptor-negative breast cancer. *Br. J. Cancer* **2012**, *106*, 1453–1459. [CrossRef]
127. Zhao, J.; Liu, J.; Lee, J.F.; Zhang, W.; Kandouz, M.; VanHecke, G.C.; Chen, S.; Ahn, Y.H.; Lonardo, F.; Lee, M.J. TGF-beta/SMAD3 Pathway Stimulates Sphingosine-1 Phosphate Receptor 3 Expression: Implication of sphingosine-1 phosphate receptor 3 in lung adenocarcinoma progression. *J. Biol. Chem.* **2016**, *291*, 27343–27353. [CrossRef] [PubMed]
128. Hsu, A.; Zhang, W.; Lee, J.F.; An, J.; Ekambaram, P.; Liu, J.; Honn, K.V.; Klinge, C.M.; Lee, M.J. Sphingosine-1-phosphate receptor-3 signaling up-regulates epidermal growth factor receptor and enhances epidermal growth factor receptor-mediated carcinogenic activities in cultured lung adenocarcinoma cells. *Int. J. Oncol.* **2012**, *40*, 1619–1626. [PubMed]
129. Kurano, M.; Yatomi, Y. Sphingosine 1-Phosphate and Atherosclerosis. *J. Atherosc. Thromb.* **2018**, *25*, 16–26. [CrossRef] [PubMed]
130. Skoura, A.; Michaud, J.; Im, D.S.; Thangada, S.; Xiong, Y.; Smith, J.D.; Hla, T. Sphingosine-1-phosphate receptor-2 function in myeloid cells regulates vascular inflammation and atherosclerosis. *Arteriosc. Thromb. Vasc. Biol.* **2011**, *31*, 81–85. [CrossRef] [PubMed]

7

Post-Craniopharyngioma and Cranial Nerve-VI Palsy Update on a MS Patient with Major Depression and Concurrent Neuroimmune Conditions

Navzer D. Sachinvala [1,*,†], Angeline Stergiou [2], Duane E. Haines [3,4,5], Armen Kocharian [6] and Andrew Lawton [7]

1 United States Department of Agriculture, Agricultural Research Service, USDA-ARS, New Orleans, Home 2261 Brighton Place, Harvey, LA 70058, USA
2 Department of Medicine, Fairfield Medical Center, 401 North Ewing, Lancaster, OH 43130, USA; drangelinestergiou@gmail.com
3 Department of Neurobiology and Anatomy, Wake Forest School of Medicine, 1 Medical Center Boulevard, Winston-Salem, NC 27157, USA; dhaines@wakehealth.edu
4 Department of Neurology, Wake Forest School of Medicine, 1 Medical Center Boulevard, Winston-Salem, NC 27157, USA
5 Department of Neurobiology and Anatomy, The University of Mississippi Medical Center, Jackson, MS 39216, USA
6 Department of Radiology, Houston Methodist Hospital, 6565 Fannin Street, Houston, TX 77030, USA; akocharian@houstonmethodist.org
7 Department of Ophthalmology, Ochsner Hospital, 1514 Jefferson Highway, New Orleans, 70121, USA; andrew.lawton@ochsner.org
* Correspondence: Sachinvala@aol.com
† This author is retired.

Abstract: We report the case of a male multiple sclerosis (MS) patient with type 2 diabetes (T2D), asthma, major depression (MD or major depressive disorder, MDD), and other chronic conditions, after his recent difficulties with craniopharyngioma and cranial nerve-VI (CN6) palsy. In addition, we show magnetic resonance image and spectroscopy (MRI, MRS), Humphrey's Visual Field (HVF), and retinal nerve fiber layer thickness (RNFLT) findings to explain the changes in the patient's health, and discuss the methods that helped/help him sustain productivity and euthymia despite long-standing problems and new CNS changes.

Keywords: major depression; multiple sclerosis; bupropion; *S*-adenosylmethionine; vitamin D3; yoga; craniopharyngioma; fractionated stereotactic radiation treatments; sphenoid sinusitis; cranial nerve-VI palsy

1. Introduction

Earlier we discussed the case of a male multiple sclerosis (MS) patient (primary author, N.D.S.) who has many concurrent conditions including asthma, type 2 diabetes (T2D), Ehlers–Danlos syndrome (EDS), infections that take long to heal, and major depression (MD or MDD), and listed the methods he learned to be euthymic, by:

- Quelling pain and disability.
- Enduring medication side effects and noting what worked and what stopped working after a while.
- Subduing MD with bupropion, and supplements *S*-adenosylmethionine (SAMe) and vitamin-D3 (vit-D3).

- Maintaining routines for all medications, self-hypnosis, yoga, and physical exercises to stay fit and lucid.
- And academically studying symptoms and potential remedies for his ailments to engage in physician-assisted autoexperiments to discover solutions that provide him lasting relief [1].

Furthermore, the same methods that helped him attain and maintain euthymia with existing illnesses were successful in enabling him to be positive and productive despite new added medical diagnoses. For example, they worked:

- During his craniopharyngioma diagnosis and bitemporal vision loss.
- Through fractionated stereotactic radiation treatments (FSRT) to shrink his perisellar tumor and regain peripheral vision.
- And in his bout with cranial nerve-VI (CN6) palsy, diplopia, and their resolution.

In this report, we update our earlier case report with magnetic resonance imaging (MRI), magnetic resonance spectroscopy (MRS), Humphrey's Visual Field (HVF), and retinal nerve fiber layer thickness (RNFLT) data to explain the patient's status with regards to his MD, MS, tumor, vision, CN6 palsy, and overall health to suggest that even with new health difficulties the above methods he chanced upon continue to keep him positive and productive [1]. We write our reports to encourage readers (scientists, physicians, and patients) to discuss their own experiences in peer-reviewed forums to create insights that could empower the chronically ill to individualize their care with physician involvement and improve the quality of their lives.

2. Case Report

In Reference [1], we reported the case of a male MS patient (primary author, N.D.S.), now 63, who has battled MD since childhood. His early disablements, which continue to date, include: amblyopia (left eye, OS), dyslexia, color blindness, asthma, urticaria, allergies to multiple foods, drugs, and narcotic pain medications, and susceptibility to infections that take weeks to resolve with antibiotics [1]. At 19, he was diagnosed selective immunoglobulin-M (IgM) deficient [2], and by his mid-40 s, required multiple rhinoplasties for apnea, lens replacements for premature cataracts, and uvula removal for swelling and apnea. He belongs to a closed Indo-Iranian minority, Zoroastrians (aka Parsees or Parsis), wherein enforced consanguineous relations for over a century have produced some children with neuroimmune maladies, e.g., Ehlers–Danlos syndrome [3], multiple sclerosis [4,5], cancer [6], and Alzheimer's, cardiovascular, and Parkinson's diseases [6–8]. Notwithstanding health limitations, he grew-up in and enjoys a stable family, and cherished a productive career as an accomplished scientist [9]. At 49 (2005), he developed fulminant MS that left him depressed (Beck Depression Inventory, BDI scores 30–40) [10], mobility impaired, and unable to balance and coordinate his hands. Despite intense therapies, three years later, he accepted disability retirement, and to-date is unable to coordinate his hands to manipulate small objects, play his piano and guitar, and tolerate hot environments [1].

Soon after MS was diagnosed, the patient received guidance from his former teachers and colleagues who were with him in graduate school in Iran (1977–1979), and to whom this paper is dedicated, to:

- Academically study his immune-related illnesses through university courses, textbooks, and journals.
- Maintain regular depression inventories.
- Have consistent routines for yoga and self-hypnosis, sleep, and fitness exercises.
- Note daily changes in serum glucose levels so that with prescribed medications (see Box 2 in Reference [1]), diet, and above routines his glucose levels are maintained between 75 and 120 mg/dL [11–14].
- Quell pain and associated anger with yoga and self-hypnosis, and use NSAIDs when pain becomes disabling.

- Judiciously use prescribed medications and note what worked and what aggravated liver enzyme levels, skin rashes, or other side reactions.
- And study new literature methods that could improve health, mood, and physical and cognitive functioning to engage in physician-assisted autoexperiments that afford sustained relief.

By employing the above approaches between 2005 and 2015, the patient with much effort regained several lost functions, e.g., emerged from bed and wheelchair to walking briskly with crutches. Likewise, after years of experiments with antidepressants, he discovered that bupropion augmented with *S*-adenosylmethionine (SAMe) and vitamin-D3 (vit-D3), in addition to other medications (see reference [1], Box 2), and routines keep him pain-free, alert, and productive.

In late April 2017, he complained of heat intolerance, dizziness, falling, headaches, and blurry vision. Tests over the year revealed that he had craniopharyngioma, a benign perisellar tumor that was growing in place, pressed against his pituitary, anterior optic chiasm, surrounding tissues, and disrupted ophthalmic functions [15]. By late November, his conjoined papillary and adamantinous tumors had enlarged to ~2.3 and 0.7 mL, respectively, caused headaches and bitemporal hemianopsia (peripheral vision loss), and deteriorated R/S vision (from 20/25 and 20/40 in Sept-2016, to 20/60 and 20/100 in Nov-2017). However, his hypothalamic pituitary and adrenal, HPA, and axis hormone levels were unaffected [1,15–18].

From April 2017 to September 2018, the patient could not operate his automobile, and to-date reads text with the Kurzweil Reading Program using ≥14-point font projected on a 140 cm TV monitor, ~1 m from him [19].

Throughout the ordeal, he kept his BDI scores as low as possible (~mid 20 s) with daily: bupropion, SAMe, vit-D3, Yoga, self-hypnosis, exercises, regular schedule for other medications (see box 2 in Reference [1]), and visual imagery of himself scuba diving among coral and marine animals, studying, publishing, lecturing, and maintaining a positive outlook [20].

Given the patient's conditions, asthma, MS, T2D, EDS, and susceptibility to infections, almost all neurosurgeons he consulted advised to ablate his tumors with 30 rounds of fractionated stereotactic radiation treatments (FSRTs), instead of surgery [21]. Gradually his difficulties lessened.

Herein we explain the before and after statuses of his tumor, vision, recent bout with CN6 palsy, and diplopia (Figure 1, Figure 2 and Table 1), and conclude by describing his overall health, mood, and the challenges he must overcome. At present, challenges from old and new ailments are managed, by first becoming free of pain and disability (or lessening them), and then, engrossing self intellectually to problem-solving, so that new and long-standing maladies become puzzles to solve rather than factors that perpetuate helplessness.

3. Materials and Methods

3.1. *Brain Imaging and Spectroscopy*

Brain images and spectra of the tumor were obtained by coauthor AK at the Houston Methodist Hospital, on a General Electric (GE) Healthcare (Waukesha, WI, USA), Model: MR750, 3Tesla instrument with software level DV 25.1 R03. Images were recorded without and with intravenous gadolinium contrast to show new lesions, changes in existing MS lesions with time, as well as postradiation size changes in the suprasellar cyst using the pituitary diffusion imaging protocol. Single voxel MRS data on the tumor were collected using short and long times to echo (TE = 35 ms, and TE = 144 ms, respectively) [15–18].

3.2. *Vision Changes*

Vision changes were studied annually by coauthor AL at the Ochsner Hospital, Jefferson Avenue, New Orleans. RNFL measurements were performed using Spectralis® Tracking Laser, Model HRA/Spectralis with 870 nm diode laser, Heidelberg Engineering, Inc. (Franklin, MA, USA). A circular scan and a 3.4 mm circle were centered around the optic disc of each eye, and RNFLTs in microns were analyzed against data from age- and sex-matched Caucasians in the database (Table 1). Humphrey's Visual Field data were recorded using Ziess Humphrey HF analyzer Model 750i, Meditec Inc., Dublin, CA, USA. After patient data, time of test, and R- or S-eye to be tested were recorded, the Swedish interactive threshold algorithm, SITA, was set to perform fast automated kinetic perimetry (duration ~3 min). The stimulus was white light of intensity 30 dB that illuminated an area of ~2 mm^2 every 200 milliseconds on a chamber screen with background light intensity set at 31.5 apostilbs (ASB). The fixation monitor was gaze at blind spot, the target was central, and threshold was set at 24-2 (which is 24 degrees-temporal, 30 degrees-nasal, to record data at 54 points). Sensitivity at foveae for right and left eyes were measured at 38 and 37 decibels (dB), respectively. Right and left pupil diameters were 4.7 and 4.5 mm, respectively, and correction for both eyes was +4.75 diopter (D). Moreover, on most occasions, fixation losses for both eyes were 2/10, which suggested data were reliable. Thereafter, patient data were compared against data from age-matched Caucasian males in the HVF database (Figure 1).

4. Results and Discussion

4.1. Brain Imaging and Spectroscopy

The patient's MRIs before and after FSRT showed occipital lobe bending (OLB), a sign of chronic MD [1,22]. His conjoined tumor volume before FSRT was ~3 mL (Figure 1A). However, 15 months after FSRT, only the papillary tumor could be seen (V = 0.18 mL), and proton (^{1}H) spectra of the papilloma, before and after FSRT, showed the same alkyl resonances of cholesterol and fatty acids at δ ~1.5 ppm and of compounds with hydroxyl groups at δ ~4 ppm, likely water and inositol. In addition, proton spectra of adamantinous tumors are undefined. Since no other perisellar tumor shows these characteristics, his CTs, MRIs, MRSs, and endocrine workup were used to tentatively diagnose craniopharyngioma without surgical biopsy. This was supported by the patient's inability to efficiently control infections and asthma, and his difficulties with EDS, T2D, MS, and other immune problems [16–18].

4.2. Vision Changes

At maximum tumor volume (ca 3 mL, Figure 1A, December 2017), his R/S vision was 20/70 and 20/100, he had bitemporal hemianopsia (Figure 1B,C), and his left-temporal retinal nerve fiber layer thickness (RNFLT) was 44 microns (Table 1), and the statistical average for RNFLT for men his age was 72 microns. This suggested that in December 2017, the patient's temporal RNFLT was (1−44/72) ×100) ~39% below average for healthy Caucasian men of his age; however, RNFLTs in other sectors were within normal range at that time [23–25]. Statistical values of age- and sex-matched RNFLTs were from the Ziess Humphrey HF analyzer Model 750i, Meditec Inc., Dublin, CA database. At minimum tumor volume 2019 (ca 0.18 mL), his R/S vision had improved to 30/40 and 20/60, respectively; however, his RNFLT was 40 microns (Table 1), which was (1−40/72) ×100) ~ 44% below average thickness, and may have been due to inflammation of his sphenoid sinuses in April 2019 (Table 1).

Figure 1B–D show Humphrey's visual field (HVF) patterns for right (OD) and left (OS) eyes. The long red arrows point to blank regions (blind spots) in the temporal hemifields in Figure 1B,D. Statistical data in 1C from the HVF database enabled comparison of the patient's retinal sensitivity to light with male subjects of his age in the HVF database. Figure 1B showed that in 2017, the patient had bitemporal hemianopsia before FSRTs (because dark patterns appeared mostly in the R and L temporal sides of the grids). It is well known that when tumors grow just above the pituitary and press against the anterior optic chiasm, patients experience bitemporal vision loss. For an excellent tutorial and discussion on visual deficits caused by lesions in visual pathways, the reader is advised to consult Reference [25], pages 264–267. After FSRT, Figure 1D data showed that the patient had central scotomas (blue arrows, points along the central meridians of retinae where vision was impaired). HVF pattern deviation maps are used to compare a patient's retinal sensitivity to 30 decibel light with statistical information from healthy age- and sex-matched subjects in the HVF database. HVF tests evaluate retinal sensitivity at 54 points, in superior (S) and inferior (I) quadrants of temporal (T) and nasal (N) hemifields. Vision losses shown in HVF maps are graded in terms of <5%, <2%, <1%, and <0.5%. So, a four-dot rectangular pattern with a <5% designation in Figure 1C, when present in the patient's maps (Figure 1B,D), indicated that in that region of his retina, 95% of age-matched men had better vision than the patient. Likewise, the blackened rectangle with a <0.5% designation, when present in his maps Figure 1B,D, showed that in that retinal region, 99.5% of age-matched men had better vision than him. A patient's HVF pattern deviation maps ascribe her/his visual field defects in terms of anopsias and scotomas. Anopsias describe vision loss in quarter (quadrantanopia) or half fields (hemianopsias, Figure 1B), and scotomas describe vision loss at individual test points (Figure 1D, blue arrows). Since the highest collection of HVF patterns shown in Figure 1C was present in both temporal S and I quadrants in Figure 1B, his data showed that he had bitemporal hemianopsia before radiation treatments. Fifteen months after FSRT, as his tumor shrank, his visual acuity improved, and he showed central scotomas in both eyes (Figure 1D), which in time could resolve as inflammation lessens [15–18,26].

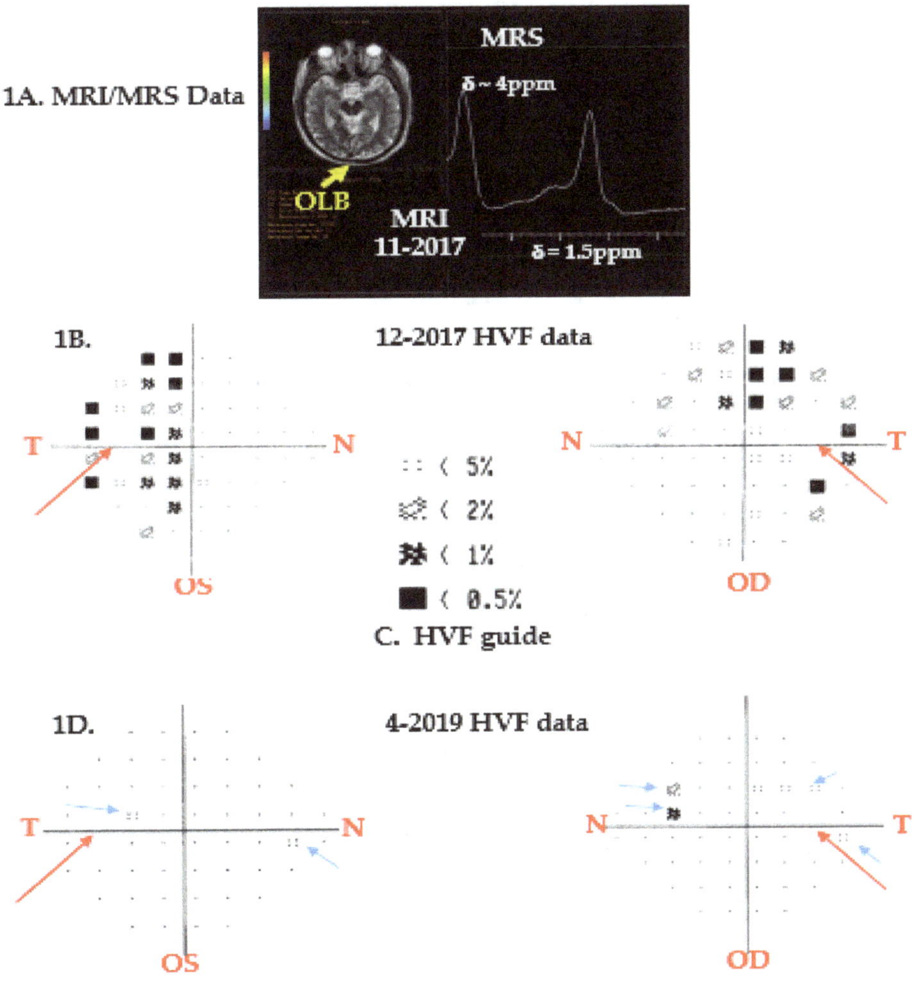

Figure 1. Patient's tumor and Humphrey's Visual Field Data.

The RNFL is a layer of retinal nerve fibers (axons) that eventually form the optic nerve, which enters the eye at the optic cup (blind spot) and proceeds to the brain. Table 1 compares the patient's RNFLTs in microns (μm) in S, I, N, and T regions (or sectors) of both retinas, with statistical data on healthy Caucasian men of his age in the RNFLT database. RNFLTs are measured using optical coherence tomography (OCT). Superior and inferior sectors of the eye are further divided into temporal superior and inferior (TS and TI), and nasal superior and inferior (NS and NI) sectors. The letter "G" in Table 1 indicates global or foveal RNFLT. Foveae are pits in retinal surfaces where visual acuity is highest due to the highest concentration of cone- and rod-shaped neuron cell bodies therein. Patient's RNFLTs that were within normal limits in comparison with statistical values from matched subjects are shown in black font. Those in **blue bold** font were borderline thicknesses, and those in **red bold** font indicated below normal retinal thicknesses (calculation shown above). Overall, his data showed that this patient could gradually lose central and temporal vision in his left eye, and needs to address the problem with a retina specialist [23–25,27].

Table 1. Patient's retinal nerve fiber layer thickness (RNFLT µm) data for December 2017 and April 2019 compared with statistical information from age- and sex-matched individuals in the database.

Right Eye (OD) Dec-2017							
Sector	**T**	**TS**	**TI**	**G**	**N**	**NS**	**NI**
Patient	85	176	136	101	72	93	91
Statistic	72	131	138	96	72	102	104
Overall Patient OD RNFLT: S = 135; I = 114; T 85; and N = 72							
Left Eye (OS) Dec-2017							
Patient	**44**	124	126	90	82	116	99
Statistic	72	131	138	96	72	102	104
Overall Patient OS RNFLT: S = 120; I = 112; T = 44; N = 82							
Right Eye (OD) Apr-2019							
Sector	**T**	**TS**	**TI**	**G**	**N**	**NS**	**NI**
Patient	55	127	128	87	70	94	94
Statistic	72	131	138	96	72	102	104
Overall Patient OD RNFLT: S = 111; I = 111; T = 55; and N = 70							
Left Eye (OS) Apr-2019							
Patient	**40**	117	119	**80**	63	102	98
Statistic	72	131	138	96	72	102	104
Overall Patient OS RNFLT: S = 109; I = 108; T = 40; and N = 63							

Numbers in **bold red** font showed that his left RNFLTs were 39% and 55% below average for years 2017 and 2019, respectively, in comparison with age-matched Caucasian men in the database. Value in **bold blue** font showed that his left foveal (G) RNFLT in April 2019 was 16% below average, but was within normal range in December 2017 (only ~6% below average). RNFLTs in black font were comparatively within normal limits.

Losses in RNFL thicknesses (Table 1) and visual fields (Figure 1) are known to occur with age in both women and men and are exacerbated in aging patients with chronic inflammatory comorbidities (obesity, diabetes, asthma, multiple sclerosis, and/or brain tumors). Furthermore, the likelihood of craniopharyngioma recurrence is also higher in obese diabetics. Therefore, it is imperative for this patient to curb inflammation, reduce weight, keep daily serum glucose values within normal ranges, and annually monitor his ophthalmic, metabolic, and CNS (brain and spine) changes to preclude recurrence of tumor and/or further retinal damage [15–18,23–25,27].

4.3. Bout with CN6 Palsy

In November 2018, the patient experienced sinus pain and intracranial pressure that did not abate with yoga, self-hypnosis, saline rinses, and naproxen. He experienced diplopia and orthostatic difficulties when fixating on vertical edges of walls to balance when standing-up, which to the patient felt like the two same vertical edges were side by side (binocular double vision). In addition, he had a slight convergent right eye squint, that is, his right eye was turning slightly inwards towards his nose. Furthermore, while driving, he saw phantom traffic lane lines obliquely cutting into his lane from the right. He stopped driving and managed diplopia with a right eye patch. Soon diplopia worsened, interfered with reading and daily functions; and by month's end (December), he was prescribed a 10-diopter base out Fresnel lens prism over his right eye (by coauthor, A.L.) after his misalignment was measured by alternate cover testing with hand-held prisms [28]. In addition, his neuro-ophthalmologist advised that the patient's diplopia might be due to right CN6 palsy, triggered by a sinus infection that might be causing his pain and intracranial pressure. Alternatively, given the patient's medical history, it could be due to his chronic diabetes and/or MS, and that such palsies are almost always temporary. At New Years, as nasal lavage thickened, appeared dark, and became more painful, the patient was prescribed amoxicillin to reduce infection. By late January, he was symptom free [22,26,28,29]. In March 2019, sinus pain, pressure, and diplopia returned, and at that time he was undergoing his postradiation therapy follow-up. His transaxial and coronal MRIs in addition to his tumor's status showed that his left sphenoid sinus was more inflamed than the right (Figure 2A and B, yellow triangles). Moreover, while MRIs showed no congestion and no legion(s) in the right pons CN6 region (Figure 2C, orange arrow), the effects of intracranial pressure on CN6 could not be ruled out. Since temporary diplopia is known to be due to ipsi- as well as contralateral CN6 palsies induced by sphenoid sinusitis and increased intracranial pressure, it was conjectured that his symptoms will subside as inflammation diminishes. Later that month, his pain and diplopia were resolved with saline rinses, naproxen, and yoga. CN3 (oculomotor nerve) palsy was ruled out because the patient's right eyelid was not droopy (no ptosis), the right pupil was not dilated, and the eye was not shifted temporally. CN4 (trochlear nerve) palsy was ruled out because diplopia did not worsen when looking down. In addition, his March MRIs showed that his tumor was greatly reduced, his MS was stable, and he had no new CNS lesions or infarctions [22–29].

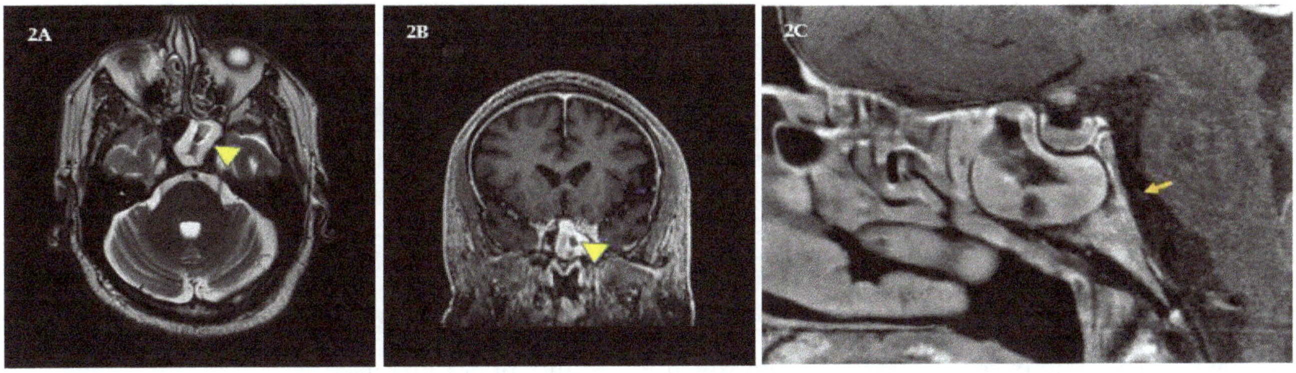

Figure 2. Sphenoid sinusitis. (**A** and **B**) shows transaxial and coronal views of inflammation in the patient's left sphenoid sinus (yellow triangles). (**C**) shows a sagittal view of his congested right sphenoid sinus and the plausible path of his right sixth cranial (abducens) nerve (orange arrow) along the pons. However, congestion in the right pons cranial nerve-VI (CN6) region was not seen, and increased intracranial pressure as cause of CN6 palsy was not ruled out.

5. Conclusions

This patient has struggled with multiple neuroimmune illnesses since childhood and as new difficulties emerge with age. Most of his maladies have a common theme, they are inflammatory, i.e., obesity, diabetes, asthma, MS, MDD, brain tumor, and the like. To control diabetes and obesity, he monitors his AM fasting glucose, which for example from January 1 to October 3, 2019, showed that his average (± standard error) serum glucose was 109.2 (± 1.3 mg/dL) and his percent glycated hemoglobin, A1C, was 5.9 (± 0.05%). Furthermore, his min–max glucose and % A1C values ranged between 71 and 188 mg/dL and 4.4% and 8.9%, respectively. These data were collected on 271 out of 275 calendar days. At present, with yoga, self-hypnosis, gym exercises, sleep, and medications (see Box 2, in Reference [1]), he manages his illnesses, weighs 231 lb (134.1 kg, BMI = 31.7), walks a mile in 20–22 min with crutches, keeps consistent routines, performs household tasks, operates his automobile, swims, scuba dives, participates in writing and editing scientific articles and reviews with former associates, and feels euthymic (BDI January 1–October 3, 2019, was between 6 and 17) [10–14]. His challenges are: reducing weight (to <200 lb, <91 kg, BMI <27), preventing tumor recurrence, not allowing further degradation of his retinae (by working with specialists), stopping exacerbation of asthma and MS symptoms, maintaining serum sugar levels between 75 and 120 mg/dL, and improving balance (to prevent falls) and hands coordination for small motor functions [23–25,27]. Important lessons he has learned to help him manage self are: to not give into overwhelm, discouragement, and anger when an existing disease is aggravated, or a new health problem arises. He understands that these will happen with age, given his background, and overall health. So, regardless the malady, he must act to quell pain, disability, and overwhelm with NSAIDs, stimulants (teas, ginko, coffee, etc.), dietary supplements, physically exhausting self in gym to sleep, and psychological methods. The patient has learned to carefully note how his prescribed medications work (i.e., absorption, distribution, metabolism, side effects, and elimination) and endures treatment hardships to heal. He enjoys working with individuals that help him discover new medications, supplements, and psychological methods to quickly emerge from illness, depression, and helplessness. He maintains routines for medications, self-hypnosis, yoga, physical exercise, mental imagery, and derives pleasure from enjoyable activities (like scuba diving). Furthermore, he academically studies symptoms and new treatments for extant and new problems, discusses them with physicians, and engages in guided autoexperiments that produce desired results.

While we have, at present, no control over our genetic inheritances, we can momentarily accept status quo, and then manage phenotype to live rewarding lives. Finally, we want to see similar case reports from readers (scientists, physicians, and patients) so much insight is created in the literature to help chronically ill patients personalize care for their health and wellbeing to live productive rewarding lives.

Author Contributions: Using his own clinical records, N.D.S. conceived, wrote, and edited the entire manuscript. A.S., D.E.H., A.K., and A.L. were invited as coauthors because of their expertise in psychiatry, neuroscience, radiology, and ophthalmology. In addition, A.K. and A.L. provided the radiology and ophthalmology data, respectively. All authors contributed toward analysis of the case and clinical data, drafting, and revising the paper, and all agree to be accountable for all aspects of this work.

Acknowledgments: We thank: Bin Teh, Steve Fung, and David Baskin, Radiation Oncology, Radiology, and Neurosurgery Departments, Houston Methodist Hospital for managing NS's craniopharyngioma; Bridget Bagert and Diana Phan, Ochsner Hospital New Orleans, for managing NS's MS and overall health; Keki and Mazda Turel, Department of Neurosurgery, Bombay University for many helpful discussions on CNS changes with craniopharyngioma, diabetes, diplopia, MS, and MDD; and Naozumi Teramoto, Chiba Institute of Technology, for help with many references and edits that improved the quality of our manuscript.

References

1. Sachinvala, N.D.; Stergiou, A.; Haines, D.E. Remitting long-standing major depression in a multiple sclerosis patient with several concurrent conditions. *Neuropsychiatr. Dis. Treat.* **2018**, *14*, 2545–2550. [CrossRef] [PubMed]
2. Chovancova, Z.; Kralickova, P.; Pejchalova, A.; Bloomfield, M.; Nechvatalova, J.; Vlkova, M.; Litzman, J. Selective IgM Deficiency: Clinical and Laboratory Features of 17 Patients and a Review of the Literature. *J. Clin. Immunol.* **2017**, *37*, 559–574. [CrossRef] [PubMed]
3. Kose-Ozlece, H.; Ilik, F.; Huseyinoglu, N. Coexistence of Ehlers-Danlos syndrome and multiple sclerosis. *Iran. J. Neurol.* **2015**, *14*, 116–117. [PubMed]
4. Tripathy, V.; Reddy, B.M. Present status of understanding on the G6PD deficiency and natural selection. *J. Postgrad. Med.* **2007**, *53*, 193–202.
5. Naser Moghadasi, A. Multiple sclerosis in Parsis: A historical issue. *Iran. J. Public Health* **2014**, *43*, 387–388.
6. López, S.; Thomas, M.G.; van Dorp, L.; Ansari-Pour, N.; Stewart, S.; Jones, A.L.; Jelinek, E.; Chikhi, L.; Parfitt, T.; Bradman, N.; et al. The Genetic Legacy of Zoroastrianism in Iran and India: Insights into Population Structure, Gene Flow, and Selection. *Am. J. Hum. Genet.* **2017**, *101*, 353–368. [CrossRef]

7. Ahmadian-Attari, M.M.; Ahmadiani, A.; Kamalinejad, M.; Dargahi, L.; Shirzad, M.; Mosaddegh, M. Treatment of Alzheimer's disease in Iranian traditional medicine. *Iran. Red Crescent Med. J.* **2014**, *17*, e18052. [CrossRef]
8. Vazquez-Vidal, I.; Chittoor, G.; Laston, S.; Puppala, S.; Kayani, Z.; Mody, K.; Comuzzie, A.G.; Cole, S.A.; Voruganti, V.S. Assessment of cardiovascular disease risk factors in a genetically homogenous population of Parsi Zoroastrians in the United States: A pilot study. *Am. J. Hum. Biol.* **2016**, *28*, 440–443. [CrossRef]
9. Available online: https://patentscope.wipo.int/search/en/andthentypeSachinvala (accessed on 12 October 2019).
10. Benedict, R.H.; Fishman, I.; McClellan, M.M.; Bakshi, R.; Weinstock-Guttman, B. Validity of the Beck Depression Inventory-Fast Screen in multiple sclerosis. *Mult. Scler. J.* **2003**, *9*, 393–396. [CrossRef]
11. Cramer, H.; Lauche, R.; Langhorst, J.; Dobos, G. Yoga for depression: A systematic review and meta-analysis. *Depress. Anxiety* **2013**, *30*, 1068–1083. [CrossRef]
12. Otani, A. Eastern meditative techniques and hypnosis: A new synthesis. *Am. J. Clin. Hypn.* **2003**, *46*, 97–108. [CrossRef] [PubMed]
13. Tiers, M. *Integrative Hypnosis a Comprehensive Course in Change*; Melissa Tiers Publisher: New York, NY, USA, 2010.
14. Stetka, B. Available online: https://www.scientificamerican.com/article/do-vitamins-and-supplements-make-antidepressants-more-effective/ (accessed on 26 April 2016).
15. Osborn, A.G.; Salzman, K.L.; Jhaveri, M.D. Craniopharyngioma. In *Diagnostic Imaging: Brain*, 3rd ed.; Elsevier: Philadelphia, PA, USA, 2016; pp. 1048–1051.
16. Einstien, A.; Virani, R.A. Clinical Relevance of Single-Voxel (1) H MRS Metabolites in Discriminating Suprasellar Tumors. *J. Clin. Diagn. Res.* **2016**, *10*, TC01–TC04. [CrossRef] [PubMed]
17. Chernov, M.F.; Kawamata, T.; Amano, K.; Ono, Y.; Suzuki, T.; Nakamura, R.; Muragaki, Y.; Iseki, H.; Kubo, O.; Hori, T.; et al. Possible role of single-voxel (1) H-MRS in differential diagnosis of suprasellar tumors. *J. Neuro-Oncology* **2009**, *91*, 191–198. [CrossRef] [PubMed]
18. Saeger, W. New aspects of tumor pathology of the pituitary. *Pathologe* **2015**, *36*, 293–300. [CrossRef] [PubMed]
19. Schmitt, A.J.; McCallum, E.; Hawkins, R.O.; Stephenson, E.; Vicencio, K. The effects of two assistive technologies on reading comprehension accuracy and rate. *Assist. Technol.* **2019**, *31*, 220–230. [CrossRef] [PubMed]
20. de Voogd, E.L.; de Hullu, E.; Burnett-Heyes, S.; Blackwell, S.E.; Wiers, R.W.; Salemink, E. Imagine the bright side of life: A randomized controlled trial of two types of interpretation bias modification procedure targeting adolescent anxiety and depression. *PLoS ONE* **2017**, *12*, e0181147. [CrossRef]
21. Barber, S.M.; Teh, B.S.; Baskin, D.S. Fractionated Stereotactic Radiotherapy for Pituitary Adenomas: Single-Center Experience in 75 Consecutive Patients. *Neurosurgery* **2016**, *79*, 406–417. [CrossRef]
22. Koch, K.; Schultz, C.C. Clinical and pathogenetic implications of occipital bending in depression. *Brain* **2014**, *137*, 1576–1578. [CrossRef]
23. Takis, A.; Alonistiotis, D.; Ioannou, N.; Mitsopoulou, M.; Papaconstantinou, D. Follow-up of the retinal nerve fiber layer thickness of diabetic patients type 2, as a predisposing factor for glaucoma compared to normal subjects. *Clin. Ophthalmol.* **2017**, *11*, 1135–1141. [CrossRef]
24. Henricsson, M.; Heijl, A. Visual fields at different stages of diabetic retinopathy. *Acta Ophthalmol.* **1994**, *72*, 560–569. [CrossRef]
25. Haines, D.E. *Neuroanatomy in Clinical Context: An Atlas of Structures, Sections, Systems, and Syndromes*; 9ED; Walter Kluwer Health: Philadelphia, PA, USA, 2015.
26. Azarmina, M.; Azarmina, H. The six syndromes of the sixth cranial nerve. *J. Ophthalmic Vis. Res.* **2013**, *8*, 160–171. [PubMed]
27. Wijnen, M.; Olsson, D.S.; van den Heuvel-Eibrink, M.M.; Hammarstrand, C.; Janssen, J.A.M.J.L.; van der Lely, A.J.; Johannsson, G.; Neggers, S.J.C.M.M. Excess morbidity and mortality in patients with craniopharyngioma: A hospital-based retrospective cohort study. *Eur. J. Endocrinol.* **2018**, *178*, 93–102. [CrossRef] [PubMed]
28. Weblink Cover Tests. Available online: https://www.aao.org/bcscsnippetdetail.aspx?id=5051fd44-4106-4b1a-bf19-00566baa0b07 (accessed on 12 October 2019).
29. Siu, J.; Sharma, S.; Sowerby, L. Unilateral isolated sphenoid sinusitis with contralateral abducens nerve palsy—A rare complication treated in a low-resource setting. *J. Otolaryngol. Head Neck Surg.* **2015**, *1*, 44–49. [CrossRef] [PubMed]

8

A Journey to the Conformational Analysis of T-Cell Epitope Peptides Involved in Multiple Sclerosis

Catherine Koukoulitsa [1], Eleni Chontzopoulou [1], Sofia Kiriakidi [1], Andreas G. Tzakos [2] and Thomas Mavromoustakos [1,*]

[1] Department of Chemistry, National and Kapodistrian University of Athens, Zographou, 15784 Athens, Greece; ckoukoulitsa@chem.uoa.gr (C.K.); elenichontzo@chem.uoa.gr (E.C.); sofki@chem.uoa.gr (S.K.)
[2] Department of Chemistry, Section of Organic Chemistry and Biochemistry, University of Ioannina, 45110e Ioannina, Greece; atzakos@uoi.gr
* Correspondence: tmavrom@chem.uoa.gr;

Abstract: Multiple sclerosis (MS) is a serious central nervous system (CNS) disease responsible for disability problems and deterioration of the quality of life. Several approaches have been applied to medications entering the market to treat this disease. However, no effective therapy currently exists, and the available drugs simply ameliorate the destructive disability effects of the disease. In this review article, we report on the efforts that have been conducted towards establishing the conformational properties of wild-type myelin basic protein (MBP), myelin proteolipid protein (PLP), myelin oligodendrocyte glycoprotein (MOG) epitopes or altered peptide ligands (ALPs). These efforts have led to the aim of discovering some non-peptide mimetics possessing considerable activity against the disease. These efforts have contributed also to unveiling the molecular basis of the molecular interactions implicated in the trimolecular complex, T-cell receptor (TCR)–peptide–major histocompatibility complex (MHC) or human leucocyte antigen (HLA).

Keywords: conformational analysis; peptides; altered peptide ligands; multiple sclerosis; MS; NMR spectroscopy; NOE-constraints; molecular dynamic; trimolecular complex; experimental autoimmune encephalomyelitis

---

1. Introduction

Multiple sclerosis (MS) is a serious disease of the central nervous system (CNS). MS affects almost 3.3 million people worldwide [1]. It affects more females than males between the ages of 20 and 40 [2]. MS-related disability significantly affects the quality of life (e.g., restraints on daily life activities) [3]. As the number of patients continuously increases, negative effects on social and economic aspects have been observed [4,5]. Factors such as genetic, environment, metabolism and viral infections considerably progress the disease [6,7].

MS is classified into four subclasses according to the increase of the neurologic deterioration of the disease:

1. Relapsing-remitting MS (RRMS): This is the most frequently occurring and affects ca. 85% of all MS patients. The patients with RRMS suffer from relapses and remissions of their neurological symptoms.
2. Secondary progressive MS (SPMS): This follows the development of RRMS and causes further worsening of the disease.
3. Primary progressive MS (PPMS): This affects 8–10% of patients and is characterized by the gradual further worsening of the disease.

4. Progressive-relapsing MS (PRMS): This is the least often occurring class, affecting less than 5% of patients and progressing from onset [8–10].

MS takes place in brain and spinal cord regions containing myelin. As shown in Figure 1, MS lesions involve demyelination and inflammation of B-cells, T-cells, macrophages and activated microglia. Then follows tissue damage, which includes loss of neurons and oligodendrocytes, astrogliosis and remyelination [11,12].

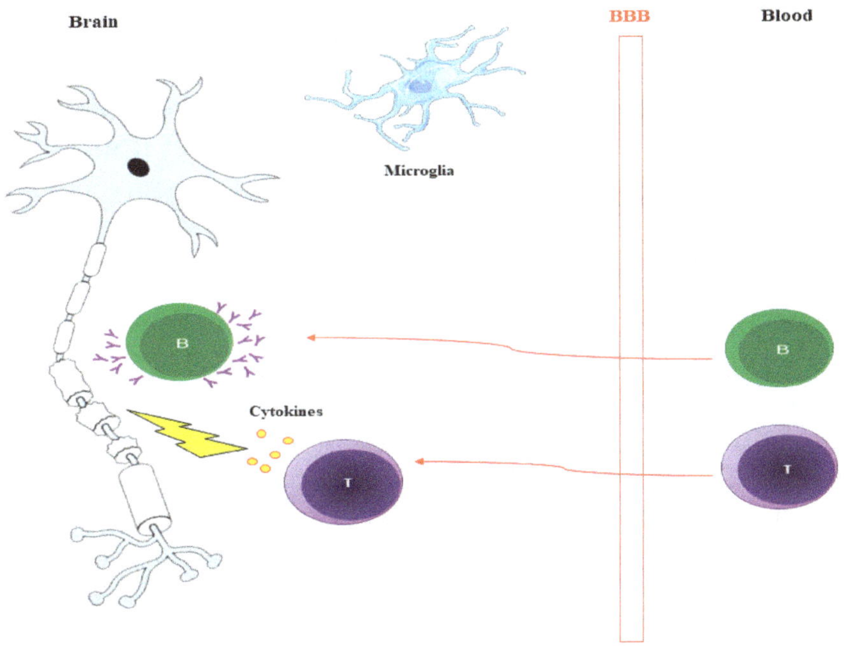

Figure 1. T-cells enter the blood brain barrier (BBB) and release cytokines which degrade the myelin. The cytokines can also recruit some other cells as B-cells. These cells enter the BBB and produce antibodies which target the myelin for further degradation. Activated microglia are also involved in myelin degradation.

The cause of autoimmune disease MS is still mostly unknown. It is hypothesized that environment induces MS in individuals prone to the disease. The molecular mimicry theory has been used to explain the pathogenesis of MS. The gathered evidence proposes that viral peptidic epitopes bearing sequence homology to protein regions of normal human tissue are responsible for the initiation of the disease. The immune response of T-cells targets mainly the viral epitopes. However, cross-reaction with the normal human tissue leads to the autoimmune disease [13,14].

The myelin basic protein (MBP), the proteolipid protein (PLP), the myelinoligodendrocyte glycoprotein (MOG), and the myelin associated oligodendrocytic basic protein (MOBP), have been associated as T-cell epitopes in MS. These peptides have been utilized to trigger experimental autoimmune encephalomyelitis (EAE). EAE is the most frequently and broadly used animal model that simulates MS [15–21].

Although advances in MS treatment have proceeded impressively, the currently available medications are not fully in line to respond to the future and emerging needs raised by the complicated nature of MS [22].

One of the major approaches for the treatment of MS is the peptidic or peptidomimetic therapeutic approach [23,24]. There are different steps involved in the development of peptidomimetic drugs in a rational design strategy. In the first step the minimal peptide amino acid sequence that exerts the activity (epitope) and serves as a lead compound is identified. In the second step the information derived from nuclear magnetic resonance (NMR) spectroscopy, and/or molecular modeling and/or x-ray crystallography is utilized in order to define a putative bioactive conformation of the minimal peptide sequence [25]. In the third step the resultant 3D architecture is used for the development of non-peptide mimetics that are prone to metabolic clearance.

Activated encephalitogenic T-cells, triggered by the formation of a trimolecular complex between the T-cell receptor (TCR), the peptide (antigen)—with identical residue sequence to a fragment of a protein of the myelin sheath—and the major histocompatibility complex (MHC) or human leukocyte antigen (HLA), initiate the onset of MS. The potential of the peptide–HLA complex to activate T-cells parallels the strength of its binding affinity with TCR [26–28]. It follows the stimulation, or not, of T-cells that cause MS [29–33].

The dimer HLA class II receptors contain two polypeptide chains named as α and β [34,35]. Their joined polypeptide chains form a single receptor suitable to form a complex with the antigen binders. This complex is recognized by the T-cell receptors on the cell surface. The formed trimolecular complex leads to the activation of T-cells through a series of biochemical alterations and the triggering of the immune response to the antigen [36].

This review summarizes the conformational analysis of peptides involved in multiple sclerosis. In addition the impact of these conformational changes on rational drug design is described.

2. Results and Discussion

Mouzaki et al. [37] pointed out that peptides constitute a class of administered molecules as immunomodulatory drugs due to their rapid and cost-effective synthesis. The peptides that can cause EAE in animals are called agonists and those that can compete the action of the agonists and treat EAE are called antagonists.

In the discussed studies peptides are used that either map to wild-type MBP, PLP [38] or MOG epitopes or are mutants (altered peptide ligands, APLs), which are linear or cyclized variants that are more resistant to in vivo enzymatic degradation [39]. APLs differ from their parent encephalitogenic peptides by single amino acid substitutions and can inhibit autoimmune mediated disease through several mechanisms.

For many years we have made an effort to explore the conformational properties that govern various epitopes related to EAE with their agonist and antagonists both in solution and in trimolecular complexes (drug:TCR:HLA). In this review we will outline the most significant results obtained from these studies.

The first step in these studies is to extract favored averaged conformations of the epitopes in solution using NMR spectroscopy. These conformations after energy minimization serve as initial conformations for applying molecular dynamics (MD) simulations in the generation of the trimolecular complex. The results will lead to the synthesis of antagonist peptides which could potentially provide useful mechanistic information to combat MS (Figure 2).

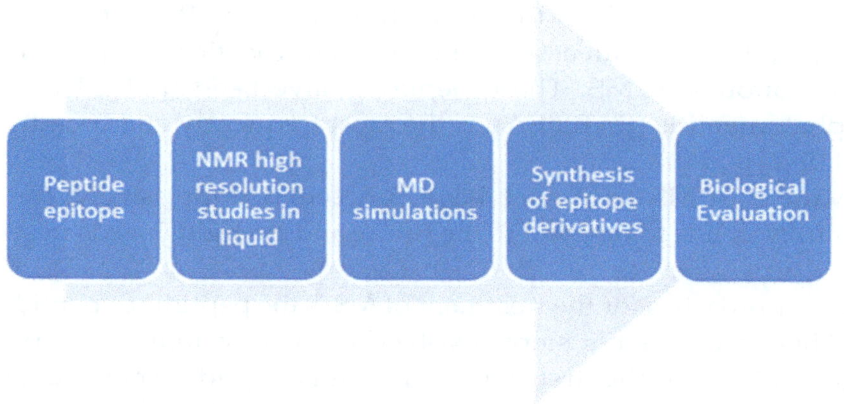

Figure 2. Steps of a rational design process aiming to aid the development of peptide mimics against multiple sclerosis (MS).

The conformational analysis of $hMOG_{35-55}$ epitope (Met_{35}-Glu-Val-Gly-Trp-Tyr-Arg-Pro^{42}-Pro-Phe-Ser-Arg-Val-Val-His-Leu-Tyr-Arg-Asn-Gly-Lys_{55}) and its mutants ($hMOG_{35-55}(Ala^{41})$ and $hMOG_{35-55}(Ala^{41,46})$) alone and in the trimolecular complex containing HLA and TCR have been studied using MD simulations [36]. The results showed that the $hMOG_{35-55}$ epitope in the MD trajectory does not retain the linear conformation. Its dominant conformation shows two bends in the polypeptide backbone between residues Trp^{39}, Tyr^{40} and Arg^{41} and Val^{48} and Arg^{52}.

This conformation is similar to that published for the rat/mouse MOG_{35-55} peptide by Ntountaniotis et al. [40] in DMSO and D_2O solvents (Figure 3).

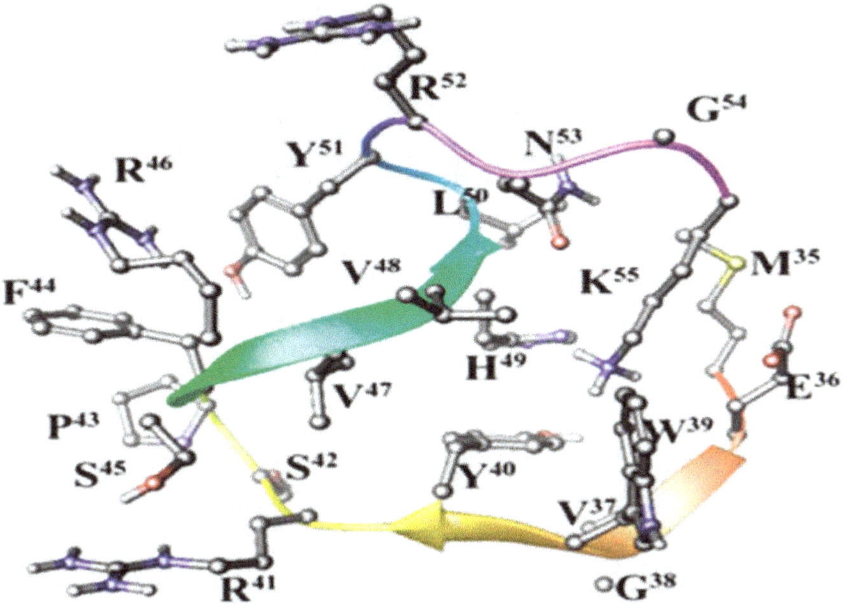

Figure 3. Low energy conformer of $hMOG_{35-55}$ (myelinoligodendrocyte glycoprotein) derived from in silico molecular synamics (MD) calculations restricted with nuclear Overhauser effect (NOE)-constraints.

During the formation of the trimolecular complex the amino acids Arg^{41} and Arg^{46} of $hMOG_{35-55}$ anchor at TCR and Tyr^{40} interacts with HLA. The amino acids Arg^{41} and Arg^{46} form an extensive hydrogen bonding (HB) network with both receptors. Substitution of Arg^{41} or Arg^{41} and Arg^{46} with Ala leads to the two mutants $hMOG_{35-55}$ (Ala^{41}) and $hMOG_{35-55}$ (Ala^{41}, Ala^{46}). These mutations lead to the elimination of key interactions with TCR but leave intact the binding affinity towards the HLA receptor. These two mutants function as EAE inhibitors. This finding is significant as it provides basic mechanistic aspects of the action of agonist versus antagonist peptides (Figure 4).

The conformational analysis of MBP_{77-89} and the antagonist altered ligands (Arg^{91}, Ala^{96}) MBP_{87-99} and ($Ala^{91,96}$) MBP_{87-99} have been studied. All the three molecules showed an extended conformation in DMSO environment with no long-range nuclear Overhauser effects (NOEs) [41] in disagreement with the observations recorded in other chemical environments [29].

Interestingly, X-ray results existed for a peptide analogue of MBP_{87-99} that formed a trimolecular complex with a human TCR and HLA-DR2b [42]. A bioactive conformation of APL that resembled that of the crystallized peptide was derived from the molecular dynamics trajectories (Root-Mean Square Deviation (RMSD) value of 0.95 Å). The two peptides were oriented similarly to the two TCR anchor residues, His^{88} and Phe^{89}, and the HLA anchor residue Phe^{90}.

These two amino acids orient variably in the trimolecular complex for (Arg^{91}, Ala^{96}) MBP_{87-99} and ($Ala^{91,96}$) MBP_{87-99}, and remain buried in HLA grooves and cannot interact with the TCR. This finding may explain the antagonism of the two altered ligands (Figure 5).

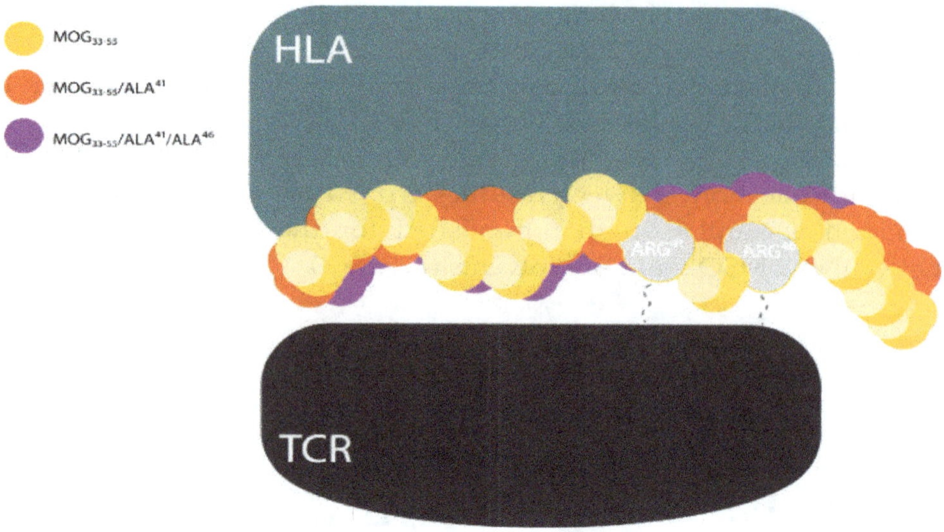

Figure 4. The replacement of Arg^{41} or Arg^{41} and Arg^{46} of $hMOG_{35-55}$ with Ala interrupts the hydrogen bonding (HB) with the amino acids Asp^{98}, Ser^{101}, and Asn^{104} of T-cell receptors (TCR). This may be due to the decrease of polarity of Ala vs. Arg (disruption of the interaction network) and may lead to a reduced bending of Ala in the low energy conformation of $hMOG_{35-55}$. HLA—Human Leukocyte Antigen.

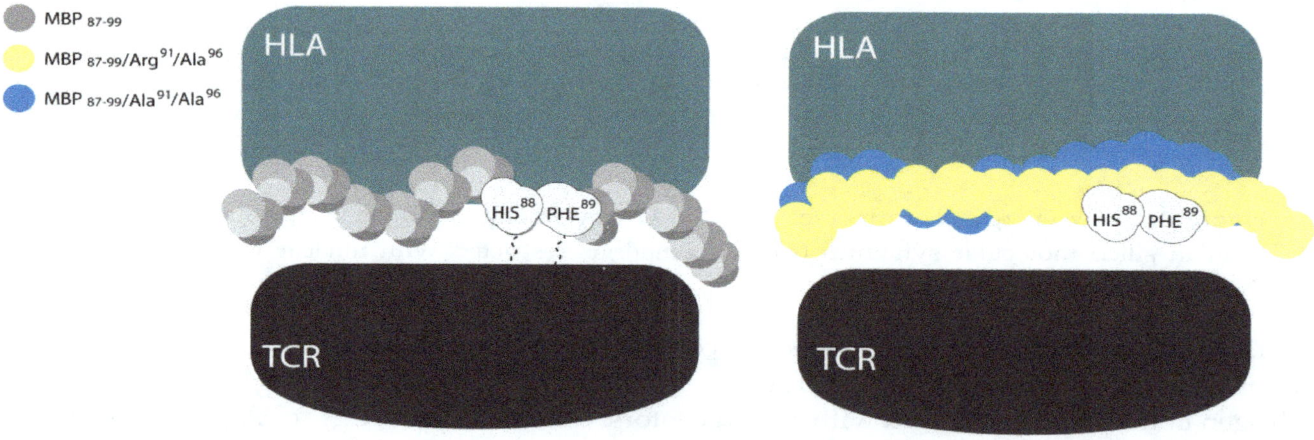

Figure 5. **(left)** His^{88} and Phe^{89} of $hMBP_{87-99}$ (myelin basic protein) interact with the TCR receptor. **(right)** In the two antagonists (Arg^{91}, Ala^{96}) MBP_{87-99} and ($Ala^{91,96}$) MBP_{87-99} this interaction is lost as the two amino acids are buried in HLA grooves.

The cyclo (91–99)(Ala^{96})MBP_{87-99}, cyclo(87–99)($Ala^{91,96}$)MBP_{87-99} and cyclo(87–99)(Arg^{91}, Ala^{96})MBP_{87-99} (Figure 6), except the wild-type linear MBP_{87-99}, were found to strongly inhibit MBP_{72-85}- induced EAE in Lewis rats. Cyclo(87–99)(Arg^{91}, Ala^{96})MBP_{87-99} provided long protection for the EAE induction [39,43,44].

Conformational analysis was achieved for the three cyclo(87–99) MBP_{87-99}, cyclo(87–99) ($Ala^{91,96}$) MBP_{87-99}, and cyclo(87–99) (Arg^{91}, Ala^{96}) MBP_{87-99} analogs using 2D NMR spectroscopy and computational analysis. The conformational analysis of the three synthetic analogues showed that their bioactivity, or its absence, may be attributed to the distinct local conformation, overall topology and exposed area after binding with MHC II. An overall larger solvent accessible area may occlude the approach and binding of the TCR on the APL-MHC complex. In contrast, more compact structures do not block weak interactions as TCR approaches and can induce EAE antagonism. These results led to the generation of the pharmacophore model described in Figure 7 [45].

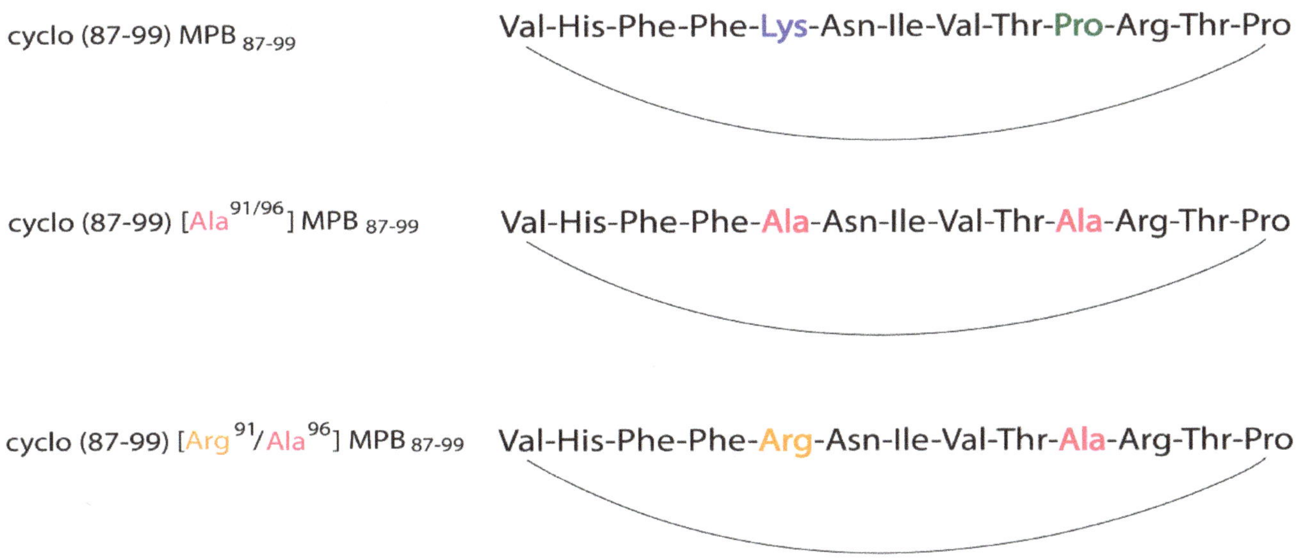

Figure 6. Structures of cyclo(91–99)(Ala^{96})MBP$_{87–99}$, cyclo(87–99)(Ala^{91},^{96})MBP$_{87–99}$ and cyclo(87–99)(Arg^{91}, Ala^{96})MBP$_{87–99}$.

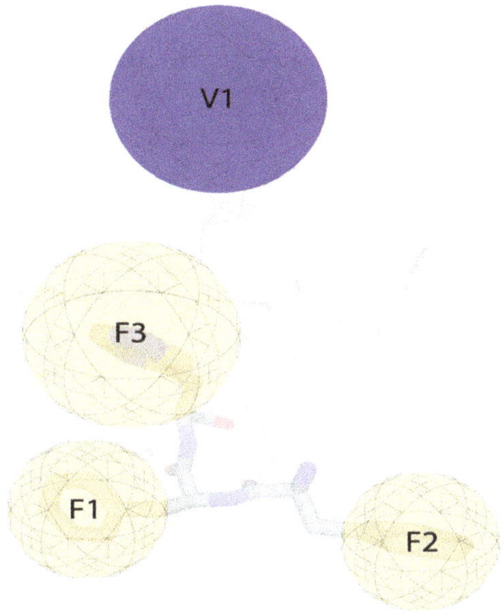

Figure 7. Pharmacophore model depicted using the conformational properties obtained from the conformational analysis for the cyclic altered peptide ligands (APLs). Exclusion volume V1 is presented with a blue sphere, feature F1 (Phe^{90}), F2 (Phe^{89}), F3 (Phe^{88}) with a yellow sphere.

Two citrullinated peptides, the linear (Cit^{91}, Ala^{96}, Cit^{97})MBP$_{87–99}$ and cyclo(87–99)(Cit^{91}, Ala^{96}, Cit^{97})MBP$_{87–99}$ have been synthesized by citrullinating the Arg residues 91 and 97 in the antagonists, linear (Arg91, Ala96)MBP$_{87–99}$ and cyclo(87–99)(Arg^{91}, Ala^{96})MBP$_{87–99}$ peptides. In contrast to the antagonists, these citrullinated molecules induced EAE. Molecular modeling results pointed out that both Cit^{91} and Cit^{97} residues are oriented toward the TCR and possibly are interacting with the complementarity-determining region (CDR3) loops of the TCR, thus triggering an altered cytokine response [46].

Another epitope which is shown to induce EAE in guinea pigs is the linear peptide MBP$_{74–85}$ (Gln^1-Lys^2-Ser^3-Gln^4-Arg^5-Ser^6-Gln^7-Asp^8-Glu^9-Asn^{10}-Pro^{11}-Val^{12}-NH$_2$). A Rotating frame Overhauser Effect Spectroscopy (ROESY) connectivity was observed for the molecule in DMSO between αVal^{12}-αGln^1, suggesting a cyclic conformation. This intriguing result prompted the synthesis of the cyclic analogue by tethering the εNH_2 of Lys and $\gamma COOH$ of Glu at positions 2 and 9, respectively. Cyclic peptides are well known to be more stable and less susceptible to enzymatic degradation than linear peptides. Moreover, cyclic peptides are an important intermediate step in the rational design and development of non-peptide mimetics [47].

This cyclic analogue illustrated comparable bioactivity with the linear one, confirming that the possible bioactive conformation of $MBP_{74–85}$ resembles that of the cyclic variant or the cyclic variant resembles more, from the available ensemble, the structure of the linear peptide that is of biological significance. The structures of the linear and cyclic analogues are shown in Figure 8. The same relationship was observed with the linear Ala^{81} $MBP_{74–85}$ and its cyclic analogue [25].

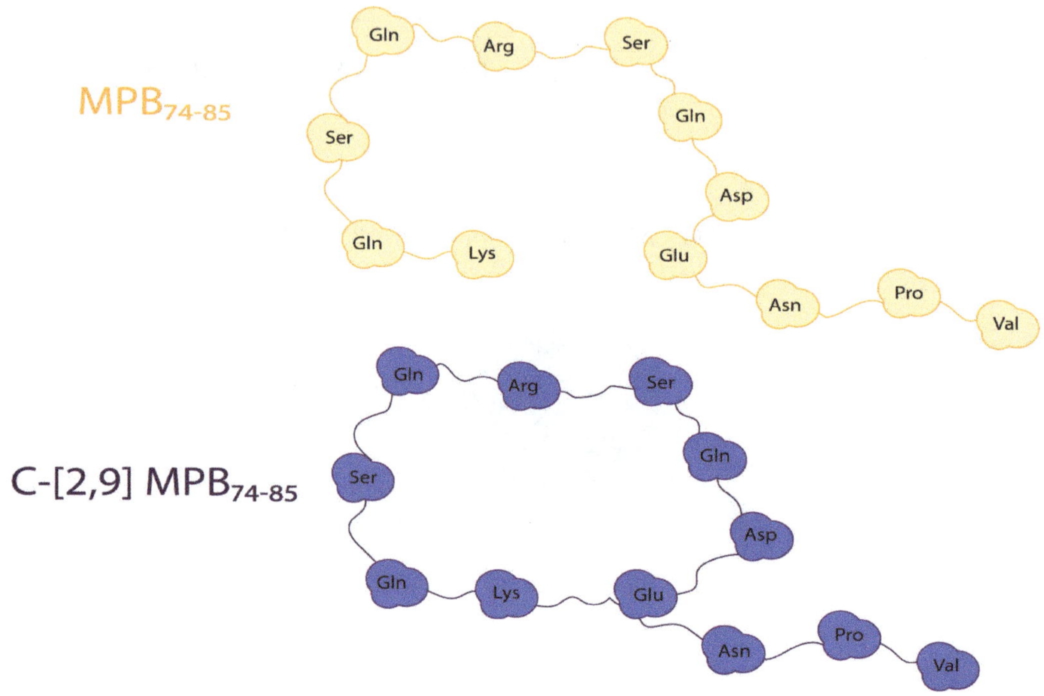

Figure 8. 2D and 3D models of linear $MBP_{74–85}$ (**top**) and its cyclic analogue (**bottom**).

Tzakos et al. [48] applied NMR and molecular dynamic simulations to study the conformational properties of agonist MBP, Gln^{74}-Lys^{75}-Ser^{76}-Gln^{77}-Arg^{78}-Ser^{79}-Gln^{80}-Asp^{81}-Glu^{82}-Asn^{83}-Pro^{84}-Val^{85} ($MBP_{(74–85)}$), and its antagonist analogue $Ala^{81}MBP_{(74–85)}$. The agonist $MBP_{(74–85)}$ adopted a compact conformation attributed to electrostatic interactions of Arg^{78} with the side chains of Asp^{81} and Glu^{82}. Arg^{78} adopted a well-defined conformation, which did not depend on the solvent. Such electrostatic interactions were not observed in the antagonist Ala^{81} $MBP_{(74–85)}$, and a high flexibility of the side chain of Arg^{78} was observed. The positively charged residue Arg^{78} is suggested to stabilize the local microdomains (epitopes) of the integral protein. Flexible docking calculations point out that Gln^{74}, Ser^{76} and Ser^{79} are MHC II anchor residues. Lys^{75}, Arg^{78} and Asp^{81} are the mainly solvent-exposed residues and this may signify their participation in the formation of the trimolecular T-cell receptor–$MBP_{(74–85)}$–MHC II complex.

In another study the conformational analysis of the immunodominant epitope of acetylated myelin basic protein residues 1–11 (Ac-MBP1–11) and its ALPs, mutated at position 4 to an alanine (Ac-MBP1–11(4A)) or a tyrosine residue (Ac-MBP1–11(4Y)), was achieved. The amino acids constituting the $MBP^{1–11}$ are Ala-Ser-Gln-Lys-Arg-Pro-Ser-Gln-Arg-His-Gly (Ac-MBP1–11). The Ac-MBP1–11(4A) analogue inhibited EAE symptoms induced by encephalitogenic Ac-MBP1–11 epitope when co-injected in (PL/J × SJL)F1 mice. These results are interpreted to suggest that Ac-MBP1–11(4A) induced immunomodulation that inhibits EAE in vivo [49]. Studies indicated that the residue at position 4 in MBP1–11 peptide plays a major role in binding of the peptide to MHC class II, I–Au [50,51].

The mutated analogue Ac-MBP1–11(4A) binds to I–Au with a minimum of 50-fold higher affinity in comparison to the native Ac-MBP1–11 [52]. In addition, the mutation at position 4 of Lys to Tyr (Ac-MBP1–11(4Y)) increases the stability of the I–Au-peptide complex by enhancing 1500-fold the affinity, which triggers Ac-MBP1–11 T-cells more effectively in relation to Ac-MBP1–11(4A) [53].

The conformational analysis of the three analogues showed that they adopt an extended conformation in deuterated DMSO solvent due to the absence of long-distance NOEs. Furthermore, they adopt a similar conformation when bound to the active site of the MHC II. Gln^3 residue is a TCR contact site and has a different orientation in the mutated analogues. Specifically, its side chain is not solvent exposed, and it is not available for interaction with the TCR. The main MHC contact residues (Ser^2, Pro^6 and Ser^7) stand in the same position for all peptides [54].

The conformational properties of $MBP_{83–99}$ have been studied using NMR spectroscopy in DMSO to simulate the biological environment. The results showed that the peptide exists in a rather extended conformation and forms a helix between Val^{87} and Phe^{90} [55].

Two analogues of the $MBP_{83–99}$ epitope substituted at Lys^{91} (primary TCR contact) with Phe ($MBP_{83–99}$ (Phe^{91})) or Tyr ($MBP_{83–99}$ (Tyr^{91})) were synthesized (Figure 9).

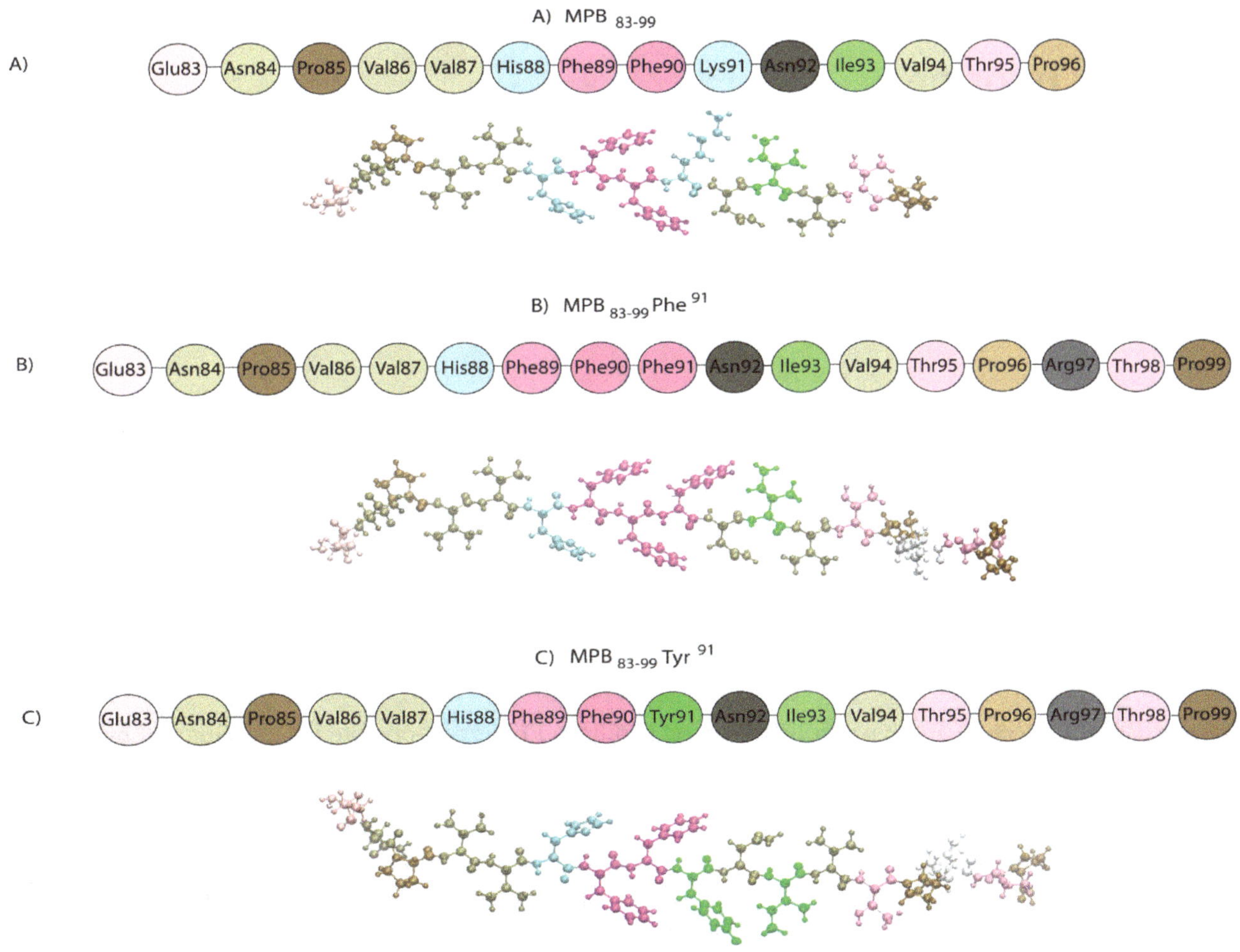

Figure 9. Sequences and 3D low energy structures of (**A**) $MBP_{83–96}$ (numbering is according to the human $MBP_{83–99}$ epitope) and the two synthetic analogs (**B**) $MBP_{83–99}$ (Phe^{91}) and (**C**) $MBP_{83–99}$ (Tyr^{91}).

The two analogues showed distinct antagonistic activity versus the agonistic activity of the $MBP_{83–99}$ epitope. The conformational analysis of the two APLs was performed using NMR spectroscopy and MD. Both synthetic analogues show an extended conformation in agreement with the structural features of the peptides that interact with the HLA-DR2 and TCR receptors. MD simulations of the two analogues in complex with HLA-DR2 (DRA, DRB1*1501) and TCR revealed their modes of interactions. MBP_{83-99} (Phe^{91}) analogue adopts more interactions during the formation of the trimolecular complex relatively to MBP_{83-99} (Tyr^{91}), as their trajectory profiles confirmed. This may explain the improved biological profile of the latter. The two analogues differ in the way of binding relatively to the wild epitope MBP_{83-96}. This is attributed to the fact that mutation of Lys^{91} by either Tyr or Phe alters their stereoelectronic properties.

This alteration of the stereoelectronic properties affects the binding mode of the regional amino acids and explains their antagonistic or agonistic activity. Such binding mode differences have been observed and outlined above with the MBP_{87-99} epitope [45,56–60].

It is important to note that although the two peptides mentioned above differ only in a small segment, they possess distinct biological profiles. The $tyrosine^{91}$ in MBP_{83-99} (Tyr^{91}) possesses a phenolic hydroxyl group that induces differential biological activity. This is in agreement with a plethora of literature data pointing out the key role of the phenolic group in drug bioactivity [61–72] (Figure 10).

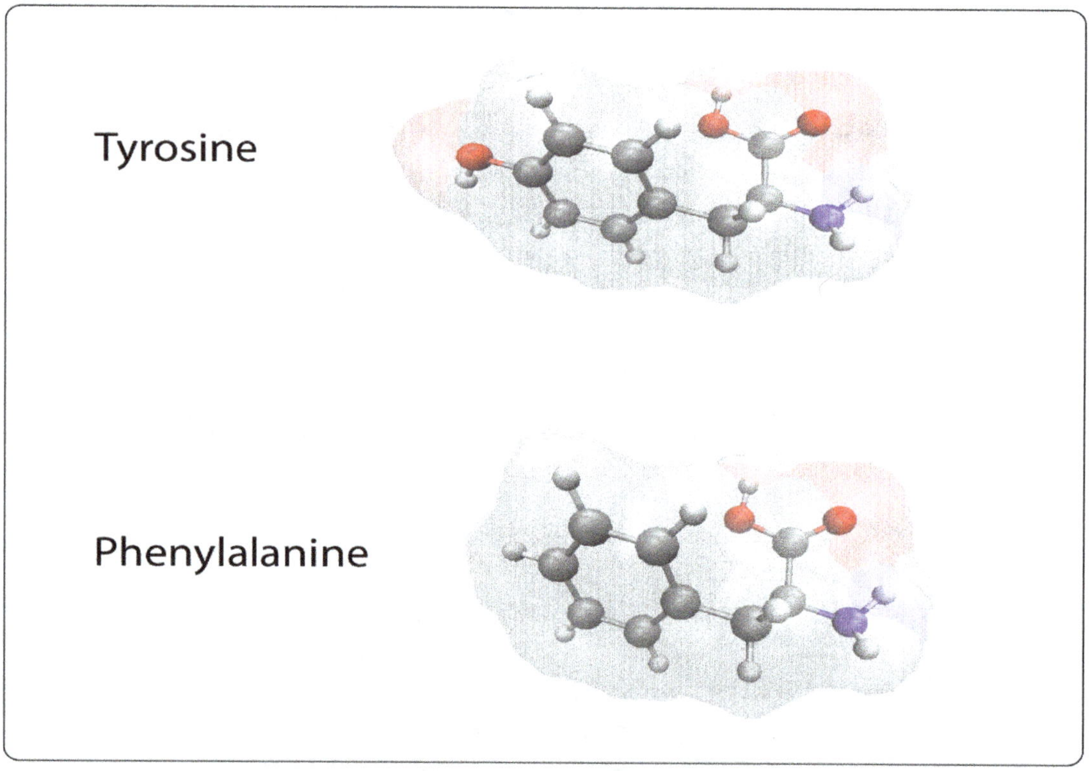

Figure 10. The absence of the phenolic hydroxyl group in Phe is responsible for the different biological properties between the two synthetic analogues MBP_{83-99} (Tyr^{91}) and MBP_{83-99} (Phe^{91}).

The superimposition of the two peptides at the binding site of the trimolecular complex shows that Phe^{91} and Tyr^{91} occupy almost identical areas. However, they induce different conformations to other vicinal amino acids Asn^{92} and Ile^{93}, as the phenolic hydroxyl group lies in a relatively hydrophobic environment. Their apparently small structural difference induces a sequence of distinct interactions that determine their fingerprint of biological action. $MBP_{(85-99)}$ is an immuno-dominant epitope of MBP which binds to the MHC haplotype HLA-DR2 and is associated with the pathogenesis of MS. The synthetic 15-mer peptide J5n (Figure 11), was designed and was found to antagonize $MBP_{(85-99)}$ through the binding of $MBP_{(85-99)}$ to soluble HLA-DR2b [73]. The therapeutic efficacy of J5 is limited, probably due to its low biological half-life or bioavailability. The structural features of J5 in relation to its parent (i.e., $MBP_{(85-99)}$) are shown in Figure 11. Phe at position P4 has been replaced with Tyr, Val at position P1 has been retained and His, Phe, and Lys at P2, P3 and P5 have been replaced with Glu, Ala and Lys, respectively.

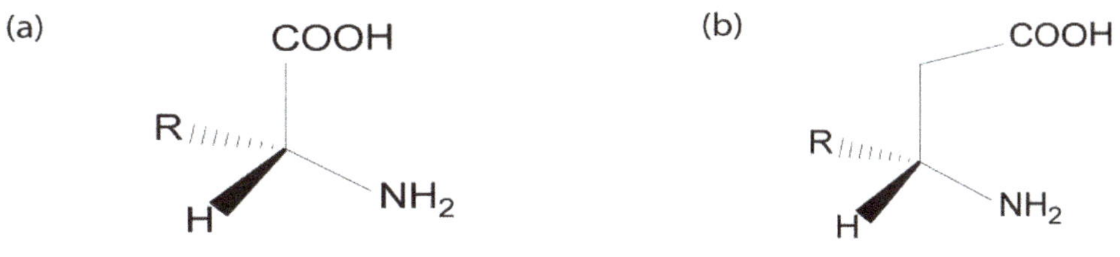

(c)

	P1 P2 P3 P4 P5
MBP $_{85\text{-}99}$	Glu-Asn-Pro-Val-Val-His-Phe-Phe-Lys-Asn-Ile-Val-Pro-Thr-Arg
J_5	Glu-Lys-Pro-Lys-Val-Glu-Ala-Tyr-Lys-Ala-Ala-Ala-Ala-Pro-Ala
S_{18}	Glu_{β}^{3}-Lys_{β}^{3}-Pro-Lys-Val-Glu-Ala-Tyr-Lys_{β}^{3}-Ala_{β}^{3}-Ala_{β}^{3}-Ala_{β}^{3}-Ala_{β}^{3}

Figure 11. (**a**) α-amino acid, (**b**) Homo-β-amino acid, (**c**) $MBP_{85\text{-}99}$, J5 and S_{18} analogue.

In another study J5 was derivatized into analogs possessing superior biological half-lives and antagonistic activities. This is achieved by substitution of some of its residues with homo-β-amino acids. S18 (Figure 11), the most active analog, ameliorated symptoms of EAE at least twice more effectively than glatiramer acetate or J5. S18 showed high resistance to proteolysis, which contributed to a delayed clinical onset of disease and prolonged therapeutic benefits [74].

The conformational analysis studies of $MBP_{83\text{–}96}$ epitope led the group of Professor T. Tselios to search for the mining and synthesis of non-peptide mimetic molecules. In particular, they sought molecules that inhibit the trimolecular complex formation and consequently the proliferation of activated T-cells. They generated a structure-based pharmacophore and used ZINC as a chemical database to extract candidates (Figure 12). Semi-empirical and density functional theory (DFT) methods were performed to predict the binding energy between the proposed non-peptide mimetics and the TCR. From the six synthesized molecules the following 15 and 16 were the most promising as they inhibited the stimulation of T-cells by the immunodominant $MBP_{83\text{–}99}$ from immunized mice [75].

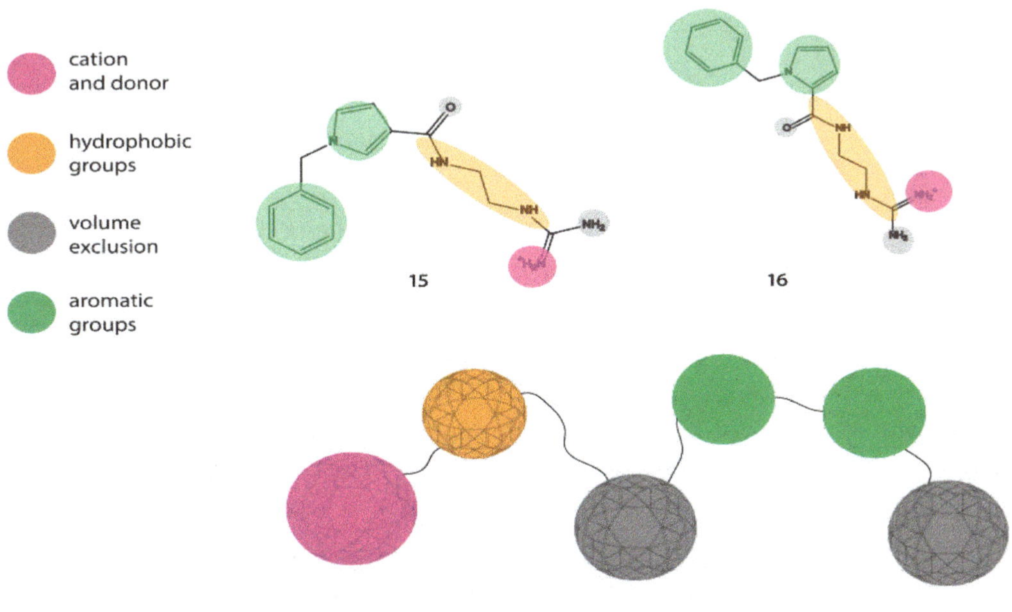

Figure 12. Structure-based pharmacophore derived from ZINC database data.

3. Conclusions

An extensive effort has been made the last years to explore the conformational properties of key peptides involved in MS. The conformational analysis of the different epitopes, consisting of in silico MD and pharmacophore studies, along with NMR spectroscopy, has led to the rational design of some bioactive non-peptide mimetics and provided some mechanistic input of the agonistic and antagonistic action of ALPs. However, there is still a long way towards the generation of more potent compounds. Interestingly, in a study it was illustrated that the extent of MHC or TCR competition does not successfully predict the EAE treatment [76]. Other routes to treat MS had also limited success [21,77].

Such an example is the immunomodulatory co-polymer 1 (Copaxone, glatiramer acetate) drug. This contains synthetic peptides composed of nonspecific sequences of four amino acids: L-alanine, L-lysine, L-glutamic acid and L-tyrosine (Figure 13). As its composition is based on the amino acid structure of MBP it exerts an antagonistic action to the 82–100 epitope of MBP [78].

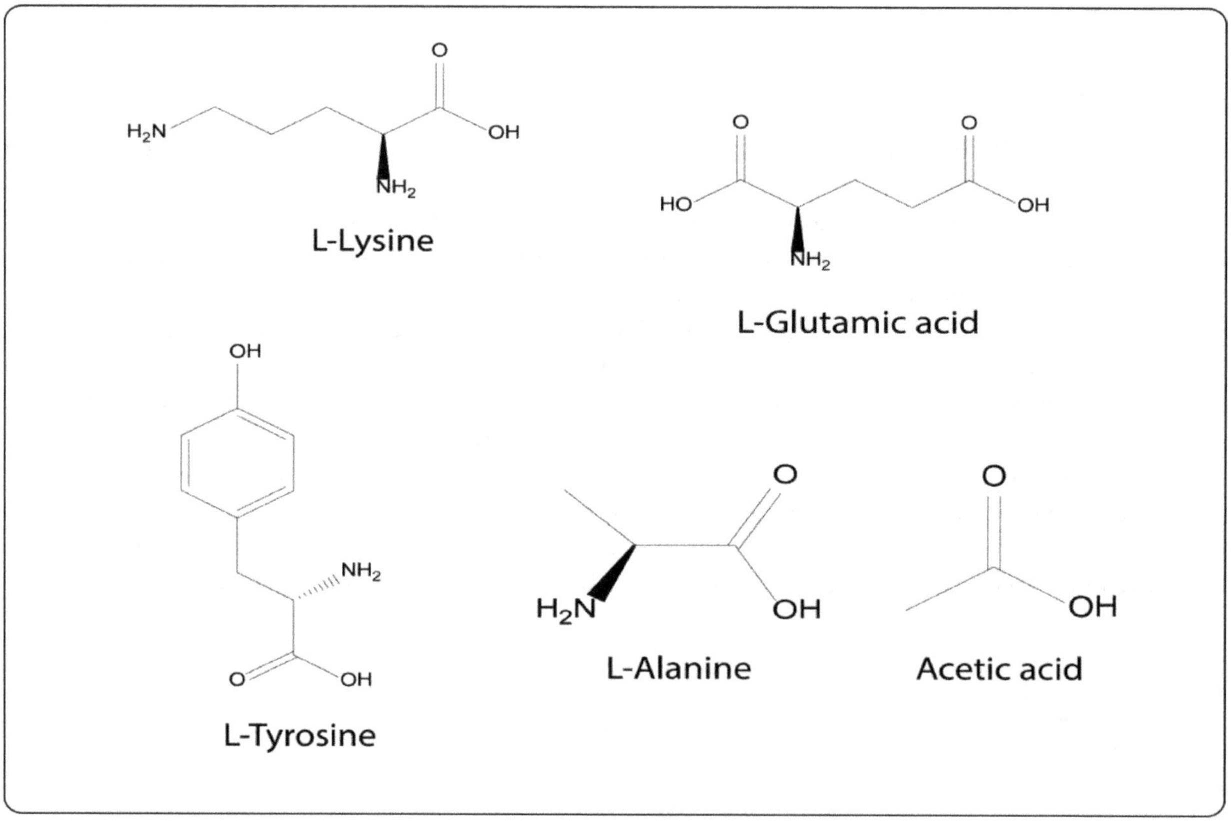

Figure 13. Synthetic peptides of Cop1 structure.

Recently, semi-empirical calculations have been applied to detect peptides associated with MS. It was found that the A_31:01 allele may be associated with the MS disease and the peptide Leu-Ile-Ile-Cys-Tyr-Asn-Trp-Leu-His-Arg may serve as a potential epitope to this allele. This finding must be confirmed by experimental evidence [79].

The multifactorial aspects of MS, especially in its severe state, makes the task of finding a drug against MS tremendously difficult. This must reinforce the efforts in order to advance the progress of understanding and treating the disease.

Author Contributions: Conceptualization, C.K., E.C., S.K., A.G.T.; writing—original draft preparation, T.M.; writing—review and editing, C.K., E.C., S.K., visualization, C.K., E.C., S.K., A.G.T.; supervision, T.M.; project administration, T.M. All authors have read and agreed to the published version of the manuscript.

References

1. Wallin, M.T.; Culpepper, W.J.; Campbell, J.D.; Nelson, L.M.; Langer-Gould, A.; Marrie, R.A.; Cutter, G.R.; Kaye, W.E.; Wagner, L.; Tremlett, H.; et al. The prevalence of MS in the United States. *Neurology* **2019**, *92*, 1029–1040. [CrossRef] [PubMed]
2. Howard, J.; Trevick, S.; Younger, D.S. Epidemiology of Multiple Sclerosis. *Neurol. Clin.* **2016**, *34*, 919–939. [CrossRef]
3. Dziedzic, A.; Miller, E.; Saluk-Bijak, J.; Bijak, M. The gpr17 receptor—A promising goal for therapy and a potential marker of the neurodegenerative process in multiple sclerosis. *Int. J. Mol. Sci.* **2020**, *21*, 1852. [CrossRef] [PubMed]
4. Jennum, P.; Wanscher, B.; Frederiksen, J.; Kjellberg, J. The socioeconomic consequences of multiple sclerosis: A controlled national study. *Eur. Neuropsychopharmacol.* **2012**, *22*, 36–43. [CrossRef]
5. Raj, R.; Kaprio, J.; Korja, M.; Mikkonen, E.D.; Jousilahti, P.; Siironen, J. Risk of hospitalization with neurodegenerative disease after moderate-to-severe traumatic brain injury in the working-age population: A retrospective cohort study using the Finnish national health registries. *PLoS Med.* **2017**, *14*, e1002316. [CrossRef] [PubMed]
6. Melchor, G.S.; Khan, T.; Reger, J.F.; Huang, J.K. Remyelination Pharmacotherapy Investigations Highlight Diverse Mechanisms Underlying Multiple Sclerosis Progression. *ACS Pharmacol. Transl. Sci.* **2019**, *2*, 372–386. [CrossRef] [PubMed]
7. Khan, F.; Amatya, B. Rehabilitation in Multiple Sclerosis: A Systematic Review of Systematic Reviews. *Arch. Phys. Med. Rehabil.* **2017**, *98*, 353–367. [CrossRef]
8. Eckstein, C.; Bhatti, M.T. Currently approved and emerging oral therapies in multiple sclerosis: An update for the ophthalmologist. *Surv. Ophthalmol.* **2016**, *61*, 318–332. [CrossRef]
9. Lublin, F.D.; Reingold, S.C. Defining the clinical course of multiple sclerosis: Results of an international survey. *Neurology* **1996**, *46*, 907–911. [CrossRef]
10. Lublin, F.D.; Baier, M.; Cutter, G. Effect of relapses on development of residual deficit in multiple sclerosis. *Neurology* **2003**, *61*, 1528–1532. [CrossRef]
11. Hemmer, B.; Archelos, J.J.; Hartung, H.P. New concepts in the immunopathogenesis of multiple sclerosis. *Nat. Rev. Neurosci.* **2002**, *3*, 291–301. [CrossRef] [PubMed]
12. Lassmann, H.; Raine, C.S.; Antel, J.; Prineas, J.W. Immunopathology of multiple sclerosis: Report on an international meeting held at the Institute of Neurology of the University of Vienna. *J. Neuroimmunol.* **1998**, 213–217. [CrossRef]
13. Tzakos, A.; Kursula, P.; Troganis, A.; Theodorou, V.; Tselios, T.; Svarnas, C.; Matsoukas, J.; Apostolopoulos, V.; Gerothanassis, I. Structure and Function of the Myelin Proteins: Current Status and Perspectives in Relation to Multiple Sclerosis. *Curr. Med. Chem.* **2005**, *12*, 1569–1587. [CrossRef] [PubMed]
14. Kouskoff, V.; Lacaud, G.; Nemazee, D. T cell-independent rescue of B lymphocytes from peripheral immune tolerance. *Science* **2000**, *287*, 2501–2513. [CrossRef]
15. Tuusa, J.; Raasakka, A.; Ruskamo, S.; Kursula, P. Myelin-derived and putative molecular mimic peptides share structural properties in aqueous and membrane-like environments. *Mult. Scler. Demyelinating Disord.* **2017**, *2*. [CrossRef]
16. Bielekova, B.; Sung, M.-H.; Kadom, N.; Simon, R.; McFarland, H.; Martin, R. Expansion and Functional Relevance of High-Avidity Myelin-Specific CD4 + T Cells in Multiple Sclerosis. *J. Immunol.* **2004**, *172*, 3893–3904. [CrossRef]
17. Greer, J.M.; Csurhes, P.A.; Cameron, K.D.; McCombe, P.A.; Good, M.F.; Pender, M.P. Increased immunoreactivity to two overlapping peptides of myelin proteolipid protein in multiple sclerosis. *Brain* **1997**, *120*, 1447–1460. [CrossRef]
18. Mendel, I.; De Rosbo, N.K.; Ben-Nun, A. Delineation of the minimal encephalitogenic epitope within the immunodominant region of myelin oligodendrocyte glycoprotein: Diverse Vβ gene usage by T cells recognizing the core epitope encephalitogenic for T cell receptor Vβb and T cell receptor Vβa H-2. *Eur. J. Immunol.* **1996**, *26*, 2470–2479. [CrossRef]

19. De Rosbo, N.K.; Kaye, J.F.; Eisenstein, M.; Mendel, I.; Hoeftberger, R.; Lassmann, H.; Milo, R.; Ben-Nun, A. The Myelin-Associated Oligodendrocytic Basic Protein Region MOBP15–36 Encompasses the Immunodominant Major Encephalitogenic Epitope(s) for SJL/J Mice and Predicted Epitope(s) for Multiple Sclerosis-Associated HLA-DRB1*1501. *J. Immunol.* **2004**, *173*, 1426–1435. [CrossRef]
20. Holz, A.; Bielekova, B.; Martin, R.; Oldstone, M.B.A. Myelin-Associated Oligodendrocytic Basic Protein: Identification of an Encephalitogenic Epitope and Association with Multiple Sclerosis. *J. Immunol.* **2000**, *164*, 1103–1109. [CrossRef]
21. Denic, A.; Johnson, A.J.; Bieber, A.J.; Warrington, A.E.; Rodriguez, M.; Pirko, I. The relevance of animal models in multiple sclerosis research. *Pathophysiology* **2011**, *18*, 21–29. [CrossRef] [PubMed]
22. Gholamzad, M.; Ebtekar, M.; Ardestani, M.S.; Azimi, M.; Mahmodi, Z.; Mousavi, M.J.; Aslani, S. A comprehensive review on the treatment approaches of multiple sclerosis: Currently and in the future. *Inflamm. Res.* **2019**, *68*, 25–38. [CrossRef]
23. Shahrizaila, N.; Yuki, N. Guillain-Barré syndrome animal model: The first proof of molecular mimicry in human autoimmune disorder. *J. Biomed. Biotechnol.* **2011**, *2011*, 829129. [CrossRef]
24. Moise, L.; Beseme, S.; Tassone, R.; Liu, R.; Kibria, F.; Terry, F.; Martin, W.; De Groot, A.S. T cell epitope redundancy: Cross-conservation of the TCR face between pathogens and self and its implications for vaccines and autoimmunity. *Expert Rev. Vaccines* **2016**, *15*, 607–617. [CrossRef] [PubMed]
25. Matsoukas, J.; Apostolopoulos, V.; Mavromoustakos, T. Designing Peptide Mimetics for the Treatment of Multiple Sclerosis. *Mini Rev. Med. Chem.* **2005**, *1*, 273–282. [CrossRef] [PubMed]
26. Compston, A.; Coles, A. Multiple sclerosis. *Lancet* **2008**, *372*, 1502–1517. [CrossRef]
27. Davis, M.M.; Boniface, J.J.; Reich, Z.; Lyons, D.; Hampl, J.; Arden, B.; Chien, Y. Ligand Recognition By alpha beta T Cell Receptors. *Annu. Rev. Immunol.* **1998**, *16*, 523–544. [CrossRef] [PubMed]
28. Wootla, B.; Eriguchi, M.; Rodriguez, M. Is multiple sclerosis an autoimmune disease? *Autoimmune Dis.* **2012**, *2012*, 969657. [CrossRef] [PubMed]
29. Hare, B.J.; Wyss, D.F.; Osburne, M.S.; Kern, P.S.; Reinherz, E.L.; Wagner, G. Structure, specificity and CDR mobility of a class II restricted single- chain T-cell receptor. *Nat. Struct. Biol.* **1999**, *6*, 574–581. [CrossRef]
30. Rudolph, M.G.; Wilson, I.A. The specificity of TCR/pMHC interaction. *Curr. Opin. Immunol.* **2002**, *14*, 52–65. [CrossRef]
31. Rudolph, M.G.; Stanfield, R.L.; Wilson, I.A. How TCRS Bind MHCS, Peptides, And Coreceptors. *Annu. Rev. Immunol.* **2006**, *24*, 419–466. [CrossRef] [PubMed]
32. Lassmann, H. Axonal and neuronal pathology in multiple sclerosis: What have we learnt from animal models. *Exp. Neurol.* **2010**, *225*, 2–8. [CrossRef] [PubMed]
33. Reuter, E.; Gollan, R.; Grohmann, N.; Paterka, M.; Salmon, H.; Birkenstock, J.; Richers, S.; Leuenberger, T.; Brandt, A.U.; Kuhlmann, T.; et al. Cross-Recognition of a myelin peptide by CD8+ T cells in the CNS is not sufficient to promote neuronal damage. *J. Neurosci.* **2015**, *35*, 4837–4850. [CrossRef] [PubMed]
34. Madden, D.R. The Three-Dimensional Structure of Peptide-MHC Complexes. *Annu. Rev. Immunol.* **1995**, *13*, 587–622. [CrossRef]
35. Adams, E.J.; Luoma, A.M. The Adaptable Major Histocompatibility Complex (MHC) Fold: Structure and Function of Nonclassical and MHC Class I–Like Molecules. *Annu. Rev. Immunol.* **2013**, *31*, 529–561. [CrossRef]
36. Yannakakis, M.P.; Tzoupis, H.; Michailidou, E.; Mantzourani, E.; Simal, C.; Tselios, T. Molecular dynamics at the receptor level of immunodominant myelin oligodendrocyte glycoprotein 35–55 epitope implicated in multiple sclerosis. *J. Mol. Graph. Model.* **2016**, *68*, 78–86. [CrossRef]
37. Mouzaki, A.; Tselios, T.; Papathanassopoulos, P.; Matsoukas, I.; Chatzantoni, K. Immunotherapy for Multiple Sclerosis: Basic Insights for New Clinical Strategies. *Curr. Neurovasc. Res.* **2005**, *1*, 325–340. [CrossRef]
38. Tselios, T.; Daliani, I.; Deraos, S.; Thymianou, S.; Matsoukas, E.; Troganis, A.; Gerothanassis, I.; Mouzaki, A.; Mavromoustakos, T.; Probert, L.; et al. Treatment of experimental allergic encephalomyelitis (EAE) by a rationally designed cyclic analogue of myelin basic protein (MBP) epitope 72-85. *Bioorg. Med. Chem. Lett.* **2000**, *10*, 2713–2717. [CrossRef]
39. Tselios, T.; Apostolopoulos, V.; Daliani, I.; Deraos, S.; Grdadolnik, S.; Mavromoustakos, T.; Melachrinou, M.; Thymianou, S.; Probert, L.; Mouzaki, A.; et al. Antagonistic effects of human cyclic MBP87-99 altered peptide ligands in experimental allergic encephalomyelitis and human T-cell proliferation. *J. Med. Chem.* **2002**, *45*, 275–283. [CrossRef]

40. Ntountaniotis, D.; Vanioti, M.; Kordopati, G.G.; Kellici, T.F.; Marousis, K.D.; Mavromoustakos, T.; Spyroulias, G.A.; Golic Grdadolnik, S.; Tselios, T.V. A combined NMR and molecular dynamics simulation study to determine the conformational properties of rat/mouse 35-55 myelin oligodendrocyte glycoprotein epitope implicated in the induction of experimental autoimmune encephalomyelitis. *J. Biomol. Struct. Dyn.* **2017**, *35*, 1559–1567. [CrossRef]
41. Mantzourani, E.D.; Platts, J.A.; Brancale, A.; Mavromoustakos, T.M.; Tselios, T.V. Molecular dynamics at the receptor level of immunodominant myelin basic protein epitope 87-99 implicated in multiple sclerosis and its antagonists altered peptide ligands: Triggering of immune response. *J. Mol. Graph. Model.* **2007**, *26*, 471–481. [CrossRef] [PubMed]
42. Willcox, B.E.; Gao, G.F.; Wyer, J.R.; Ladbury, J.E.; Bell, J.I.; Jakobsen, B.K.; Van der Merwe, P.A. TCR binding to peptide-MHC stabilizes a flexible recognition interface. *Immunity* **1999**, *10*, 357–365. [CrossRef]
43. Matsoukas, J.; Apostolopoulos, V.; Kalbacher, H.; Papini, A.M.; Tselios, T.; Chatzantoni, K.; Biagioli, T.; Lolli, F.; Deraos, S.; Papathanassopoulos, P.; et al. Design and synthesis of a novel potent myelin basic protein epitope 87-99 cyclic analogue: Enhanced stability and biological properties of mimics render them a potentially new class of immunomodulators. *J. Med. Chem.* **2005**, *48*, 1470–1480. [CrossRef] [PubMed]
44. Emmanouil, M.; Tseveleki, V.; Triantafyllakou, I.; Nteli, A.; Tselios, T.; Probert, L. A cyclic altered peptide analogue based on myelin basic protein 87-99 provides lasting prophylactic and therapeutic protection against acute experimental autoimmune encephalomyelitis. *Molecules* **2018**, *23*, 304. [CrossRef] [PubMed]
45. Spyranti, Z.; Dalkas, G.A.; Spyroulias, G.A.; Mantzourani, E.D.; Mavromoustakos, T.; Friligou, I.; Matsoukas, J.M.; Tselios, T.V. Putative bioactive conformations of amide linked cyclic myelin basic protein peptide analogues associated with experimental autoimmune encephalomyelitis. *J. Med. Chem.* **2007**, *50*, 6039–6047. [CrossRef] [PubMed]
46. Deraos, G.; Chatzantoni, K.; Matsoukas, M.T.; Tselios, T.; Deraos, S.; Katsara, M.; Papathanasopoulos, P.; Vynios, D.; Apostolopoulos, V.; Mouzaki, A.; et al. Citrullination of linear and cyclic altered peptide ligands from myelin basic protein (MBP87-99) epitope elicits a Th1 polarized response by T cells isolated from multiple sclerosis patients: Implications in triggering disease. *J. Med. Chem.* **2008**, *51*, 7834–7842. [CrossRef] [PubMed]
47. Matsoukas, J.; Apostolopoulos, V.; Lazoura, E.; Deraos, G.; Matsoukas, M.-T.; Katsara, M.; Tselios, T.; Deraos, S. Round and Round we Go: Cyclic Peptides in Disease. *Curr. Med. Chem.* **2006**. [CrossRef]
48. Tzakos, A.G.; Fuchs, P.; Van Nuland, N.A.J.; Troganis, A.; Tselios, T.; Deraos, S.; Matsoukas, J.; Gerothanassis, I.P.; Bonvin, A.M.J.J. NMR and molecular dynamics studies of an autoimmune myelin basic protein peptide and its antagonist: Structural implications for the MHC II (I-A u)-peptide complex from docking calculations. *Eur. J. Biochem.* **2004**, *271*, 3399–3413. [CrossRef]
49. Wraith, D.C.; Smilek, D.E.; Mitchell, D.J.; Steinman, L.; McDevitt, H.O. Antigen recognition in autoimmune encephalomyelitis and the potential for peptide-mediated immunotherapy. *Cell* **1989**, *59*, 247–255. [CrossRef]
50. Lee, C.; Liang, M.N.; Tate, K.M.; Rabinowitz, J.D.; Beeson, C.; Jones, P.P.; McConnell, H.M. Evidence that the autoimmune antigen myelin basic protein (MBP) Ac1-9 binds towards one end of the major histocompatibility complex (MHC) cleft. *J. Exp. Med.* **1998**, *187*, 1505–1516. [CrossRef]
51. He, X.L.; Radu, C.; Sidney, J.; Sette, A.; Ward, E.S.; Garcia, K.C. Structural snapshot of aberrant antigen presentation linked to autoimmunity: The immunodominant epitope of MBP complexed with I-Au. *Immunity* **2002**, *17*, 83–94. [CrossRef]
52. Fugger, L.; Liang, J.; Gautam, A.; Rothbard, J.B.; McDevitt, H.O. Quantitative analysis of peptides from myelin basic protein binding to the MHC class II protein, I-A(u), which confers susceptibility to experimental allergic encephalomyelitis. *Mol. Med.* **1996**, *2*, 181–188. [CrossRef] [PubMed]
53. Metzler, B.; Wraith, D.C. Inhibition of experimental autoimmune encephalomyelitis by inhalation but not oral administration of the encephalitogenic peptide: Influence of MHC binding affinity. *Int. Immunol.* **1993**, *5*, 1159–1165. [CrossRef] [PubMed]
54. Laimou, D.; Lazoura, E.; Troganis, A.N.; Matsoukas, M.T.; Deraos, S.N.; Katsara, M.; Matsoukas, J.; Apostolopoulos, V.; Tselios, T.V. Conformational studies of immunodominant myelin basic protein 1-11 analogues using NMR and molecular modeling. *J. Comput. Aided. Mol. Des.* **2011**, *25*, 1019–1032. [CrossRef]
55. Spyranti, Z.; Tselios, T.; Deraos, G.; Matsoukas, J.; Spyroulias, G.A. NMR structural elucidation of myelin basic protein epitope 83-99 implicated in multiple sclerosis. *Amino Acids* **2010**, *38*, 929–936. [CrossRef]

56. Mantzourani, E.; Mavromoustakos, T.; Platts, J.; Matsoukas, J.; Tselios, T. Structural Requirements for Binding of Myelin Basic Protein (MBP) Peptides to MHC II: Effects on Immune Regulation. *Curr. Med. Chem.* **2005**, *12*, 1521–1535. [CrossRef]
57. Mantzourani, E.D.; Tselios, T.V.; Grdadolnik, S.G.; Platts, J.A.; Brancale, A.; Deraos, G.N.; Matsoukas, J.M.; Mavromoustakos, T.M. Comparison of proposed putative active conformations of myelin basic protein epitope 87-99 linear altered peptide ligands by spectroscopic and modelling studies: The role of positions 91 and 96 in T-cell receptor activation. *J. Med. Chem.* **2006**, *49*, 6683–6691. [CrossRef]
58. Mantzourani, E.D.; Tselios, T.V.; Grdadolnik, S.G.; Brancale, A.; Platts, J.A.; Matsoukas, J.M.; Mavromoustakos, T.M. A putative bioactive conformation for the altered peptide ligand of myelin basic protein and inhibitor of experimental autoimmune encephalomyelitis [Arg91, Ala96] MBP87-99. *J. Mol. Graph. Model.* **2006**, *25*, 17–29. [CrossRef]
59. Mantzourani, E.; Laimou, D.; Matsoukas, M.; Tselios, T. Peptides as Therapeutic Agents or Drug Leads for Autoimmune, Hormone Dependent and Cardiovascular Diseases. *Antiinflamm. Antiallergy Agents Med. Chem.* **2008**, *7*, 294–306. [CrossRef]
60. Mantzourani, E.D.; Blokar, K.; Tselios, T.V.; Matsoukas, J.M.; Platts, J.A.; Mavromoustakos, T.M.; Grdadolnik, S.G. A combined NMR and molecular dynamics simulation study to determine the conformational properties of agonists and antagonists against experimental autoimmune encephalomyelitis. *Bioorg. Med. Chem.* **2008**, *16*, 2171–2182. [CrossRef]
61. Martel, P.; Makriyannis, A.; Mavromoustakos, T.; Kelly, K.; Jeffrey, K.R. Topography of tetrahydrocannabinol in model membranes using neutron diffraction. *BBA Biomembr.* **1993**, *1151*, 51–58. [CrossRef]
62. Mavromoustakos, T.; Daliani, I. Effects of cannabinoids in membrane bilayers containing cholesterol. *Biochim. Biophys. Acta Biomembr.* **1999**, *1420*, 252–265. [CrossRef]
63. Mavromoustakos, T.; Theodoropoulou, E. A combined use of 13C-cross polarization/magic angle spinning, 13C-magic angle spinning and 31P-nuclear magnetic resonance spectroscopy with differential scanning calorimetry to study cannabinoid-membrane interactions. *Chem. Phys. Lipids* **1998**, *92*, 37–52. [CrossRef]
64. Mavromoustakos, T.; De-Ping, Y.; Broderick, W.; Fournier, D.; Makriyannis, A. Small angle X-ray diffraction studies on the topography of cannabinoids in synaptic plasma membranes. *Pharmacol. Biochem. Behav.* **1991**, *40*, 547–552. [CrossRef]
65. Mavromoustakos, T.; Yang, D.P.; Makriyannis, A. Topography of alphaxalone and Δ16-alphaxalone in membrane bilayers containing cholesterol. *BBA Biomembr.* **1994**, *1194*, 69–74. [CrossRef]
66. Mavromoustakos, T.; Yang, D.P.; Makriyannis, A. Small angle X-ray diffraction and differential scanning calorimetric studies on O-methyl-(-)-Δ8-tetrahydrocannabinol and its 5′ iodinated derivative in membrane bilayers. *BBA Biomembr.* **1995**, *1237*, 183–188. [CrossRef]
67. Mavromoustakos, T.; Yang, D.P.; Makriyannis, A. Effects of the anesthetic steroid alphaxalone and its inactive Δ16-analog on the thermotropic properties of membrane bilayers. A model for membrane perturbation. *BBA Biomembr.* **1995**, *1239*, 257–264. [CrossRef]
68. Mavromoustakos, T.; Yang, D.P.; Makriyannis, A. Topography and thermotropic properties of cannabinoids in brain sphingomyelin bilayers. *Life Sci.* **1996**, *59*, 1969–1979. [CrossRef]
69. Mavromoustakos, T.; Theodoropoulou, E.; Papahatjis, D.; Kourouli, T.; Yang, D.P.; Trumbore, M.; Makriyannis, A. Studies on the thermotropic effects of cannabinoids on phosphatidylcholine bilayers using differential scanning calorimetry and small angle X-ray diffraction. *Biochim. Biophys. Acta Biomembr.* **1996**, *1281*, 235–244. [CrossRef]
70. Mavromoustakos, T.; Theodoropoulou, E.; Yang, D.P. The use of high-resolution solid-state NMR spectroscopy and differential scanning calorimetry to study interactions of anaesthetic steroids with membrane. *Biochim. Biophys. Acta Biomembr.* **1997**, *1328*, 65–73. [CrossRef]
71. Mavromoustakos, T.; Papahatjis, D.; Laggner, P. Differential membrane fluidization by active and inactive cannabinoid analogues. *Biochim. Biophys. Acta Biomembr.* **2001**, *1512*, 183–190. [CrossRef]
72. Koukoulitsa, C.; Durdagi, S.; Siapi, E.; Villalonga-Barber, C.; Alexi, X.; Steele, B.R.; Micha-Screttas, M.; Alexis, M.N.; Tsantili-Kakoulidou, A.; Mavromoustakos, T. Comparison of thermal effects of stilbenoid analogs in lipid bilayers using differential scanning calorimetry and molecular dynamics: Correlation of thermal effects and topographical position with antioxidant activity. *Eur. Biophys. J.* **2011**, *40*, 865–875. [CrossRef] [PubMed]

73. Stern, J.N.H.; Illés, Z.; Reddy, J.; Keskin, D.B.; Fridkis-Hareli, M.; Kuchroo, V.K.; Strominger, J.L. Peptide 15-mers of defined sequence that substitute for random amino acid copolymers in amelioration of experimental autoimmune encephalomyelitis. *Proc. Natl. Acad. Sci. USA* **2005**, *102*, 1620–1625. [CrossRef] [PubMed]
74. Kant, R.; Pasi, S.; Surolia, A. Homo-β-amino acid containing MBP(85-99) analogs alleviate experimental autoimmune encephalomyelitis. *Sci. Rep.* **2015**, *3*, 8205. [CrossRef]
75. Yannakakis, M.P.; Simal, C.; Tzoupis, H.; Rodi, M.; Dargahi, N.; Prakash, M.; Mouzaki, A.; Platts, J.A.; Apostolopoulos, V.; Tselios, T.V. Design and synthesis of non-peptide mimetics mapping the immunodominant myelin basic protein (MBP83-96) epitope to function as T-cell receptor antagonists. *Int. J. Mol. Sci.* **2017**, *18*, 1215. [CrossRef]
76. Karin, N.; Mitchell, D.J.; Brocke, S.; Ling, N.; Steinman, L. Reversal of experimental autoimmune encephalomyelitis by a soluble peptide variant of a myelin basic protein epitope: T cell receptor antagonism and reduction of interferon γ and tumor necrosis factor α production. *J. Exp. Med.* **1994**, *180*, 2227–2237. [CrossRef]
77. Katsara, M.; Matsoukas, J.; Deraos, G.; Apostolopoulos, V. Towards immunotherapeutic drugs and vaccines against multiple sclerosis. *Acta Biochim. Biophys. Sin.* **2008**, *40*, 636–642. [CrossRef]
78. Aharoni, R.; Teitelbaum, D.; Arnon, R.; Sela, M. Copolymer 1 acts against the immunodominant epitope 82-100 of myelin basic protein by T cell receptor antagonism in addition to major histocompatibility complex blocking. *Proc. Natl. Acad. Sci. USA* **1999**, *96*, 634–639. [CrossRef]
79. Mohammadi-Milasi, F.; Mahnam, K.; Shakhsi-Niaei, M. In silico study of the association of the HLA-A*31:01 allele (human leucocyte antigen allele 31:01) with neuroantigenic epitopes of PLP (proteolipid protein), MBP (myelin basic protein) and MOG proteins (Myelin oligodendrocyte glycoprotein) for studying t. *J. Biomol. Struct. Dyn.* **2020**, 1–17. [CrossRef]

9

Diagnosis and Management of Progressive Multiple Sclerosis

Gabrielle Macaron and Daniel Ontaneda *

Mellen Center for Multiple Sclerosis, Neurological Institute, Cleveland Clinic Foundation, Cleveland, OH 44195, USA
* Correspondence: ontaned@ccf.org;

Abstract: Multiple sclerosis is a chronic autoimmune disease of the central nervous system that results in varying degrees of disability. Progressive multiple sclerosis, characterized by a steady increase in neurological disability independently of relapses, can occur from onset (primary progressive) or after a relapsing–remitting course (secondary progressive). As opposed to active inflammation seen in the relapsing–remitting phases of the disease, the gradual worsening of disability in progressive multiple sclerosis results from complex immune mechanisms and neurodegeneration. A few anti-inflammatory disease-modifying therapies with a modest but significant effect on measures of disease progression have been approved for the treatment of progressive multiple sclerosis. The treatment effect of anti-inflammatory agents is particularly observed in the subgroup of patients with younger age and evidence of disease activity. For this reason, a significant effort is underway to develop molecules with the potential to induce myelin repair or halt the degenerative process. Appropriate trial methodology and the development of clinically meaningful disability outcome measures along with imaging and biological biomarkers of progression have a significant impact on the ability to measure the efficacy of potential medications that may reverse disease progression. In this issue, we will review current evidence on the physiopathology, diagnosis, measurement of disability, and treatment of progressive multiple sclerosis.

Keywords: progressive multiple sclerosis; neurodegeneration; remyelination; outcome measures; biomarkers

---

1. Introduction

Multiple sclerosis (MS) is a chronic inflammatory disease of the central nervous system that affects over 2.3 million people globally, with an estimated prevalence of approximately 310 per 100,000 population in the United States [1,2]. Most patients (~90%) have relapsing–remitting disease at onset, which typically is followed by a secondary progressive course, while a minority of patients have a primary progressive course from onset (~10%). Relapsing–remitting MS (RRMS) is characterized by frequent formation of inflammatory lesions in the brain and spinal cord. Approved disease-modifying therapies (DMTs) target the inflammatory component of the disease, and strong evidence support their effectiveness in RRMS. However, trials evaluating their efficacy in slowing disease progression have shown mixed results, or have shown only modest effects in slowing progression. The goal of this review is to provide a comprehensive overview on the current knowledge of the pathogenesis, diagnosis, and treatment of progressive MS, as well as future directions in the field.

2. Pathogenesis

The pathogenesis of MS is incompletely elucidated. This is particularly the case for progressive MS, for which various and sometimes conflicting data have been proposed to explain the underlying pathogenic process of progression [3]. In RRMS, actively demyelinating plaques are the most prominent lesion type, and are characterized by inflammatory demyelination and axonal transection within the lesions [4–6]. However, active lesions are rare in progressive MS, and axonal transection is not seen as frequently within inactive lesions compared to highly inflammatory recently developed lesions [3–5]. Whole brain atrophy, smoldering and enlarging lesions, cortical demyelination (specifically subpial lesions), and diffuse axonal injury and microglial activation in normal appearing grey and white matter are prominent in patients with progressive MS compared to patients with early RRMS [6–10]. Disability in progressive MS is thought to be related to secondary neurodegeneration of chronically demyelinating axons, which is thought to be driven by a series of factors, including: (1) inflammation and lesion accumulation, with subsequent retrograde and anterograde degeneration, (2) mitochondrial damage and subsequently virtual hypoxia and oxidative stress, (3) iron accumulation in myelin sheath and oligodendrocytes with subsequent amplification of oxidative stress, (4) lymphoid follicle-like structures that might contribute to sustaining cortical pathology, and [5] age-related neurodegeneration and reduced neuronal reserve (loss of the ability to compensate for axonal loss) [3,11–15]. A recent paper by Brown et al. [16], among others, showed that the early use of DMTs, specifically highly-effective DMTs, decreases the odds of conversion to secondary progressive MS (SPMS), which supports the role of early disease activity in the development of long-term disability progression [16–21]. The role of age-related mechanisms is supported by the fact that children with MS rarely present with progressive disease and have a longer time to reach secondary progression and disability milestones compared to adult-onset MS, and that certain disability milestones are acquired at certain ages independently of the duration of the disease [22,23]. However, for primary progressive MS (PPMS), the time course of irreversible damage is not clearly affected by the presence or absence of superimposed relapses [24]. Recent observations support a change in the natural history of MS with earlier use of highly-effective DMTs; however, this effect seems to be more clearly evidenced in RRMS [25]. Despite the wide variability of clinical and radiological presentations and the inherent pathological differences between RRMS, SPMS, and PPMS, the consensus is that PPMS is biologically part of the MS spectrum [13].

3. Diagnostic Criteria and Disease Course Definitions

The diagnosis of progressive MS is based on patient-reported clinical history, and should be confirmed based on objective physical examination findings. Based on the 2017 McDonald diagnostic criteria, PPMS can be diagnosed in patients with a 1-year history of disability progression, which can be retrospectively or prospectively determined, independent of clinical relapses, plus two of the following criteria: (1) One or more T2 lesions characteristic of MS in one or more typical brain regions (periventricular, cortical or juxtacortical, infratentorial); (2) two or more T2 lesions in the spinal cord, and (3) the presence of CSF-specific oligoclonal bands. Unlike the 2010 McDonald criteria, both symptomatic and asymptomatic MRI lesions are taken into account [26,27]. The panel also recommends specifying a provisional disease course at the time of diagnosis, and whether disease activity and/or progression are present or not based on the previous year's history, which can then be revisited based on periodic re-evaluation [27]. Providing a clinical definition of disease progression, however, is somewhat harder. Progression is characterized by a steady increase in neurological disability occurring independently of relapses [27,28]. Symptoms can fluctuate (i.e., pseudo relapses), and bona fide superimposed relapses might occur. Detailed history taking is key in differentiating events suggestive of disease activity from worsening of previously experienced symptoms in the context of fatigue, heat, or stress. PPMS is defined by a progressive course from onset and SPMS by a progressive course following an initial relapsing–remitting course. The 2013 revisions of MS clinical course definitions aimed at standardizing the terminology across clinicians and researchers, for prognostication, design of clinical trials, and treatment decisions purposes [28]. These definitions included the presence or absence of clinical or radiological activity, and the presence or absence of disability progression into the phenotypic description of the disease. Figure 1 illustrates the currently used description of different progressive MS phenotypes. The distinction between "active" and "inactive" progressive disease, whether primary or secondary, has important therapeutic implications. This will be discussed in the treatment section of this manuscript.

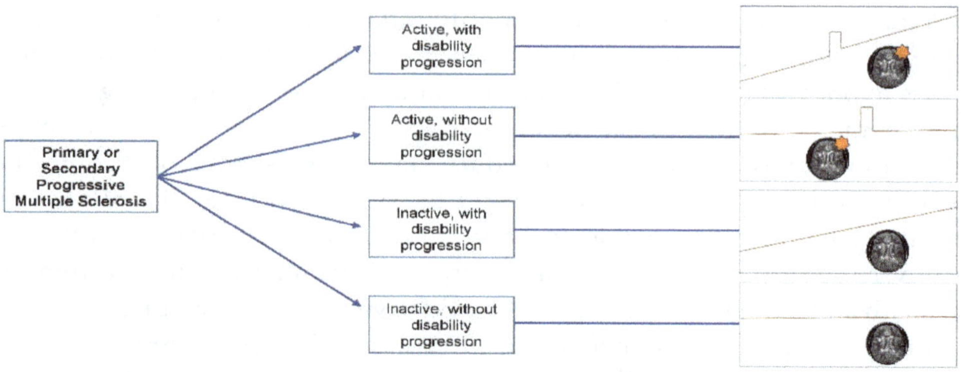

Figure 1. Clinical course of progressive multiple sclerosis. The orange star indicates the presence of radiological activity (new/enlarging T2 lesions or gadolinium enhancing lesions).

4. Disability Outcome Measures

Disability progression in MS affects multiple functional domains, occurs insidiously over time, and can be difficult to quantify in an objective, comprehensive, and reproducible manner. Reliable detection of clinical and sub-clinical progression is key to interpreting treatment efficacy in trials and in clinical practice of DMT and repair promoting strategies in progressive MS. The expanded disability status scale (EDSS) is the most commonly used clinical outcome measure in trials for quantification of physical disability in MS. However, the EDSS does not comprehensively reflect disability status, and is particularly restricted in assessing cognitive and upper extremity functions [29]. Other limitations of the EDSS include poor intra and inter-rater variability especially for lower scores. The test also shows little sensitivity to detect change, especially in patients with scores of 6.0 or more, and the EDSS is difficult to administer in routine care [30–32]. Since it is an ordinal scale, changes in EDSS scores are not equivalent across the range of the scale. Finally, the most commonly used outcome measure in progressive MS trials is the 3 or 6-month confirmed disability progression, which might be insufficient to predict long-term disability worsening [33]. Evaluating multiple functional domains improves the likelihood of observing a change in patients with MS. The multiple sclerosis functional composite (MSFC) [34,35] was developed as a quantitative clinical measure of neurologic disability to overcome some of the shortcomings of the EDSS. Cognitive function was evaluated originally using the paced auditory serial addition test (PASAT), but more recently using the symbol–digit modalities test (SDMT), and upper extremity function is evaluated using the 9-hole peg test (9HPT) [36,37]. Walking speed is usually evaluated using the timed-25-foot walk test (T25FW). The MSFC has proven to be more sensitive to change than the EDSS, and correlates with subsequent changes in EDSS [34] T1 and T2 lesion load on brain MRI [38], and patient reported physical and emotional functioning and quality of life [39]. In the interferon beta (IFN-β)-1a SPMS trial, there was some benefit of treatment on the MSFC z-scores but not on the EDSS [40]. This benefit was mainly driven by two of the components of the MSFC, the 9HPT and the PASAT, which further illustrates the importance of a comprehensive neurological evaluation to assess disability progression. The low contrast letter acuity testing using a low-contrast Sloan letter chart was later proposed as an additional component of the MSFC to capture visual dysfunction with a high sensitivity, and also correlates with other components of the MSFC and the EDSS [37,41,42]. In addition, internal consistency (reliability) is higher for the MSFC (Cronbach's alpha coefficient 0.93–0.96) than for the EDSS (Cronbach's alpha 0.7) [43,44]. Although the MSFC has been used as an outcome measure in clinical trials [40,45,46], administration in routine clinical practice is time consuming, and requires personnel to administer the test properly [47]. Recently, there has been increasing interest in developing tools to facilitate and standardize testing in MS patients. For example, a technology-enabled version of the MSFC has been developed and was incorporated into routine clinical practice. This tool, called the multiple sclerosis performance test (MSPT), comprises a battery of quantitative neuroperformance assessments administered using a suite of iPad® applications modeled after the MSFC approach, and has allowed the gathering of large-scale comprehensive and standardized measures of disability from routine care [48,49]. A limitation of these outcome measures is the uncertainty of what constitutes a clinically meaningful change, although a threshold of ± 20% change in T25FW [50,51] ±15–20% in the 9HPT [52,53] ±10% (or 4 points) in the SDMT [53,54] and ±7 letters in the low contrast letter acuity test [55] have been suggested as clinically meaningful in MS.

5. Measuring Disease Progression

Numerous imaging biomarkers that have been proposed for the monitoring of progressive disease in MS trials, whole brain atrophy being the most widely used. Monitoring of T1 hypointensity evolution over time on conventional imaging has also been suggested. Other more advanced MRI techniques that can reflect axonal loss in progressive MS include thalamic volume, spinal cord atrophy, hippocampal volume, gray matter fraction, cortical lesion quantification, and sodium imaging, among others [56,57]. Several additional advanced MRI measures have been used as exploratory outcomes [58] as well as neurophysiological measures, such as evoked potentials [59]. Optical coherence tomography (OCT) is a non-invasive tool that allows the measurements of retinal nerve fiber layer thickness, ganglion cell/inner plexiform layer thickness, and macular volume. Since these measurements correlate with whole brain and gray matter atrophy and physical disability, OCT can serve as an outcome measure of axonal loss in phase 2 proof of concept clinical trials of progressive MS [60]. Other imaging and non-imaging techniques are used in remyelination trials as biomarkers of myelin repair, and include magnetization transfer ratio, diffusion-weighted imaging, myelin water imaging, and visual evoked potentials [56].

There has been increasing interest in the use of serum neurofilament light chain (NfL) as a biomarker in MS over the past few years [61]. Serum NfL levels correlate with CSF NfL levels and reflect disease activity and response to therapy [61]. In progressive MS, NfL levels appear to be associated with superimposed clinical or radiological activity, as well as T1-hypointense lesion volume [62]. Recent data suggests that CSF NfL correlates with disease activity rather than progression, irrespective of the disease subtype, and does not reflect disease severity [63,64], whereas previous data report a strong correlation between NfL levels and future worsening on the EDSS and brain and cervical spinal volume loss [65,66]. Serum NfL levels can be easily obtained, and are being further investigated and used as an outcome measure in newer progressive MS trials.

6. Treatment

6.1. *Anti-Inflammatory Disease-Modifying Therapies*

6.1.1. Approved Therapies

Ocrelizumab (*Ocrevus*®) a humanized monoclonal antibody targeting the CD20 antigen on B-cells. Ocrelizumab exerts its anti-inflammatory effects by causing rapid and profound depletion of B cells. Ocrelizumab has been studied in patients with RRMS in two phase 3 double-blind, placebo-controlled randomized clinical trial (OPERA I and II) [67] and in patients with PPMS (ORATORIO trial) [68], but not in patients with SPMS. Participants with PPMS were required to have positive oligoclonal bands to enroll in the study. In the ORATORIO trial ocrelizumab significantly reduced the risk of 24-week confirmed disability progression compared to placebo (29.6% with ocrelizumab versus 35.7% with placebo). Treatment with ocrelizumab in PPMS also decreased worsening on the timed-25-foot walk, T2 lesion volume, and brain atrophy at 120 weeks compared to placebo. In a pre-specified subgroup analysis, the magnitude of the effect of ocrelizumab was larger in patients with baseline enhancing lesions and younger patients; however, older patients without enhancing lesions at baseline also derived benefit across primary and secondary endpoints [68]. The ENCORE study evaluated the effect of ocrelizumab on upper limb function in the ORATORIO cohort, and also showed positive results (reduction in time—to 12- and 24-week confirmed ≥15% increase on 9HPT by 37% (hazard ratio 0.627; $p = 0.001$) and 39% (HR = 0.607; $p = 0.002$) for both-hands) [69]. Ocrelizumab was approved by the FDA and the EMA to treat PPMS in 2017. Ongoing trials aim at evaluating the effect of ocrelizumab on hand function in patients with more advanced disability (ORATORIO-HAND, NCT03562975), and in a broader range of patients (with PPMS and SPMS, up to 65 years old) (CONSONNANCE, NCT03523858). It is important to note that previous trials using the chimeric monoclonal antibody rituximab, which has a similar mechanism of action as ocrelizumab, yielded results in one pivotal trial that shaped the inclusion criteria for the ORATORIO study. In the OLYMPUS trial of rituximab, the primary endpoint was negative but sub-group analysis found that younger patients with clinical or radiological evidence of disease activity did derive treatment benefit. The subgroup of patients who were older and did not have gadolinium-enhancing lesions had faster disability progression than those on placebo [70]. This indicates a potential harm of treating with a B-cell therapy in this population. Another recent observational study using retrospective data from three European centers and propensity score matching, analyzed the effect of rituximab treatment on disability progression in patients with SPMS. In this study, patients with SPMS treated with rituximab had significantly delayed confirmed progression compared with matched untreated controls at up to 10 years [71]. The difference in effects seen between ocrelizumab and rituximab are most likely related to trial design; however, biological differences may exist as well, given that ocrelizumab appears to promote cell death via greater antibody-dependent cellular cytotoxicity (ADCC) activity and less complement-dependent cytotoxicity (CDC) activity compared to rituximab, and has a more favorable antigenic profile compared to rituximab [72–74].

Siponimod (*Mayzent*®) is a selective sphingosine-1-phosphate receptor 1 and 5 modulator, which inhibits the egress of lymphocytes from lymph nodes, thus decreasing their entry into the CNS. In addition to its anti-inflammatory effects, siponimod has been found to have putative neuroprotective and repair properties in preclinical studies. It was recently approved for the treatment of SPMS based on the results of the EXPAND trial [75]. Compared to the placebo group, a significant reduction in time to 3 and 6-month confirmed disability progression (relative risk reductions of 21% and 26%, respectively) was observed in the siponimod group, and this trend was consistent in subgroup analysis with respect to pre-treatment relapse activity, disease progression rate, and disease severity. Significant reduction in markers of disease activity were also observed in the siponimod group, including annualized relapse rate, time to relapse, and gadolinium-enhancing lesions, and new/enlarging T2 lesions. Brain volume change from baseline was lower in the siponimod group at both months 12 and 24 compared to placebo [75]. Pre-clinical data also suggest that sphingosine-1-phosphate modulators cross the blood–brain barrier, and have the potential to improve morphological markers of remyelination [76]. In addition, modulation of sphingosine-1-phosphate receptor 5 has been shown to promote remyelination in vitro [76]. Interestingly, fingolimod, a sphingosine-1-phosphate receptor 1 to 5 modulator, failed to show significant reduction in confirmed disability worsening in patients with PPMS in the INFORMS trial [77]. The fact that other DMTs with a similar mechanism of action to siponimod and ocrelizumab failed to show benefit in PMS can be due to different patient population and sub-optimal trial designs, but also illustrates the lack of efficacy of anti-inflammatory strategies in the prevention of disability worsening in inactive PMS, and the need to develop molecules with a potential effect on neurodegeneration.

Mitoxantrone is a DNA intercalating agent that interferes with the replication and proliferation of B and T lymphocytes. Its use is nowadays limited due to the well-known serious adverse events (including cardio-toxicity, leukemia, amenorrhea, infections, alopecia, leucopenia, anemia, and hepatotoxicity) [78], and the availability of safer DMTs. The mitoxantrone in progressive multiple sclerosis (MIMS) trial was a double-blind, multicenter, phase 3 trial that randomized patients with worsening RRMS or SPMS to placebo or low (5 mg/m^2) or high (12 mg/m^2) dose mitoxantrone for 2 years [79]. About half of the participants had SPMS, with or without clinical activity in the year prior to enrollment. The primary outcome was a combination of five clinical measures: change from baseline EDSS at 24 months, change from baseline ambulation index at 24 months, number of relapses treated with corticosteroids, time to first treated relapse, and change from baseline standardized neurological status at 24 months [79]. In the cohort as a whole, a beneficial effect on the primary outcome clinical composite measure was observed for the mitoxantrone, with comparable treatment effects in patients with and without relapses in the year prior to enrollment. A few years later, the MIMS trial group analyzed the effect of low and high-dose mitoxantrone on measures of radiological activity in a subgroup of patients with worsening RRMS or SPMS, and surprisingly did not show a consistent effect of mitoxantrone on the presence of gadolinium-enhancing lesions for up to 24 months compared to placebo [80]. Mitoxantrone is approved by the FDA for the treatment of RRMS, SPMS, and what was previously referred to as "progressive relapsing MS". There is no evidence that supports a benefit of mitoxantrone in PPMS without clinical or radiological activity [81,82]. Single-nucleotide polymorphism in the ATP-binding cassette transporter genes may serve as pharmacogenetic markers associated with clinical response to mitoxantrone in RRMS and SPMS [83]; however, this association was not observed in patients with PPMS [81].

Cladibine produces rapid and long-lasting reductions in T-lymphocytes and rapid but transient reduction in B-lymphocytes, by disrupting cellular metabolism, inhibiting DNA synthesis and repair, and subsequent apoptosis of affected cells. The oral formulation of cladribine (*Mavenclad®*) has recently received FDA approval for the treatment of active RRMS and SPMS based on the results of the CLARITY and ORACLE MS trials, and post-hoc analysis of the ONWARD trial [84–87]. Intravenous formulations of cladribine have been mainly studied in progressive MS. An initial small trial (24 matched patients with clinically definite progressive MS as defined at the time of the study, baseline EDSS of 4.7, randomized to receive IV cladribine or placebo) showed a significant benefit of cladribine on EDSS worsening, with some patients even experiencing improvement on EDSS at month 12 [88]. There was also a positive effect on T2 lesion volume in this study. Another larger trial was then conducted in light of these results. Patients with SPMS or PPMS and a median baseline EDSS score of 6.0 were randomly assigned to receive either placebo or cladribine 0.07 mg/kg/day for 5 consecutive days every 4 weeks for 2 or 6 cycles, followed by placebo, for 8 cycles [89]. No benefit of cladribine on the primary outcome (mean change in EDSS at month 12) was observed compared to placebo. As expected, there was a significant effect of cladribine on gadolinium-enhancing lesions and T2 lesion accumulation, and a somewhat marginal benefit in a subgroup analysis of SPMS patients. Similarly, in another study, cladribine did not have a beneficial effect on whole brain volumes compared to placebo [90].

In the ONWARD trial, the effect of oral cladribine as an add-on to IFN-β in patients with active RRMS or SPMS was studied [87]. As expected, cladribine + IFN-β was superior to placebo + IFN-β in reducing annualized relapse rate and gadolinium-enhancing lesions. However, the confirmed EDSS progression over 96 weeks was similar between the two groups. In a post-hoc analysis of subgroups in the intention-to-treat population, cladribine + IFN-β was superior to placebo + IFN-β in reduction of annualized relapse rate (relative risk ratio of 0.11, 95% CI 0.01–0.94) in patients with active SPMS. Hence, oral cladribine was approved by the FDA for the treatment of active SPMS, but not for progressive MS without evidence of clinical or radiological activity.

6.1.2. Therapies with Negative or Weak Effect in Progressive MS

Studies of other anti-inflammatory DMTs in progressive MS have yielded deceiving results. Interferon-beta (IFN-β) has complex immunomodulatory effects (downregulation of pro-inflammatory and upregulation of anti-inflammatory cytokines). There is no robust evidence of the beneficial effect of IFN-β on progression, although early treatment in RRMS decreases conversion to SPMS, which is attributable to its anti-inflammatory properties [16–19]. In SPMS, IFN-β significantly delayed time to confirmed disability progression compared to those receiving placebo in the European SPMS IFN-β-1b trial [91]. However, discrepant results were observed in the North American SPMS IFN-β-1b trial, which did not show a difference in time to 6-month sustained EDSS progression compared to placebo [92]. A post hoc pooled analysis of the clinical trial data of both groups was performed to better clarify this discrepancy, and showed that patients in the European studies who benefited from treatment were significantly younger (41 vs. 46.9 years, $p < 0.001$), with shorter disease duration (13.1 vs. 14.7 years, $p < 0.001$), and more active disease (number of relapses in the last 2 years 1.7 vs. 0.8, contrast-enhancing lesions 2.6 vs. 1.5, $p < 0.001$) [93]. The lack of benefit of IFN-β-1b in patients with SPMS with less active disease was confirmed in other SPMS trials as well [94,95].

IFN-β trials in PPMS have also been largely mixed, with negative results on primary (confirmed disability progression) and most secondary endpoints [96–98], although significant differences in MSFC scores, MRI T2 lesion volume, and MRI T1 lesion volume after 2 years of treatment favoring IFN-β-1a was observed in one trial [98].

Glatiramer acetate (GA), a synthetic polypeptide with a complex and incompletely understood immunomodulatory mechanism of action, was studied in patients with PPMS in the PROMiSe trial, a multicenter, placebo-controlled, double-blind randomized clinical trial comparing GA to placebo over a 3-year period [99]. This trial was successful in including a large majority of patients without signs of disease activity. GA decreased markers of radiological activity (gadolinium enhancing lesions and accumulation of T2 lesions), and had some benefit on disability progression in males, but there was no effect on the primary outcome and the study was terminated early [99,100].

As discussed earlier in this manuscript, the INFORMS trial failed to show a positive effect of fingolimod (*Gilenya*®) on reduction in confirmed disability worsening in patients with PPMS [77]. The primary endpoint was defined by a composite of outcomes including the EDSS, T25FW, and 9HPT. There was no benefit of fingolimod on the disability composite (HR = 0.95, 95%FW CI 0.80–1.10, $p = 0.544$). Fingolimod has not been studied in SPMS.

Natalizumab (*Tysabri*®) is a monoclonal antibody that exerts its potent anti-inflammatory effect by inhibiting the alpha-4 integrin and subsequently preventing the migration of T-lymphocytes across the blood–brain barrier. The ASCEND trial evaluated the effect of natalizumab on a composite score including the EDSS, T25FW, and 9HPT in patients with SPMS [101]. No benefit was observed on the composite primary outcome, and individually on the EDSS and 9HPT, although in a post hoc analysis, there was a 44% reduction in hand function progression measured by the 9HPT (OR 0.56, 95% CI 0.40–0.80, $p = 0.001$).

Rituximab is a chimeric monoclonal antibody targeting the CD20 antigen on pre-B-cells and mature B-cells that has been used in many autoimmune neurological disorders of the central and peripheral nervous systems for decades [102]. Similarly to ocrelizumab, it causes rapid and profound depletion of B-cells via antibody-dependent cellular cytotoxicity (ADCC) and complement-dependent cytotoxicity (CDC) mechanisms leading to B-cell death [73,74]. Rituximab has been used off-label to treat progressive MS in certain countries, and there has been long-standing evidence of its efficacy to control inflammatory disease activity in observational studies [103]. Furthermore, as discussed above, a recent study also suggests that rituximab significantly delayed confirmed progression in SPMS [71]. The OLYMPUS trial evaluated the effect of rituximab on disability progression in patients with PPMS [70]. This was a phase 2/3 multicenter, placebo-controlled trial involving 439 patients with PPMS for 96 weeks. There were no differences in the primary endpoint in the overall cohort (time to 12-week confirmed disability progression using the EDSS at 96 weeks). There was a significant effect on T2 lesion volume, which was lower with rituximab. An important point of this trial is the result of the subgroup analysis, which showed a significant difference on the primary endpoint in the subgroup of patients who were <51 years old and who had baseline enhancing lesions (hazard ratio 0.52 ($p = 0.010$) and 0.41 ($p = 0.007$), respectively), whereas rituximab-treated patients who were older than 51 years and had no enhancing lesions at baseline had non-significant but worse outcomes than the placebo group (hazard ratio 1.27 ($p = 0.425$)). This highlights the predominantly anti-inflammatory effect of B-cell therapies in MS.

There has been evidence of the presence of lymphoid follicle-like structures in the cerebral meninges that are typically adjacent to large subpial lesions, and associated with more severe cortical pathology and accelerated disability progression in patients with SPMS [14,15]. Based on these observations, the eventual role of these lymphoid follicles in sustaining cortical injury and accelerating clinical worsening was hypothesized, and the effect of intrathecal rituximab was evaluated since IV rituximab does not cross the blood–brain barrier [104–107]. The RIVITALISE trial, a randomized, double-blind trial study of intravenous and intrathecal rituximab in patients with SPMS, showed that intrathecal rituximab transiently decreased the B cell counts in the CSF and did not induce consistent effects on CSF biomarkers [104].

A very recent trial evaluated the safety and efficacy of intrathecal rituximab in eight patients with progressive MS who had focal leptomeningeal contrast-enhancement on contrast-enhanced T2-FLAIR [105]. Transient reduction in CSF B cells and biomarkers (reduction in chemokine ligand 13 (CXCL-13) levels with an increase in B cell-activating factor belonging to the TNF family (BAFF) levels), along with profound peripheral B cell depletion was observed; however, the number of leptomeningeal lesions did not change.

Other immunomodulating and immunosuppressive therapies have been investigated in PMS. Examples include azathioprine [108–110], cyclophosphamide [111–114], intravenous immunoglobulins [110,115], methotrexate [116–118], cyclosporine [109,119], mycophenolate mofetil [120], laquinimod [121], and MBP8298 [122]. Results from these trials have been largely negative, with no or modest benefit on markers of disability progression.

6.2. Remyelination and Neuroprotection in Progressive MS

While some agents have shown to be beneficial on slowing disability progression, no molecules have shown to have an effect on halting progression or reversing neurological damage in well-powered clinical trials. There are two therapeutic approaches that are thought to be promising to achieve the latter: remyelination and neuroprotection. Remyelinating agents can theoretically repair damage and neuroprotective agents can theoretically prevent axonal loss. High-throughput methods have generated many promising remyelinating molecules to test in pre-clinical studies, to be followed by phase 1, 2, and 3 trials. Unfortunately, studies have been mostly negative or have shown only modest benefits on measures of brain atrophy for which clinical significance still needs to be better elucidated. Table 1 provides an overview of positive trials of molecules with a putative remyelinating and neuroprotective effect. Some agents such as biotin and mesenchymal stem cells may have both remyelinating and neuroprotective effects; these medications are discussed under neuroprotection.

Table 1. Potential remyelinating and neuroprotective molecules studied in multiple sclerosis.

Therapy	Potential Mechanism of Action	Trials	Primary Endpoint	Results
Remyelination strategies				
Clemastine fumarate	First-generation anti-histamine, promotes remyelination and oligodendrocyte differentiation via anti-muscarinic effect [123,124]	ReBUILD [125]	Shortening of P100 latency delay on visual-evoked potentials at 150 days	Improvement in P100 latency of 1.7 ms/eye (95% CI 0.5 to 2.9, $p = 0.0048$) with clemastine
Opicinumab	Anti-LINGO-1 antibody, promotes remyelination and oligodendrocyte differentiation via blocking of inhibitory adhesion molecule [126,127]	RENEW [128] (in acute unilateral optic neuritis)	24-week change in optic nerve conduction latency using full-field visual evoked potential	Non-significant trend towards improvement in the intention-to-treat analysis, modest but significant benefit at week 32 in the per-protocol analysis
		SYNERGY [129,130] (in RRMS and SPMS with active disease)	Percentage of participants with ≥3 month confirmed improvement of composite endpoint (EDSS, T25FW, 9HPT, PASAT) over 72 weeks	Benefit seen in those receiving the 30 mg/kg dose.
Neuroprotection strategies				
Ibudilast	Phosphodiesterase-inhibitor, inhibits macrophage migration inhibitory factor, and toll-like receptor 4 [131]	SPRINT-MS [132]	Progression of whole brain atrophy over 96 weeks	48% slowing in the rate of atrophy progression with ibudilast compared to placebo

Table 1. *Cont.*

Therapy	Potential Mechanism of Action	Trials	Primary Endpoint	Results
Simvastatin	HMG-CoA reductase inhibitor, inhibit MHCII-restricted antigen presentation, shifts cytokine production from a pro- to an anti-inflammatory response, decreases T-cell proliferation [133]	MS-STAT [134]	Progression of whole-brain atrophy, change in EDSS and total MS Impact Scale-29 at 24 months	Decrease in annualized rate of whole brain atrophy compared to placebo, benefit on EDSS and MS Impact Scale-29 as well
Lipoic acid	Endogenous antioxidant, various potential mechanisms, including free radical scavenging, oxidative damage repair, downregulation of inflammatory cytokines, T-cell migration in CNS inhibition [135,136]	Spain et al. [137].	Annual percent change of brain volume	68% reduction in the rate of brain atrophy compared to placebo over 24 months
Phenytoin	Selective sodium-channel inhibitor, reverses sodium influx, which drives calcium influx via reverse operation of the sodium/calcium exchanger after axonal injury [138]	Raftopoulos et al. [139].	RNFL thickness in the affected eye	30% reduction in the extent of RNFL loss with phenytoin compared with placebo at 6 months
Mesenchymal stem cells *	Pluripotent non-hematopoietic precursor cells (isolated from bone marrow or adipose tissue), release of soluble trophic factors that promote intrinsic tissue repair mechanisms [140]	Multiple small clinical trials and open label studies using variable route of administration and dosing regimens [141–149]	Variable endpoints depending on trial	Good safety and tolerability, efficacy not yet established [150]
		Phase II randomized, double-blind trial, MESEMS (NCT01854957) [151]	Safety, reduction in the total number of contrast-gadolinium enhancing lesions	Ongoing
		Open-label study, MSC-NTF Cells (NCT03799718)	Safety, T25FW change from baseline, changes in neurotrophic factors	Ongoing

Table 1. *Cont.*

Therapy	Potential Mechanism of Action	Trials	Primary Endpoint	Results
High-dose biotin (MD 1003) *	Essential co-factor for five carboxylases involved in fatty acid synthesis and energy production, promotes remyelination, and reduces axonal hypoxia [152]	Sedel et al. (pilot study) [153]	Shortening of P100 latency on visual-evoked potentials	Improvement or normalization of P100 latency
		Tourbah et al. (randomized, double-blind placebo-controlled trial) [154]	Proportion of patients with disability reversal on EDSS or T25FW at month 9, confirmed at month 12	2.6% of treated patients achieved the primary endpoint versus none of the placebo-treated patients ($p = 0.005$)
		Birnbaum et al. (open-label study of compound medication, not MD 1003) [155]	EDSS worsening or improvement while on treatment (3 to 12 months)	No benefits observed

* possibly dual effect on remyelination and neuroprotection. 9HPT: 9-hole-peg test, EDSS: Expanded disability status scale, LINGO-1: Leucine-rich repeat and immunoglobulin domain-containing neurite outgrowth inhibitor receptor interacting protein-1, PASAT: Paced auditory serial addition test, RRMS: Relapsing–remitting multiple sclerosis, RNFL: Retinal nerve fiber layer, SPMS: Secondary progressive multiple sclerosis, T25FW: Timed-25-foot walk.

In MS, progression secondary to neurodegeneration is thought to be secondary to chronic demyelination [3]. While neuronal cell bodies and axons have a low potential of regeneration, myelin may have a potential for repair. Remyelination can be seen in shadow plaques, which supports this potential repair property likely mediated by oligodendrocytes [3,6]. A few compounds promoting endogenous oligodendrocyte progenitor cell differentiation have been found in pre-clinical work to be promising remyelinating agents [156]. Out of thousands of compounds identified through high-volume screening of existing drugs [124], opicinumab [128–130], and clemastine [125] have been studied in phase 2 trials. Clemastine demonstrated improvement in P100 latency on visual evoked potential in patients with chronic optic neuropathy compared to placebo [125]. Opicinumab showed a similar effect in patients with acute optic neuritis [128,129] (Table 1). Other potentially effective molecules are currently being evaluated, including domperidone (in SPMS, NCT02308137), quetiapine (in RRMS and progressive MS, NCT02087631), liothyronine (in RRMS and progressive MS, NCT02760056), among others. Miconazole and clobetazol have recently been identified as agents with a potential to produce mature oligodendrocytes from progenitor cells [157].

Most of the trials of molecules with a potential for axonal repair have been deceiving. The SPRINT-MS study results were promising; however, phase 3 trials are needed to confirm this result before considering ibudilast as a therapy for progressive MS [132]. Similarly, lipoic acid and simvastatin [134] appear to be potentially beneficial in slowing brain atrophy, and further studies are needed to confirm the results of the phase 2 trials. In a randomized placebo-controlled phase 2 trial, phenytoin was found to have neuroprotective effects after acute optic neuritis compared to placebo [139]. The MS-SMART trial (NCT01910259) failed to show a benefit of amiloride, fluoxetine, or riluzole on brain atrophy in progressive MS (results presented at ECTRIMS 2018). High-dose biotin [153–155] and mesenchymal stem cells appear to have a dual effect on neuroprotection and remyelination, and have been studied in multiple small trials and open-label studies in progressive MS, with promising results (Table 1). It is important to note that treatment with autologous hematopoietic stem cell transplantation is reserved for patients with treatment-refractory highly active MS, specifically those who have poor prognostic factors of future disability, including ongoing clinical or radiological activity despite treatment with potent DMT [158], and is out of the scope of this review. Other compounds that are being investigated in phase 2 or 3 trials, include idebenone (NCT01854359), masitinib (NCT01433497), hormone-based therapies (ACTH (NCT01950234)), and erythropoietin (NCT01144117), lithium (NCT01259388), and T-cell receptor vaccines (NCT02057159), among others.

6.3. Symptomatic Management

Optimal symptom management is essential to improve quality of life of patients and to complement the beneficial effect of long-term maintenance therapies in MS. The most commonly encountered symptoms in MS include fatigue, spasticity-related symptoms, neuropathic pain, urinary dysfunction, sleep disturbances, and mood changes. A high number of patients complain of more than one symptom, many of which may be interrelated. For example, poor sleep and depression worsens diurnal fatigue, which can hence not solely be attributed to the disease. Routine evaluations should include screening for persistent symptoms, preferably using validated scales. A general rule in our experience is to start by treating the most disabling or consequential symptom, titrate medications up slowly, use molecules that have a potential to address more than one symptom, and avoid polypharmacy. Combining pharmacological and non-pharmacological approaches to address specific symptoms is important. For example, gait difficulties can be addressed with physical therapy (with a focus on improving ataxia or muscle strength depending on presentation), spasticity management (stretching, anti-spasticity medications, botulinum toxin injections, baclofen pump), and fatigue with dalfampridine. A significant emphasis should also be placed on physical, occupational, and speech therapy. Evaluation and treatment by a multi-disciplinary team is key to provide optimal care across the range of dysfunction in progressive MS. General wellness measures and management of comorbidities should always be discussed with patients, most importantly hyperlipidemia, hypertension, and diabetes control, consuming a healthy diet, weight loss, smoking cessation, vitamin D supplementation, osteoporosis management, and emotional wellness [159].

7. Challenges in Progressive MS Treatment and Research

There are many unmet needs in the field of progressive MS. First, our experience with anti-inflammatory medications like ocrelizumab and siponimod has shown positive but modest results. These medications work on the inflammatory component of the disease, and their potential mechanism of action on the neurodegenerative aspect of MS is probably minimal, if any. As discussed above, the rituximab/ocrelizumab and fingolimod/siponimod experiences in progressive MS provide evidence that therapeutic approaches for progressive MS should probably focus on a different pathophysiological aspect of the disease. Second, trial methodology has significant implications for the effect of agents in progressive MS. Study population selection and amount of disease activity (pre-trial and in-trial annualized relapse rates, presence or absence of baseline gadolinium enhancing lesions) in enrolled subjects are key in driving these efficacy differences between therapies. The definition of progressive MS also varies between trials, and often but not always, a minimum confirmed EDSS step of three at trial entry is required in progressive MS trials, which makes the study populations somewhat heterogeneous and trial results inconsistent and difficult to compare across studies [57].

Third, the selection of appropriate clinical outcome measures plays an important role in capturing treatment effects in progressive MS trials, as discussed earlier in this manuscript [160]. Non-ambulatory patients are typically excluded from progressive MS trials, and the benefit of different therapies on functional domains other than gait function could yield more promising results, specifically in this patient population. For example, studying hand and cognitive function or using composite outcomes like the MSFC rather than relying solely on ambulation as a primary endpoint could inform treatment effects in a more sensitive way. Hand function might be more amenable to treatment compared to lower extremity function in patients with more advanced disability. In the ASCEND trial for instance, natalizumab was associated with a 44% reduction in the relative risk of confirmed upper limb disability progression measured by the 9HPT (adjusted OR 0·56 (95% CI 0·40–0·80); $p = 0{\cdot}001$), whereas no benefit was observed on other measures of disability like the EDSS and the T25FW [101]. In a pre-specified baseline subgroup analysis of patients with EDSS ≥6.0 and age >45 years from the OROTARIO trial, ocrelizumab also reduced disability progression as measured by the 12-week confirmed 9HPT in older non-ambulatory patients [161]. Moreover, despite the high prevalence of cognitive dysfunction in progressive MS, there are methodological gaps in outcome measures of cognition in MS, and cognitive function is not adequately and comprehensively evaluated in trials [57,162]. The use of composite outcome measures has been used increasingly in progressive MS trials, and appear to have higher sensitivity to changes. For example, the primary endpoint of the INFORMS trial was a novel composite outcome measure that was defined as a 3-month confirmed change from baseline of the EDSS, the T25FW, or the 9HPT, and although the trial was negative, this outcome measure detected changes with excellent sensitivity in this population [77] Trials evaluating therapies with a remyelinating or repair potential are expected to have a modest clinical effect and can particularly benefit from using composite measures to enhance detection of changes. This approach was used in the opicinimab (SYNERGY) [129] and ibudilast (SPRINT-MS) [132] trials. MRI outcome measures also have some limitations. For example, measures of whole brain atrophy are mostly used as primary endpoints, and have the issue of being variable, which is a concern for interpretability. Other measures like cortical atrophy or magnetization transfer ratio might be more useful depending on the population and mechanism of action of the investigational product.

Finally, the efficacy of molecules with a potential for remyelination and/or neuroprotection needs to be confirmed in large trials with clinically meaningful outcome measures, which will require time and resources. Ultimately, for FDA approval, an agent that can demonstrate clinically meaningful changes in disability measures in large multicenter phase 3 trials is needed. To be able to achieve that, research on the optimal outcome markers is needed. Moreover, many of these molecules are old drugs that do not generate interest in the pharmaceutical industry.

Overall, optimal and novel trial methodology and development of sensitive and clinically meaningful outcome measures and biomarkers are needed in the near-future. The International Progressive MS Alliance and the UK Expert Consortium for Progression in MS Clinical Trials have a mission to expedite development of therapies for progressive forms of MS, which includes the development of optimal trial designs and more responsive outcome measures.

8. Conclusions

A significant amount of effort is delivered to improve knowledge in the field of progressive MS. Future trials will incorporate lessons from previous trials, and hopefully, therapies that halt or even stop neurodegeneration in MS will be available in the future.

Author Contributions: G.M. drafted the manuscript. D.O. reviewed and edited the manuscript for scientific content.

References

1. Wallin, M.T.; Culpepper, W.J.; Campbell, J.D.; Nelson, M.L.; Langer-Gould, A.; Marrie, R.A.; Cutter, G.R.; Kaye, W.E.; Wagner, L.; Tremlett, H.; et al. The prevalence of MS in the United States: A population-based estimate using health claims data. *Neurology* **2019**, *92*, e1019–e1024. [CrossRef] [PubMed]
2. Browne, P.; Chandraratna, D.; Angood, C.; Tremlett, H.; Baker, C.; Taylor, B.V.; Thompson, A.J. Atlas of Multiple Sclerosis 2013: A growing global problem with widespread inequity. *Neurology* **2014**, *83*, 1022–1024. [CrossRef] [PubMed]
3. Mahad, D.H.; Trapp, B.D.; Lassmann, H. Pathological mechanisms in progressive multiple sclerosis. *Lancet Neurol.* **2015**, *14*, 183–193. [CrossRef]
4. Trapp, B.D.; Peterson, J.; Ransohoff, R.M.; Rudick, R.; Mörk, S.; Bö, L. Axonal Transection in the Lesions of Multiple Sclerosis. *N. Engl. J. Med.* **1998**, *338*, 278–285. [CrossRef] [PubMed]
5. Kornek, B.; Storch, M.K.; Weissert, R.; Wallstroem, W.; Stefferl, A.; Olsson, T.; Linington, C.; Schmidbauer, M.; Lassmann, H. Multiple sclerosis and chronic autoimmune encephalomyelitis: A comparative quantitative study of axonal injury in active, inactive, and remyelinated lesions. *Am. J. Pathol.* **2000**, *157*, 267–276. [CrossRef]
6. Frischer, J.M.; Weigand, S.D.; Guo, Y.; Kale, N.; Parisi, J.E.; Pirko, I.; Mandrekar, J.; Bramow, S.; Metz, I.; Bruck, W.; et al. Clinical and Pathological Insights into the Dynamic Nature of the White Matter Multiple Sclerosis Plaque. *Ann. Neurol.* **2015**, *78*, 710–721. [CrossRef]
7. De Stefano, N.; Giorgio, A.; Battaglini, M.; Rovaris, M.; Sormani, M.P.; Barkhof, F.; Korteweg, T.; Enzinger, C.; Fazekas, F.; Calabrese, M.; et al. Assessing brain atrophy rates in a large population of untreated multiple sclerosis subtypes. *Neurology* **2010**, *74*, 1868–1876. [CrossRef] [PubMed]
8. Lucchinetti, C.F.; Rauschka, H.; Bergmann, M.; Schmidbauer, M.; Kutzelnigg, A.; Parisi, J.E.; Stadelmann, C.; Brück, W.; Lassmann, H. Cortical demyelination and diffuse white matter injury in multiple sclerosis. *Brain* **2005**, *128*, 2705–2712.
9. Amato, M.P.; Portaccio, E.; Goretti, B.; Zipoli, V.; Battaglini, M.; Bartolozzi, M.L.; Stromillo, M.L.; Guidi, L.; Siracusa, G.; Sorbi, S.; et al. Association of Neocortical Volume Changes with Cognitive Deterioration in Relapsing-Remitting Multiple Sclerosis. *Arch. Neurol.* **2007**, *64*, 1157–1161. [CrossRef]
10. Calabrese, M.; Agosta, F.; Rinaldi, F.; Mattisi, I.; Grossi, P.; Favaretto, A.; Atzori, M.; Bernardi, V.; Barachino, L.; Rinaldi, L.; et al. Cortical Lesions and Atrophy Associated with Cognitive Impairment in Relapsing-Remitting Multiple Sclerosis. *Arch. Neurol.* **2009**, *66*, 1144–1150. [CrossRef]
11. Mahad, D.J.; Ziabreva, I.; Campbell, G.; Lax, N.; White, K.; Hanson, P.S.; Lassmann, H.; Turnbull, D.M. Mitochondrial changes within axons in multiple sclerosis. *Brain* **2009**, *132*, 1161–1174. [CrossRef] [PubMed]
12. Trapp, B.D.; Stys, P.K. Virtual hypoxia and chronic necrosis of demyelinated axons in multiple sclerosis. *Lancet Neurol.* **2009**, *8*, 280–291. [CrossRef]

13. Ontaneda, D.; Thompson, A.J.; Fox, R.J.; ACohen, J. Progressive multiple sclerosis: Prospects for disease therapy, repair, and restoration of function. *Lancet* **2017**, *389*, 1357–1366. [CrossRef]
14. Howell, O.W.; Reeves, C.A.; Nicholas, R.; Carassiti, D.; Radotra, B.; Gentleman, S.M.; Serafini, B.; Aloisi, F.; Roncaroli, F.; Magliozzi, R.; et al. Meningeal inflammation is widespread and linked to cortical pathology in multiple sclerosis. *Brain* **2011**, *134*, 2755–2771. [CrossRef] [PubMed]
15. Magliozzi, R.; Howell, O.; Vora, A.; Serafini, B.; Nicholas, R.; Puopolo, M.; Reynolds, R.; Aloisi, F. Meningeal B-cell follicles in secondary progressive multiple sclerosis associate with early onset of disease and severe cortical pathology. *Brain* **2007**, *130*, 1089–1104. [CrossRef]
16. Brown, J.W.L.; Coles, A.; Horakova, D.; Havrdova, E.; Izquierdo, G.; Prat, A.; Girard, M.; Duquette, P.; Trojano, M.; Lugaresi, A.; et al. Association of Initial Disease-Modifying Therapy with Later Conversion to Secondary Progressive Multiple Sclerosis. *JAMA* **2019**, *321*, 175–187. [CrossRef] [PubMed]
17. Bergamaschi, R.; Quaglini, S.; Tavazzi, E.; Amato, M.P.; Paolicelli, D.; Zipoli, V.; Romani, A.; Tortorella, C.; Portaccio, E.; D'Onghia, M.; et al. Immunomodulatory therapies delay disease progression in multiple sclerosis. *Mult. Scler. J.* **2016**, *22*, 1732–1740. [CrossRef]
18. Trojano, M.; Pellegrini, F.; Paolicelli, D.; Fuiani, A.; Zimatore, G.B.; Tortorella, C.; Simone, I.L.; Patti, F.; Ghezzi, A.; Zipoli, V.; et al. Real-life impact of early interferon beta therapy in relapsing multiple sclerosis. *Ann. Neurol.* **2009**, *66*, 513–520. [CrossRef]
19. Trojano, M.; Pellegrini, F.; Fuiani, A.; Paolicelli, D.; Zipoli, V.; Zimatore, G.B.; Monte, E.D.; Portaccio, C.; Lepore, V.; Livrea, P.; et al. New natural history of interferon-beta-treated relapsing multiple sclerosis. *Ann. Neurol.* **2007**, *61*, 300–306. [CrossRef]
20. Haider, L.; Simeonidou, C.; Steinberger, G.; Hametner, S.; Grigoriadis, N.; Deretzi, G.; Kovacs, G.G.; Kutzelnigg, A.; Lassmann, H.; Frischer, J.M. Multiple sclerosis deep grey matter: The relation between demyelination, neurodegeneration, inflammation and iron. *J. Neurol. Neurosurg. Psychiatry* **2014**, *85*, 1386–1395. [CrossRef]
21. Hametner, S.; Wimmer, I.; Haider, L.; Pfeifenbring, S.; Brück, W.; Lassmann, H. Iron and neurodegeneration in the multiple sclerosis brain. *Ann. Neurol.* **2013**, *74*, 848–861. [CrossRef]
22. Harding, K.E.; Liang, K.; Cossburn, M.D.; Ingram, G.; Hirst, C.; Pickersgill, T.; Te Water, N.; Johann, W.; Ben-Shlomo, M.; Robertson, Y.; et al. Long-term outcome of paediatric-onset multiple sclerosis: A population-based study. *J Neurol. Neurosurg. Psychiatry* **2013**, *84*, 141–147. [CrossRef]
23. Leray, E.; Yaouanq, J.; Le Page, E.; Coustans, M.; Laplaud, D.; Oger, J.; Edan, G. Evidence for a two-stage disability progression in multiple sclerosis. *Brain* **2010**, *133*, 1900–1913. [CrossRef]
24. Confavreux, C.; Moreau, T.; Vukusic, S.; Adeleine, P. Relapses and Progression of Disability in Multiple Sclerosis. *N. Engl. J. Med.* **2000**, *343*, 1430–1438. [CrossRef]
25. Beiki, O.; Frumento, P.; Bottai, M.; Manouchehrinia, A.; Hillert, J. Changes in the Risk of Reaching Multiple Sclerosis Disability Milestones in Recent Decades: A Nationwide Population-Based Cohort Study in Sweden. *JAMA Neurol.* **2019**, 1–7. [CrossRef]
26. Polman, C.H.; Reingold, S.C.; Banwell, B.; Clanet, M.; Cohen, J.A.; Filippi, M.; Fujihara, K.; Havrdova, E.K.; Hutchinson, M.; Kappos, L.; et al. Diagnostic criteria for multiple sclerosis: 2010 Revisions to the McDonald criteria. *Ann. Neurol.* **2011**, *69*, 292–302. [CrossRef]
27. Thompson, A.J.; Banwell, B.L.; Barkhof, F.; Carroll, W.; Coetzee, T.; Comi, G.; Correale, J.; Fazekas, F.; Filippi, M.; Freedman, M.; et al. Diagnosis of multiple sclerosis: 2017 revisions of the McDonald criteria. *Lancet Neurol.* **2018**, *17*, 162–173. [CrossRef]
28. Lublin, F.; Stephen, C.; Reingold, P.; Cohen, J.A.; Cutter, G.; Sørensen, P.S.; Thompson, A.J.; Wolinsky, J.S.; Balcer, L.J.; Banwell, B.; et al. Defining the clinical course of multiple sclerosis: The 2013 revisions. *Neurology* **2014**, *83*, 278–286. [CrossRef]
29. Whitaker, J.N.; McFarland, H.F.; Rudge, P.; Reingold, R.S. Outcomes assessment in multiple sclerosis trials. *Mult. Scler.* **1995**, *1*, 37–47. [CrossRef]
30. Noseworthy, J.H.; Vandervoort, M.K.; Wong, C.J.; Ebers, G.C. Interrater variability with the Expanded Disability Status Scale (EDSS) and Functional Systems (FS) in a multiple sclerosis clinical trial. *Neurology* **1990**, *40*, 971. [CrossRef]

31. Goodkin, D.E.; Cookfair, D.; Wende, K.; Bourdette, D.; Pullicino, P.; Scherokman, B.; Whitham, R. Inter- and intrarater scoring agreement using grades 1.0 to 3.5 of the Kurtzke Expanded Disability Status Scale (EDSS). *Neurology* **1992**, *42*, 859. [CrossRef]
32. Kragt, J.J.; Nielsen, J.M.; Van Der Linden, F.A.; Uitdehaag, B.M.; Polman, C.H. How similar are commonly combined criteria for EDSS progression in multiple sclerosis? *Mult. Scler. J.* **2006**, *12*, 782–786. [CrossRef]
33. Ontaneda, D.; ACohen, J.; Amato, M.P. Clinical outcome measures for progressive MS trials. *Mult. Scler. J.* **2017**, *23*, 1627–1635. [CrossRef]
34. Cutter, G.R.; Baier, M.L.; Rudick, R.A.; Cookfair, D.L.; Fischer, J.S.; Petkau, J.; Syndulko, K.; Weinshenker, B.G.; Antel, J.P.; Confavreux, C.; et al. Development of a multiple sclerosis functional composite as a clinical trial outcome measure. *Brain* **1999**, *122*, 871–882. [CrossRef]
35. Fischer, J.; Rudick, R.; Cutter, G.; Reingold, S. The Multiple Sclerosis Functional Composite measure (MSFC): An integrated approach to MS clinical outcome assessment. *Mult. Scler. J.* **1999**, *5*, 244–250. [CrossRef]
36. Cohen, J.A.; Cutter, G.R.; Fischer, J.S.; Goodman, A.D.; Heidenreich, F.R.; Jak, A.J.; Kniker, J.E.; Kooijmans, M.F.; Lull, J.M.; Sandrock, A.W.; et al. Use of the Multiple Sclerosis Functional Composite as an Outcome Measure in a Phase 3 Clinical Trial. *Arch. Neurol.* **2001**, *58*, 961–967. [CrossRef]
37. Polman, C.H.; Rudick, R.A. The Multiple Sclerosis Functional Composite: A clinically meaningful measure of disability. *Neurology* **2010**, *74*, 8–15. [CrossRef]
38. Kalkers, N.; Bergers, L.; De Groot, V.; Lazeron, R.; Van Walderveen, M.; Uitdehaag, B.; Polman, C.; Barkhof, F. Concurrent validity of the MS Functional Composite using MRI as a biological disease marker. *Neurology* **2001**, *56*, 215–219. [CrossRef]
39. Miller, D.M.; Rudick, R.A.; Cutter, G.; Baier, M.; Fischer, J.S. Clinical Significance of the Multiple Sclerosis Functional Composite. *Arch. Neurol.* **2000**, *57*, 1319–1324. [CrossRef]
40. Cohen, J.A.; Cutter, G.R.; Fischer, J.S.; Goodman, A.; Heidenreich, F.R.; Kooijmans, M.F.; Sandrock, A.W.; Rudick, R.A.; Simon, J.H.; Simonian, N.A.; et al. Benefit of interferon -1a on MSFC progression in secondary progressive multiple sclerosis. *Neurology* **2002**, *59*, 679–687. [CrossRef]
41. Baier, M.L.; Cutter, G.R.; Rudick, R.A.; Miller, D.; Cohen, J.A.; Weinstock-Guttman, B.; Mass, M.; Balcer, L.J. Low-contrast letter acuity testing captures visual dysfunction in patients with multiple sclerosis. *Neurology* **2005**, *64*, 992–995. [CrossRef]
42. Balcer, L.J.; Baier, M.L.; Cohen, J.A.; Kooijmans, M.F.; Sandrock, A.W.; Nano-Schiavi, M.L.; Pfohl, D.C.; Mills, M.; Bowen, J.; Ford, C.; et al. Contrast letter acuity as a visual component for the Multiple Sclerosis Functional Composite. *Neurology* **2003**, *61*, 1367–1373. [CrossRef]
43. Freeman, J.; Hobart, J.; Thompson, A. Kurtzke scales revisited: The application of psychometric methods to clinical intuition. *Brain* **2000**, *123*, 1027–1040.
44. Rasova, K.; Martinkova, P.; Vyskotova, J.; Sedova, M. Assessment set for evaluation of clinical outcomes in multiple sclerosis: Psychometric properties. *Patient Relat. Outcome Meas.* **2012**, *3*, 59–70. [CrossRef]
45. ACohen, J.; Coles, A.J.; Arnold, D.L.; Confavreux, C.; Fox, E.J.; Hartung, H.-P.; Havrdova, E.K.; Selmaj, K.W.; Weiner, H.L.; Fisher, E.; et al. Alemtuzumab versus interferon beta 1a as first-line treatment for patients with relapsing-remitting multiple sclerosis: A randomised controlled phase 3 trial. *Lancet* **2012**, *380*, 1819–1828.
46. Polman, C.; Hohlfeld, R.; Agoropoulou, C.; Leyk, M.; Zhang-Auberson, L.; Burtin, P.; Kappos, L.; Radue, E.-W.; O'Connor, P.; Calabresi, P.; et al. A Placebo-Controlled Trial of Oral Fingolimod in Relapsing Multiple Sclerosis. *N. Engl. J. Med.* **2010**, *362*, 387–401.
47. Meyer-Moock, S.; Feng, Y.-S.; Maeurer, M.; Dippel, F.-W.; Kohlmann, T. Systematic literature review and validity evaluation of the Expanded Disability Status Scale (EDSS) and the Multiple Sclerosis Functional Composite (MSFC) in patients with multiple sclerosis. *BMC Neurol.* **2014**, *14*, 58. [CrossRef]
48. Rudick, R.A.; Miller, D.; Bethoux, F.; Rao, S.M.; Lee, J.-C.; Stough, D.; Reece, C.; Schindler, D.; Mamone, B.; Alberts, J. The Multiple Sclerosis Performance Test (MSPT): An iPad-Based Disability Assessment Tool. *J. Vis. Exp.* **2014**, e51318. [CrossRef]
49. Macaron, G.; Moss, B.P.; Li, H.; Baldassari, L.; Rao, S.; Schindler, D.; Alberts, J.; Weber, M.; Ayers, M.; Bethoux, F.; et al. Technology-enabled assessments to enhance multiple sclerosis clinical care and research. *Neurol. Clin. Pract.* **2019**, in press.

50. Motl, R.W.; A Cohen, J.; Benedict, R.; Phillips, G.; LaRocca, N.; Hudson, L.D.; Rudick, R. Multiple Sclerosis Outcome Assessments Consortium Validity of the timed 25-foot walk as an ambulatory performance outcome measure for multiple sclerosis. *Mult. Scler. J.* **2017**, *23*, 704–710. [CrossRef]
51. Feng, J.; Qu, J.; Felix, C.; McGinley, M.; Nakamura, K.; Macaron, G.; Moss, B.; Li, H.; Jones, S.; Rao, S.; et al. Quantitative MRI and patient-reported outcomes validate clinically meaningful changes on tests of ambulation and hand function. *ACTRIMS* **2019**, P050.
52. Feys, P.; Lamers, I.; Francis, G.; Benedict, R.; Phillips, G.; LaRocca, N.; Hudson, L.D.; Rudick, R. Multiple Sclerosis Outcome Assessments Consortium the Nine-Hole Peg Test as a manual dexterity performance measure for multiple sclerosis. *Mult. Scler. J.* **2017**, *23*, 711–720. [CrossRef]
53. Benedict, R.H.; DeLuca, J.; Phillips, G.; LaRocca, N.; Hudson, L.D.; Rudick, R. Multiple Sclerosis Outcome Assessments Consortium Validity of the Symbol Digit Modalities Test as a cognition performance outcome measure for multiple sclerosis. *Mult. Scler. J.* **2017**, *23*, 721–733. [CrossRef]
54. Macaron, G.; Moss, B.; Baldassari, L.E.; Conway, D.; McGinley, M.; Alshehri, E.; Feng, J.; Bermel, R.; Boissy, A.; Cohen, J.A.; et al. Cross-sectional predictive value of clinically meaningful change in processing speed on self-reported cognition and MRI metrics. *ACTRIMS* **2019**, P034.
55. Balcer, L.J.; Raynowska, J.; Nolan, R.; Galetta, S.L.; Kapoor, R.; Benedict, R.; Phillips, G.; LaRocca, N.; Hudson, L.; Rudick, R.; et al. Validity of low-contrast letter acuity as a visual performance outcome measure for multiple sclerosis. *Mult. Scler. J.* **2017**, *23*, 734–747. [CrossRef]
56. Oh, J.; Ontaneda, D.; Azevedo, C.; Klawiter, E.; Absinta, M.; Arnold, D.; Bakshi, R.; Calabresi, P.; Crainiceanu, C.; Dewey, B.; et al. Imaging outcome measures of neuroprotection repair in MS: A consensus statement from NAIMS. *Neurology* **2019**, *92*, 519–533. [CrossRef]
57. Ontaneda, D.; Fox, R.J.; Chataway, J. Clinical trials in progressive multiple sclerosis: Lessons learned and future perspectives. *Lancet Neurol.* **2015**, *14*, 208–223. [CrossRef]
58. Mahajan, K.R.; Ontaneda, D. The Role of Advanced Magnetic Resonance Imaging Techniques in Multiple Sclerosis Clinical Trials. *Neurotherapeutics* **2017**, *14*, 905–923. [CrossRef]
59. Hardmeier, M.; Leocani, L.; Fuhr, P. A new role for evoked potentials in MS? Repurposing evoked potentials as biomarkers for clinical trials in MS. *Mult. Scler. J.* **2017**, *23*, 1309–1319. [CrossRef]
60. Saidha, S.; Al-Louzi, O.; Ratchford, J.N.; Bhargava, P.; Oh, J.; Newsome, S.D.; Prince, J.L.; Pham, D.; Roy, S.; Van Zijl, P.; et al. Optical Coherence Tomography Reflects Brain Atrophy in Multiple Sclerosis: A Four-Year Study. *Ann. Neurol.* **2015**, *78*, 801–813. [CrossRef]
61. Novakova, L.; Zetterberg, H.; Sundström, P.; Axelsson, M.; Khademi, M.; Gunnarsson, M.; Malmeström, C.; Svenningsson, A.; Olsson, T.; Piehl, F.; et al. Monitoring disease activity in multiple sclerosis using serum neurofilament light protein. *Neurology* **2017**, *89*, 2230–2237. [CrossRef]
62. Damasceno, A.; Dias-Carneiro, R.P.C.; Moraes, A.S.; Boldrinib, V.O.; Quintilianob, R.P.S.; de Paula Galdino da Silvab, V.A.; Fariasb, A.S.; Brandãob, C.O.; Damascenoa, B.P.; dos Santos, L.M.B.; et al. Clinical MRI correlates of CSF neurofilament light chain levels in relapsing progressive multiple sclerosis. *Mult. Scler. Relat. Disord.* **2019**, *30*, 149–153. [CrossRef]
63. Martin, S.J.; McGlasson, S.; Hunt, D.; Overell, J. Cerebrospinal fluid neurofilament light chain in multiple sclerosis and its subtypes: A meta-analysis of case-control studies. *J. Neurol. Neurosurg. Psychiatry* **2019**. [CrossRef]
64. Pawlitzki, M.; Schreiber, S.; Bittner, D.; Kreipe, J.; Leypoldt, F.; Rupprecht, K.; Carare, R.O.; Meuth, S.G.; Vielhaber, S.; Körtvélyessy, P. CSF Neurofilament Light Chain Levels in Primary Progressive MS: Signs of Axonal Neurodegeneration. *Front. Neurol.* **2018**, *9*, 9. [CrossRef]
65. Barro, C.; Naegelin, Y.; Schädelin, S.; Giardiello, A.; Zecca, C.; Blennow, K.; Zetterberg, H.; Leppert, D.; Gobbi, C.; Kuhle, J.; et al. Serum Neurofilament light: A biomarker of neuronal damage in multiple sclerosis. *Ann. Neurol.* **2017**, *81*, 857–870.
66. Barro, C.; Benkert, P.; Disanto, G.; Tsagkas, C.; Amann, M.; Naegelin, Y.; Leppert, D.; Gobbi, C.; Granziera, C.; Yaldizli, O.; et al. Serum neurofilament as a predictor of disease worsening and brain and spinal cord atrophy in multiple sclerosis. *Brain* **2018**, *141*, 2382–2391. [CrossRef]

67. Hauser, S.L.; Bar-Or, A.; Comi, G.; Giovannoni, G.; Hartung, H.-P.; Hemmer, B.; Lublin, F.; Montalban, X.; Rammohan, K.W.; Selmaj, K.; et al. Ocrelizumab versus Interferon Beta-1a in Relapsing Multiple Sclerosis. *N. Engl. J. Med.* **2017**, *376*, 221–234. [CrossRef]
68. Montalban, X.; Hauser, S.L.; Kappos, L.; Arnold, D.L.; Bar-Or, A.; Comi, G.; De Seze, J.; Giovannoni, G.; Hartung, H.-P.; Hemmer, B.; et al. Ocrelizumab versus Placebo in Primary Progressive Multiple Sclerosis. *N. Engl. J. Med.* **2017**, *376*, 209–220. [CrossRef]
69. Fox, E.; Markowitz, C.; Applebee, A.; Montalban, X.; Wolinsky, J.S.; Belachew, S.; Damian, F.; Han, J.; Musch, B.; Giovannoni, G. Effect of ocrelizumab on upper limb function in patients with primary progressive multiple sclerosis (PPMS) in the oratorio study (ENCORE). *J. Neurol. Neurosurg. Psychiatry* **2018**, *89*, A14. [CrossRef]
70. Hawker, K.; O'Connor, P.; Freedman, M.S.; Calabresi, P.A.; Antel, J.; Simon, J.; Hauser, S.; Waubant, E.; Vollmer, T.; Panitch, H.; et al. Rituximab in patients with primary progressive multiple sclerosis: Results of a randomized double-blind placebo-controlled multicenter trial. *Ann. Neurol.* **2009**, *66*, 460–471. [CrossRef]
71. Naegelin, Y.; Naegelin, P.; Von Felten, S.; Lorscheider, J.; Sonder, J.; Uitdehaag, B.M.J.; Scotti, B.; Zecca, C.; Gobbi, C.; Kappos, L.; et al. Association of Rituximab Treatment with Disability Progression Among Patients With Secondary Progressive Multiple Sclerosis. *JAMA Neurol.* **2019**, *76*, 274. [CrossRef]
72. Gelfand, J.M.; Cree, B.A.C.; Hauser, S.L. Ocrelizumab and Other CD20+ B-Cell-Depleting Therapies in Multiple Sclerosis. *Neurotherapeutics* **2017**, *14*, 835–841. [CrossRef]
73. Klein, C.; Lammens, A.; Schäfer, W.; Georges, G.; Schwaiger, M.; Mössner, E.; Hopfner, K.-P.; Umana, P.; Niederfellner, G. Epitope interactions of monoclonal antibodies targeting CD20 and their relationship to functional properties. *mAbs* **2013**, *5*, 22–33. [CrossRef]
74. Feng, J.J.; Ontaneda, D. Treating primary-progressive multiple sclerosis: Potential of ocrelizumab and review of B-cell therapies. *Degener. Neurol. Neuromuscul. Dis.* **2017**, *7*, 31–45. [CrossRef]
75. Kappos, L.; Bar-Or, A.; Cree, B.A.C.; Fox, R.J.; Giovannoni, G.; Gold, R.; Vermersch, P.; Arnold, D.L.; Arnould, S.; Scherz, T.; et al. Siponimod versus placebo in secondary progressive multiple sclerosis (EXPAND): A double-blind, randomised, phase 3 study. *Lancet* **2018**, *391*, 1263–1273. [CrossRef]
76. Jackson, S.J.; Giovannoni, G.; Baker, D. Fingolimod modulates microglial activation to augment markers of remyelination. *J. Neuroinflamm.* **2011**, *8*, 76. [CrossRef]
77. Lublin, F.; Miller, D.H.; Freedman, M.S.; Cree, B.A.C.; Wolinsky, J.S.; Weiner, H.; Lubetzki, C.; Hartung, H.-P.; Montalban, X.; Uitdehaag, B.M.J.; et al. Oral fingolimod in primary progressive multiple sclerosis (INFORMS): A phase 3, randomised, double-blind, placebo-controlled trial. *Lancet* **2016**, *387*, 1075–1084. [CrossRef]
78. Martinelli Boneschi, F.; Vacchi, L.; Rovaris, M.; Capra, R.; Comi, G. Mitoxantrone for multiple sclerosis. *Cochrane Database Syst. Rev.* **2013**, *5*, CD002127. [CrossRef]
79. Hartung, H.P.; Gonsette, R.; König, N.; Kwiecinski, H.; Guseo, A.; Morrissey, S.; Krapf, S.; Zwingers, T. Mitoxantrone in Multiple Sclerosis Study Group. Mitoxantrone in progressive multiple sclerosis: A placebo-controlled, double-blind, randomised, multicentre trial. *Lancet* **2002**, *28*, 2018–2025. [CrossRef]
80. Krapf, H.; Morrissey, S.P.; Zenker, O.; Zwingers, T.; Gonsette, R.; Hartung, H.-P. Effect of mitoxantrone on MRI in progressive MS: Results of the MIMS trial. *Neurology* **2005**, *65*, 690–695. [CrossRef]
81. Grey Née Cotte, S.; Salmen Née Stroet, A.; Von Ahsen, N.; Starck, M.; Winkelmann, A.; Zettl, U.K.; Comabella, M.; Montalban, X.; Zipp, F.; Fleischer, V.; et al. Lack of efficacy of mitoxantrone in primary progressive Multiple Sclerosis irrespective of pharmacogenetic factors: A multi-center, retrospective analysis. *J. Neuroimmunol.* **2015**, *278*, 277–279. [CrossRef]
82. Pelfrey, C.M.; Cotleur, A.C.; Zamor, N.; Lee, J.C.; Robert, R.J. Immunological studies of mitoxantrone in primary progressive multiple sclerosis. *J. Neuroimmunol.* **2006**, *175*, 192–199. [CrossRef]
83. Cotte, S.; Von Ahsen, N.; Kruse, N.; Huber, B.; Winkelmann, A.; Zettl, U.K.; Starck, M.; König, N.; Téllez, N.; Dorr, J.; et al. ABC-transporter gene-polymorphisms are potential pharmacogenetic markers for mitoxantrone response in multiple sclerosis. *Brain* **2009**, *132*, 2517–2530. [CrossRef]
84. US Food and Drug Administration. Press Announcement–FDA Approves New Oral Drug to Treat Multiple Sclerosis. Office of the Commissioner. Available online: https://www.fda.gov/NewsEvents/Newsroom/PressAnnouncements/ucm634469.htm (accessed on 2 April 2019).
85. Giovannoni, G.; Comi, G.; Cook, S.; Rammohan, K.; Rieckmann, P.; Sørensen, P.S.; Vermersch, P.; Chang, P.; Hamlett, A.; Musch, B.; et al. A Placebo-Controlled Trial of Oral Cladribine for Relapsing Multiple Sclerosis. *N. Engl. J. Med.* **2010**, *362*, 416–426. [CrossRef]

86. Montalban, X.; Leist, T.P.; Cohen, B.A.; Moses, H.; Campbell, J.; Hicking, C.; Dangond, F. Cladribine tablets added to IFN-β in active relapsing multiple sclerosis. *Neurol. Neuroimmunol. NeuroInflamm.* **2018**, *5*, 477. [CrossRef]
87. Leist, T.P.; Comi, G.; Cree, B.A.C.; Coyle, P.K.; Freedman, M.S.; Hartung, H.-P.; Vermersch, P.; Casset-Semanaz, F.; Scaramozza, M. Effect of oral cladribine on time to conversion to clinically definite multiple sclerosis in patients with a first demyelinating event (ORACLE MS): A phase 3 randomised trial. *Lancet Neurol.* **2014**, *13*, 257–267. [CrossRef]
88. Sipe, J. Cladribine in treatment of chronic progressive multiple sclerosis. *Lancet* **1994**, *344*, 9–13. [CrossRef]
89. Rice, G.P.A.; Filippi, M.; Comi, G. Cladribine and progressive MS: Clinical and MRI outcomes of a multicenter controlled trial. *Neurology* **2000**, *54*, 1145–1155. [CrossRef]
90. Filippi, M.; Rovaris, M.; Iannucci, G.; Mennea, S.; Sormani, M.P.; Comi, G. Whole brain volume changes in patients with progressive multiple sclerosis treated with cladribine. *Neurology* **2000**, *55*, 1714–1718. [CrossRef]
91. Polman, C.; Pozzilli, C.; Thompson, A.; Beckmann, K.; Dahlke, F. Final analysis of the European multicenter trial on IFNbeta-1b in secondary-progressive multiple sclerosis. *Neurology* **2001**, *57*, 1969–1975.
92. The North American Study Group. Interferon beta-1b in secondary progressive MS: Results from a 3-year controlled study. *Neurology* **2004**, *63*, 1788–1795. [CrossRef]
93. Kappos, L.; Weinstock-Guttman, B.; Pozzilli, C.; Thompson, A.J.; Dahlke, F.; Beckmann, K.; Polman, C.; McFarland, H.; European (EU-SPMS) Interferon beta-1b in Secondary Progressive Multiple Sclerosis Trial Steering Committee and Independent Advisory Board; North American (NA-SPMS) Interferon beta-1b in Secondary Progressive Multiple Sclerosis Trial Steering Committee and Independent Advisory Board. Interferon beta-1b in secondary progressive multiple sclerosis. A combined analysis of the two trials. *Neurology* **2004**, *63*, 1779–1787. [CrossRef]
94. Secondary Progressive Efficacy Clinical Trial of Recombinant Interferon-Beta-1a in MS (SPECTRIMS) Study Group. Randomized controlled trial of interferon- beta-1a in secondary progressive MS: Clinical results. *Neurology* **2001**, *56*, 1496–1504. [CrossRef]
95. Andersen, O.; Elovaara, I.; Färkkilä, M.; Hansen, H.J.; Mellgren, S.; Myhr, K.-M.; Sandberg-Wollheim, M.; Soelberg, S. Multicentre, randomised, double blind, placebo controlled, phase III study of weekly, low dose, subcutaneous interferon beta-1a in secondary progressive multiple sclerosis. *J. Neurol. Neurosurg. Psychiatry* **2004**, *75*, 706–710. [CrossRef]
96. Leary, S.M.; Miller, D.H.; Stevenson, V.L.; Brex, P.A.; Chard, D.T.; Thompson, A.J. Interferon beta-1a in primary progressive MS: An exploratory, randomized, controlled trial. *Neurology* **2003**, *60*, 44–51. [CrossRef]
97. Montalban, X. Overview of European pilot study of interferon beta-Ib in primary progressive multiple sclerosis. *Mult. Scler.* **2004**, *10*, S62–S64.
98. Montalban, X.; Garriga, J.S.; Tintoré, M.; Brieva, L.; Aymerich, F.; Rio, J.; Porcel, J.; Borràs, C.; Nos, C.; Rovira, À.; et al. A single-center, randomized, double-blind, placebo-controlled study of interferon beta-1b on primary progressive and transitional multiple sclerosis. *Mult. Scler. J.* **2009**, *15*, 1195–1205. [CrossRef]
99. Wolinsky, J.S.; Narayana, P.A.; O'Connor, P.; Coyle, P.K.; Ford, C.; Johnson, K.; Miller, A.; Pardo, L.; Kadosh, S.; Ladkani, D.; et al. Glatiramer acetate in primary progressive multiple sclerosis: Results of a multinational, multicenter, double-blind, placebo-controlled trial. *Ann. Neurol.* **2007**, *61*, 14–24. [CrossRef]
100. Wolinsky, J.S.; Shochat, T.; Weiss, S.; Ladkani, D. Glatiramer acetate treatment in PPMS: Why males appear to respond favorably. *J. Neurol. Sci.* **2009**, *286*, 92–98. [CrossRef]
101. Ho, P.-R.; Campbell, N.; Chang, I.; Deykin, A.; Forrestal, F.; Lucas, N.; Yu, B.; Arnold, D.L.; Hartung, H.-P.; Miller, A.; et al. Effect of natalizumab on disease progression in secondary progressive multiple sclerosis (ASCEND): A phase 3, randomised, double-blind, placebo-controlled trial with an open-label extension. *Lancet Neurol.* **2018**, *17*, 405–415.
102. Graves, D.; Vernino, S. Immunotherapies in Neurologic Disorders. *Med. Clin. N. Am.* **2012**, *96*, 497–523. [CrossRef]
103. Salzer, J.; Svenningsson, R.; Alping, P.; Novakova, L.; Bjorck, A.; Fink, K.; Islam-Jakobsson, P.; Malmestrom, C.; Axelsson, M.; Vagberg, M. Rituximab in multiple sclerosis: A retrospective observational study on safety and efficacy. *Neurology* **2016**, *87*, 2074–2081. [CrossRef]
104. Komori, M.; Lin, Y.C.; Cortese, I.; Blake, A.; Ohayon, J.; Cherup, J.; Maric, D.; Kosa, P.; Wu, T.; Bielekova, B. Insufficient disease inhibition by intrathecal rituximab in progressive multiple sclerosis. *Ann. Clin. Transl. Neurol.* **2016**, *3*, 166–179. [CrossRef]

105. Bhargava, P.; Wicken, C.; Smith, M.D.; Strowd, R.E.; Cortese, I.; Reich, D.S.; Calabresi, P.A.; Mowry, E.M. Trial of intrathecal rituximab in progressive multiple sclerosis patients with evidence of leptomeningeal contrast enhancement. *Mult. Scler. Relat. Disord.* **2019**, *30*, 136–140. [CrossRef]
106. Bergman, J.; Burman, J.; Gilthorpe, J.D.; Zetterberg, H.; Jiltsova, E.; Bergenheim, T.; Svenningsson, A. Intrathecal treatment trial of rituximab in progressive MS: An open-label phase 1b study. *Neurology* **2018**, *91*, e1893–e1901. [CrossRef]
107. Topping, J.; Dobson, R.; Lapin, S.; Maslyanskiy, A.; Kropshofer, H.; David, L.; Giovannoni, G.; Evdoshenko, E. The effects of intrathecal rituximab on biomarkers in multiple sclerosis. *Mult. Scler. Relat. Disord.* **2016**, *6*, 49–53. [CrossRef]
108. British and Dutch Multiple Sclerosis Azathioprine Trial Group. Double-masked trial of azathioprine in multiple sclerosis. *Lancet* **1988**, *2*, 179–183.
109. Kappos, L.; Pätzold, U.; Dommasch, D.; Poser, S.; Haas, J.; Krauseneck, P.; Malin, J.-P.; Fierz, W.; Graffenried, B.U.; Gugerli, U.S. Cyclosporine versus azathioprine in the long-term treatment of multiple sclerosis? results of the german multicenter study. *Ann. Neurol.* **1988**, *23*, 56–63. [CrossRef]
110. Uccelli, A.; Capello, E.; Fenoglio, D.; Incagliato, M.; Valbonesi, M.; Mancardi, G.L. Intravenous immunoglobulin, plasmalymphocytapheresis and azathioprine in chronic progressive multiple sclerosis. *Neurol. Sci.* **1994**, *15*, 49–53. [CrossRef]
111. Perini, P.; Calabrese, M.; Tiberio, M.; Ranzato, F.; Battistin, L.; Gallo, P. Mitoxantrone versus cyclophosphamide in secondary-progressive multiple sclerosis: A comparative study. *J. Neurol.* **2006**, *253*, 1034–1040. [CrossRef]
112. Zephir, H.; De Seze, J.; Duhamel, A.; Debouverie, M.; Hautecoeur, P.; Lebrun, C.; Malíková, I.; Pelletier, J.; Sénéchal, O.; Vermersch, P. Treatment of progressive forms of multiple sclerosis by cyclophosphamide: A cohort study of 490 patients. *J. Neurol. Sci.* **2004**, *218*, 73–77. [CrossRef]
113. Brochet, B.; Deloire, M.S.A.; Perez, P.; Loock, T.; Baschet, L.; Debouverie, M.; Pittion, S.; Ouallet, J.-C.; Clavelou, P.; De Seze, J.; et al. Double-Blind Controlled Randomized Trial of Cyclophosphamide versus Methylprednisolone in Secondary Progressive Multiple Sclerosis. *PLoS ONE* **2017**, *12*, e0168834. [CrossRef]
114. Weiner, H.L.; Mackin, G.A.; Orav, E.J.; Hafler, D.A.; Dawson, D.M.; Lapierre, Y.; Herndon, R.; Lehrich, J.R.; Hauser, S.L.; Turel, A.; et al. Intermittent cyclophosphamide pulse therapy in progressive multiple sclerosis: Final report of the Northeast Cooperative Multiple Sclerosis Treatment Group. *Neurology* **1993**, *43*, 910. [CrossRef]
115. Hommes, O.R.; Sørensen, P.S.; Fazekas, F.; Enriquez, M.M.; Koelmel, H.W.; Fernández, Ó.; Pozzilli, C.; O'Connor, P. Intravenous immunoglobulin in secondary progressive multiple sclerosis: Randomised placebo-controlled trial. *Lancet* **2004**, *364*, 1149–1156. [CrossRef]
116. Goodkin, D.; Rudick, R.; Medendorp, S.V.; Daughtry, M.; Van Dyke, C. Low-dose oral methotrexate in chronic progressive multiple sclerosis: Analyses of serial MRIs. *Neurology* **1996**, *47*, 1153–1157. [CrossRef]
117. Goodkin, D.E.; Rudick, R.A.; Medendorp, S.V.; Daughtry, M.M.; Schwetz, K.M.; Fischer, J.; Van Dyke, C. Low-dose (7.5 mg) oral methotrexate reduces the rate of progression in chronic progressive multiple sclerosis. *Ann. Neurol.* **1995**, *37*, 30–40. [CrossRef]
118. Lugaresi, A.; Caporale, C.; Farina, D.; Marzoli, F.; Bonanni, L.; Muraro, P.A.; De Luca, G.; Iarlori, C.; Gambi, D. Low-dose oral methotrexate treatment in chronic progressive multiple sclerosis. *Neurol. Sci. Off. J. Ital. Neurol. Soc. Ital. Soc. Clin. Neurophysiol.* **2001**, *22*, 209–210. [CrossRef]
119. The Multiple Sclerosis Study Group. Efficacy and toxicity of cyclosporine in chronic progressive multiple sclerosis: A randomized, double-blinded, placebo-controlled clinical trial. *Ann Neurol.* **1990**, *27*, 591–605. [CrossRef]
120. Fakih, R.; Matiello, M.; Chitnis, T.; Stankiewicz, J.M. Efficacy and safety of mycophenolate mofetil in progressive multiple sclerosis patients. *J. Neurol.* **2018**, *265*, 2688–2694. [CrossRef]
121. Barkhof, F.; Giovannoni, G.; Hartung, H.P.; Cree, B.; Uccelli, A.; Sormani, M.P.; Krieger, S.; Uitdehaag, B.; Vollmer, T.; Montalban, X. ARPEGGIO: A randomized, placebo-controlled study to evaluate oral laquinimod in patients with primary progressive multiple sclerosis (PPMS) (P7.210). *Neurology* **2015**, *84*, P7.210.
122. Freedman, M.S.; Bar-Or, A.; Oger, J.; Traboulsee, A.; Patry, D.; Young, C.; Olsson, T.; Li, D.; Hartung, H.P.; Krantz, M.; et al. A phase III study evaluating the efficacy safety of MBP8298 in secondary progressive multiple sclerosis. *Neurology* **2011**, *77*, 1551–1560. [CrossRef]

123. Deshmukh, V.A.; Tardif, V.; Lyssiotis, C.A.; Green, C.C.; Kerman, B.; Kim, H.J.; Padmanabhan, K.; Swoboda, J.G.; Ahmad, I.; Kondo, T.; et al. A regenerative approach to the treatment of multiple sclerosis. *Nature* **2013**, *502*, 327–332. [CrossRef]
124. Mei, F.; Fancy, S.P.J.; Shen, Y.A.; Niu, J.; Zhao, C.; Presley, B.; Miao, E.; Lee, S.; Mayoral, S.R.; Redmond, S.A.; et al. Micropillar arrays as a high-throughput screening platform for therapeutics in multiple sclerosis. *Nat. Med.* **2014**, *20*, 954–960. [CrossRef]
125. Green, A.J.; Gelfand, J.M.; Cree, B.A.; Bevan, C.; Boscardin, W.J.; Mei, F.; Inman, J.; Arnow, S.; Devereux, M.; Abounasr, A.; et al. Clemastine fumarate as a remyelinating therapy for multiple sclerosis (ReBUILD): A randomised, controlled, double-blind, crossover trial. *Lancet* **2017**, *390*, 2481–2489. [CrossRef]
126. Jepson, S.; Vought, B.; Gross, C.H.; Gan, L.; Austen, D.; Frantz, J.D.; Zwahlen, J.; Lowe, D.; Markland, W.; Krauss, R. LINGO-1, a Transmembrane Signaling Protein, Inhibits Oligodendrocyte Differentiation and Myelination through Intercellular Self-interactions. *J. Boil. Chem.* **2012**, *287*, 22184–22195. [CrossRef]
127. Mi, S.; Miller, R.H.; Lee, X.; Scott, M.L.; Shulag-Morskaya, S.; Shao, Z.; Chang, J.; Thill, G.; Levesque, M.; Zhang, M.; et al. LINGO-1 negatively regulates myelination by oligodendrocytes. *Nat. Neurosci.* **2005**, *8*, 745–751. [CrossRef]
128. Cadavid, D.; Balcer, L.; Galetta, S.; Aktas, O.; Ziemssen, T.; Vanopdenbosch, L.; Frederiksen, J.; Skeen, M.; Jaffe, G.J.; Butzkueven, H.; et al. Safety and efficacy of opicinumab in acute optic neuritis (RENEW): A randomised, placebo-controlled, phase 2 trial. *Lancet Neurol.* **2017**, *16*, 189–199. [CrossRef]
129. Mellion, M.; Edwards, K.R.; Hupperts, R.; Drulović, J.; Montalban, X.; Hartung, H.P.; Brochet, B.; Calabresi, P.A.; Rudick, R.; Ibrahim, A. Efficacy Results from the Phase 2b SYNERGY Study: Treatment of Disabling Multiple Sclerosis with the Anti-LINGO-1 Monoclonal Antibody Opicinumab (S33.004). *Neurology* **2017**, *88*, S33.004.
130. .McCroskery, P.; Selmaj, K.; Fernandez, O.; Grimaldi, L.; Silber, E.; Pardo, G.; Freedman, M.S.; Zhang, Y.; Xu, L.; Cadavid, D. Safety and Tolerability of Opicinumab in Relapsing Multiple Sclerosis. *Neurology* **2017**, *88*, P5.369.
131. Cho, Y.; Crichlow, G.V.; Vermeire, J.J.; Leng, L.; Du, X.; Hodsdon, M.E.; Bucala, R.; Cappello, M.; Gross, M.; Gaeta, F.; et al. Allosteric inhibition of macrophage migration inhibitory factor revealed by ibudilast. *Proc. Natl. Acad. Sci. USA* **2010**, *107*, 11313–11318. [CrossRef]
132. Fox, R.J.; Coffey, C.S.; Conwit, R.; Cudkowicz, M.E.; Gleason, T.; Goodman, A.; Klawiter, E.C.; Matsuda, K.; McGovern, M.; Naismith, R.T.; et al. Phase 2 Trial of Ibudilast in Progressive Multiple Sclerosis. *N. Engl. J. Med.* **2018**, *379*, 846–855. [CrossRef]
133. Greenwood, J.; Steinman, L.; Zamvil, S.S. Statin therapy and autoimmune disease: From protein prenylation to immunomodulation. *Nat. Rev. Immunol.* **2006**, *6*, 358–370. [CrossRef]
134. Chataway, J.; Schuerer, N.; Alsanousi, A.; Chan, D.; MacManus, D.; Hunter, K.; Anderson, V.; Bangham, C.R.M.; Clegg, S.; Nielsen, C.; et al. Effect of high-dose simvastatin on brain atrophy and disability in secondary progressive multiple sclerosis (MS-STAT): A randomised, placebo-controlled, phase 2 trial. *Lancet* **2014**, *383*, 2213–2221. [CrossRef]
135. Rocamonde, B.; Paradells, S.; Barcia, J.; Barcia, C.; García-Verdugo, J.M.; Miranda, M.; Gómez, F.R.; Soria, J. Neuroprotection of lipoic acid treatment promotes angiogenesis and reduces the glial scar formation after brain injury. *Neuroscience* **2012**, *224*, 102–115. [CrossRef]
136. Rochette, L.; Ghibu, S.; Richard, C.; Zeller, M.; Cottin, Y.; Vergely, C. Direct and indirect antioxidant properties of alpha-lipoic acid and therapeutic potential. *Mol. Nutr. Food Res.* **2013**, *57*, 114–125. [CrossRef]
137. Spain, R.; Powers, K.; Murchison, C.; Heriza, E.; Winges, K.; Yadav, V.; Cameron, M.; Kim, E.; Horak, F.; Simon, J.; et al. Lipoic acid in secondary progressive multiple sclerosis: A randomized controlled pilot trial. *Neur. Neuroimmunol. Neuroinflamm.* **2017**, *4*, e374. [CrossRef]
138. Lo, A.C.; Saab, C.Y.; Black, J.A.; Waxman, S.G. Phenytoin Protects Spinal Cord Axons and Preserves Axonal Conduction and Neurological Function in a Model of Neuroinflammation in Vivo. *J. Neurophysiol.* **2003**, *90*, 3566–3571. [CrossRef]
139. Raftopoulos, R.; Hickman, S.J.; Toosy, A.; Sharrack, B.; Mallik, S.; Paling, D.; Altmann, D.R.; Yiannakas, M.C.; Malladi, P.; Sheridan, R.; et al. Phenytoin for neuroprotection in patients with acute optic neuritis: A randomised, placebo-controlled, phase 2 trial. *Lancet Neurol.* **2016**, *15*, 259–269. [CrossRef]
140. Cohen, J.A. Mesenchymal Stem Cell Transplantation in Multiple Sclerosis. *J. Neurol. Sci.* **2013**, *333*, 43–49. [CrossRef]

141. Bonab, M.M.; Yazdanbakhsh, S.; Lotfi, J.; Alimoghaddom, K.; Talebian, F.; Hooshmand, F.; Ghavamzadeh, A.; Nikbin, B. Does mesenchymal stem cell therapy help multiple sclerosis patients? Report of a pilot study. *Iran. J. Immunol. IJI* **2007**, *4*, 50–57.
142. Bonab, M.M.; Sahraian, M.A.; Aghsaie, A.; Karvigh, S.A.; Hosseinian, S.M.; Nikbin, B.; Lotfi, J.; Khorramnia, S.; Motamed, M.R.; Togha, M.; et al. Autologous mesenchymal stem cell therapy in progressive multiple sclerosis: An open label study. *Curr. Stem Cell Res. Ther.* **2012**, *7*, 407–414. [CrossRef]
143. Yamout, B.; Hourani, R.; Salti, H.; Barada, W.; El-Hajj, T.; Al-Kutoubi, A.; Herlopian, A.; Baz, E.K.; Mahfouz, R.; Khalil-Hamdan, R.; et al. Bone marrow mesenchymal stem cell transplantation in patients with multiple sclerosis: A pilot study. *J. Neuroimmunol.* **2010**, *227*, 185–189. [CrossRef]
144. Lublin, F.D.; Bowen, J.D.; Huddlestone, J.; Kremenchutzky, M.; Carpenter, A.; Corboy, J.R.; Freedman, M.S.; Krupp, L.; Paulo, C.; Hariri, R.J.; et al. Human placenta-derived cells (PDA-001) for the treatment of adults with multiple sclerosis: A randomized, placebo-controlled, multiple-dose study. *Mult. Scler. Relat. Disord.* **2014**, *3*, 696–704. [CrossRef]
145. Karussis, D.; Karageorgiou, C.; Vaknin-Dembinsky, A.; Gowda-Kurkalli, B.; Gomori, J.M.; Kassis, I.; Bulte, J.W.M.; Petrou, P.; Ben-Hur, T.; Abramsky, O.; et al. Safety and Immunological Effects of Mesenchymal Stem Cell Transplantation in Patients with Multiple Sclerosis and Amyotrophic Lateral Sclerosis. *Arch. Neurol.* **2010**, *67*, 1187–1194. [CrossRef]
146. Harris, V.K.; Vyshkina, T.; Sadiq, S.A. Clinical safety of intrathecal administration of mesenchymal stromal cell–derived neural progenitors in multiple sclerosis. *Cytotherapy* **2016**, *18*, 1476–1482. [CrossRef]
147. Harris, V.K.; Stark, J.; Vyshkina, T.; Blackshear, L.; Joo, G.; Stefanova, V.; Sara, G.; Sadiq, S.A. Phase I Trial of Intrathecal Mesenchymal Stem Cell-derived Neural Progenitors in Progressive Multiple Sclerosis. *EBioMedicine* **2018**, *29*, 23–30. [CrossRef]
148. Li, J.-F.; Zhang, D.-J.; Geng, T.; Chen, L.; Huang, H.; Yin, H.-L.; Zhang, Y.-Z.; Lou, J.-Y.; Cao, B.; Wang, Y.-L. The Potential of Human Umbilical Cord-Derived Mesenchymal Stem Cells as a Novel Cellular Therapy for Multiple Sclerosis. *Cell Transplant.* **2014**, *23*, 113–122. [CrossRef]
149. Liang, J.; Zhang, H.; Hua, B.; Wang, H.; Wang, J.; Han, Z.; Sun, L. Allogeneic mesenchymal stem cells transplantation in treatment of multiple sclerosis. *Mult. Scler. J.* **2009**, *15*, 644–646. [CrossRef]
150. Cohen, J.A.; Atkins, H.; Banwell, B.; Bar-Or, A.; Bebo, B.; Bowen, J.; Burt, R.; Calabresi, P.; Cohen, J.; Comi, G.; et al. Cell-based therapeutic strategies for multiple sclerosis. *Brain* **2017**, *140*, 2776–2796.
151. Uccelli, A.; Brundin, L.; Clanet, M.; Fernandez, O.; Nabavi, S.M.; Muraro, P.A.; Oliveri, R.S.; Radue, E.W.; Sellner, J.; Sorensen, P.S.; et al. MEsenchymal StEm cells for Multiple Sclerosis (MESEMS): A randomized, double blind, cross-over phase I/II clinical trial with autologous mesenchymal stem cells for the therapy of multiple sclerosis. *Trials* **2019**, *20*, 263. [CrossRef]
152. Sedel, F.; Bernard, D.; Mock, D.M.; Tourbah, A. Targeting demyelination and virtual hypoxia with high-dose biotin as a treatment for progressive multiple sclerosis. *Neuropharmacology* **2016**, *110*, 644–653. [CrossRef]
153. Sedel, F.; Papeix, C.; Bellanger, A.; Touitou, V.; Lebrun-Frenay, C.; Galanaud, D.; Gout, O.; Lyon-Caen, O.; Tourbah, A. High doses of biotin in chronic progressive multiple sclerosis: A pilot study. *Mult. Scler. Relat. Disord.* **2015**, *4*, 159–169. [CrossRef]
154. Tourbah, A.; Lebrun-Frenay, C.; Edan, G.; Clanet, M.; Papeix, C.; Vukusic, S.; De Sèze, J.; Debouverie, M.; Gout, O.; Clavelou, P.; et al. MD1003 (high-dose biotin) for the treatment of progressive multiple sclerosis: A randomised, double-blind, placebo-controlled study. *Mult. Scler. J.* **2016**, *22*, 1719–1731. [CrossRef]
155. Birnbaum, G.; Stulc, J. High dose biotin as treatment for progressive multiple sclerosis. *Mult. Scler. Relat. Disord.* **2017**, *18*, 141–143. [CrossRef]
156. Baldassari, L.E.; Feng, J.; Clayton, B.L.; Oh, S.-H.; Sakaie, K.; Tesar, P.J.; Wang, Y.; Cohen, J.A. Developing therapeutic strategies to promote myelin repair in multiple sclerosis. *Expert Rev. Neurother.* **2019**, 1–17. [CrossRef]
157. Najm, F.J.; Madhavan, M.; Zaremba, A.; Shick, E.; Karl, R.T.; Factor, D.C.; Miller, T.E.; Nevin, Z.S.; Kantor, C.; Sargent, A.; et al. Drug-based modulation of endogenous stem cells promotes functional remyelination in vivo. *Nature* **2015**, *522*, 216–220. [CrossRef]
158. Cohen, J.A.; Baldassari, L.E.; Atkins, H.L.; Bowen, J.D.; Bredeson, C.; Carpenter, P.A.; Corboy, J.R.; Freedman, M.S.; Griffith, L.M.; Lowsky, R.; et al. Autologous Hematopoietic Cell Transplantation for Treatment-Refractory Relapsing Multiple Sclerosis: Position Statement from the American Society for Blood and Marrow Transplantation. *Boil. Blood Marrow Transplant.* **2019**, *25*, 845–854. [CrossRef]

159. Marrie, R.A.; Hanwell, H. General health issues in multiple sclerosis: Comorbidities, secondary conditions, and health behaviors. *Continuum* **2013**, *19*, 1046–1057. [CrossRef]
160. Ontaneda, D. Inadequate outcome measures are the biggest impediment to successful clinical trials in progressive MS-Commentary. *Mult. Scler.* **2017**, *23*, 508–509. [CrossRef]
161. Giovannoni, G.; Airas, L.; Bove, R.; Boyko, A.; Cutter, G.; Hobart, J.; Kuhle, J.; Oh, J.; Tur, C.; Garas, M.; et al. *Ocrelizumab Treatment Effect on Upper Limb Function in PPMS Patients with Disability: Subgroup Results of the ORATORIO Study to Inform the ORATORIO-HAND Study Design*; ECTRIMS Online Library: London, UK, 2018; p. 619.
162. Sumowski, J.F.; Benedict, R.; Enzinger, C.; Filippi, M.; Geurts, J.J.; Hamalainen, P.; Hulst, H.; Inglese, M.; Leavitt, V.M.; Rocca, M.A.; et al. Cognition in multiple sclerosis State of the field and priorities for the future. *Neurology* **2018**, *90*, 278–288. [CrossRef]

10

Promising Nanotechnology Approaches in Treatment of Autoimmune Diseases of Central Nervous System

Maria Chountoulesi and Costas Demetzos *

Section of Pharmaceutical Technology, Department of Pharmacy, School of Health Sciences, National and Kapodistrian University of Athens, Panepistimioupolis Zografou, 15771 Athens, Greece; mchountoules@pharm.uoa.gr

* Correspondence: demetzos@pharm.uoa.gr;

Abstract: Multiple sclerosis (MS) is a chronic, autoimmune, neurodegenerative disease of the central nervous system (CNS) that yields to neuronal axon damage, demyelization, and paralysis. Although several drugs were designed for the treatment of MS, with some of them being approved in the last few decades, the complete remission and the treatment of progressive forms still remain a matter of debate and a medical challenge. Nanotechnology provides a variety of promising therapeutic tools that can be applied for the treatment of MS, overcoming the barriers and the limitations of the already existing immunosuppressive and biological therapies. In the present review, we explore literature case studies on the development of drug delivery nanosystems for the targeted delivery of MS drugs in the pathological tissues of the CNS, providing high bioavailability and enhanced therapeutic efficiency, as well as nanosystems for the delivery of agents to facilitate efficient remyelination. Moreover, we present examples of tolerance-inducing nanocarriers, being used as promising vaccines for antigen-specific immunotherapy of MS. We emphasize on liposomes, as well as lipid- and polymer-based nanoparticles. Finally, we highlight the future perspectives given by the nanotechnology field toward the improvement of the current treatment of MS and its animal model, experimental autoimmune encephalomyelitis (EAE).

Keywords: multiple sclerosis; nanotechnology; drug delivery nanosystems; lipids; polymers; vaccines; nanoparticles; antigen-specific immunotherapy; experimental autoimmune encephalomyelitis; neurodegeneration

1. Introduction

Multiple sclerosis (MS) is a chronic, autoimmune, demyelinating disease of the central nervous system (CNS), accompanied by a relapsing/remitting (RR) or a progressive course that is followed by axon damage and paralysis, including symptoms of muscle weakness, weak reflexes, muscle spasm, difficulty in movement, miscoordination, unbalance, vertigo, fatigue, and pain. Other symptoms that are usually referred are optic nerve dysfunction, loss of vision, diplopia, pyramidal tract dysfunction, ataxia, tremor, bladder and bowel dysfunction, sexual dysfunction, depression, anxiety, swallowing dysfunction, memory loss, sleep disturbance, and obstructive sleep apnea [1–5]. Unfortunately, the exact etiology of MS remains unknown, while many different risk factors were referred, characterizing MS as a heterogeneous, multifactorial disease. The occurrence is 2–3 times higher in females than males. MS is the most common neurologically disabling disease in young adults, while older people and children can also acquire MS [4,6]. Our understanding of the immune processes that contributes to MS led to the approval or clinical development of some disease-modifying therapies (DMTs) that are effective in relapsing forms of MS. However, few treatments are effective for the progressive forms of the disease [7,8].

Nanotechnology provides a variety of promising therapeutic tools that can be applied for the treatment of CNS-related disorders, such as MS, overcoming the barriers and the restrictions of the already existing conventional therapies. Extensive research is being carried out for the development of drug delivery nanosystems for the targeted delivery of MS drugs in the pathological tissues of CNS, providing high bioavailability and enhanced therapeutic efficiency. In addition, remyelination is an attractive, innovative strategy toward MS therapy [9], where nanoparticles can also contribute, via the targeted delivery of remyelinating agents to specific cells, leading to the improvement of their therapeutic performance. Moreover, tolerance-inducing vaccines, based on tolerance-inducing nanocarriers for antigen-specific immunotherapies, are considered to be another promising strategy toward the treatment of MS [10,11].

In the present review study, literature examples of the aforementioned nanocarriers that were designed for MS treatment are presented, highlighting the future perspectives given by the nanotechnology field toward the improvement of the current treatment of MS. We focus on liposomes, as well as lipid- and polymer- based nanocarriers.

2. Multiple Sclerosis (MS)

MS is an autoimmune, chronic, neurodegenerative disorder, targeting the myelin sheaths (a protective layer surrounding the nerve fibers) of the CNS. The caused damage of myelin sheaths provokes nerve demyelination, followed by axon damage and, thus, interruption of signal transmission to and from the CNS. As with many other neurodegenerative diseases, the real and exact origin of MS is still unidentified, although the literature describes many different potential triggering factors that may stimulate the autoimmune responses, which harm the brain tissues and spinal cord. More particularly, genetic predisposition and environmental factors, as well as microbial and viral infections, smoking, toxins, low concentrations of vitamin D, and circadian rhythm disruption, can contribute to the onset of this disorder [12–16]. Regarding genetic predisposition, the major histocompatibility complex (MHC) class II phenotype, the human leukocyte antigen (HLA)-DR2, and HLA-DR4 are reported as the most commonly affected, while the incidence of MS is also increased 10-fold in monozygotic twins, as compared to siblings of patients with MS [17,18].

MS is categorized into three distinct types, primarily based on its clinical course, which are characterized by increasing severity. Relapsing/remitting MS (RRMS) is the most common form, which involves relapses followed by silent remission with any MS symptoms. RRMS generally switches to a chronic progressive course several years after onset, while a minor number of patients display primary chronic progressive course without the RR phase. Subsequently, we have secondary progressive MS (SPMS), which develops over time following diagnosis of RRMS, and primary progressive MS (PPMS), noted as gradual continuous neurologic deterioration, which provides continuous disease progression [19–21].

The symptoms may vary person-to-person and produce temporary, long-lasting, or even permanent losses due to the disrupted signal transmission, including mood swings, memory-related issues, tingling, fatigue, numbness, partial or complete blindness, pain, and partial or even whole-body paralysis, depending upon the severity of disease. The disrupted signal transmission is responsible for various complex and erratic indications. MS broadly presents three stages, starting from a pre-clinical stage, followed by a relapsing/remitting stage and a progressive clinical stage, in which, after typically 10–20 years, neurologic dysfunction progressively worsens, eventually leading to impaired mobility, cognition, and a progressive loss of nerve functions [22–25].

2.1. Immunopathophysiology of MS

Myelin sheath damage and inflammation contribute to the formation of lesions [26]. MS lesions appear in the white matter inside the visual neuron, brain stem, and spinal cord [26]. In MS, the immune system starts to recognize myelin components as foreign, leading to its destruction [12]. Plaque formation and disease symptoms are widely accepted as the result of immune cell infiltration, with the release of cytokines and inflammatory mediators, leading to inflammation, myelin destruction, oligodendrocyte loss, and loss of neuronal function and eventual axonal degeneration. On the other hand, demyelination further increases the activation of inflammatory processes, causing damage of the blood–brain barrier (BBB), stimulation of oxidative stress pathways, and macrophage activation [27]. Microglial cells upregulate MHC class I and II molecules, as well as cell surface co-stimulatory molecules, while they also secrete cytokines and chemokines. Several types of immune infiltrates can be found in the white matter lesions, where myelin is damaged, including monocytes, B cells, T cells (for example, TH cells and myelin-reactive auto-T cells), and dendritic cells [25,28–32]. Substantial fractions of cluster of differentiation 4 (CD4)+ and CD8+ T cells being isolated from MS lesions and cerebrospinal fluid (CSF) indicate that antigen-specific T-cell responses contribute to the disease process [33]. It seems that T helper 1 (TH1) and TH17 cells are the main pathogenic populations in the immunopathogenesis of MS, along with regulatory T cells (Treg) and natural killer T (NKT) cells [34–37]. The pro-inflammatory state of macrophages is correlated with MS because macrophages interact with T and B cells, instructing demyelination, axonal loss, and degeneration, and they are presented as of the most predominant cell type in patient lesions [38,39]. In Figure 1, there is a detailed presentation of the cells that are involved in the immune process of MS [25].

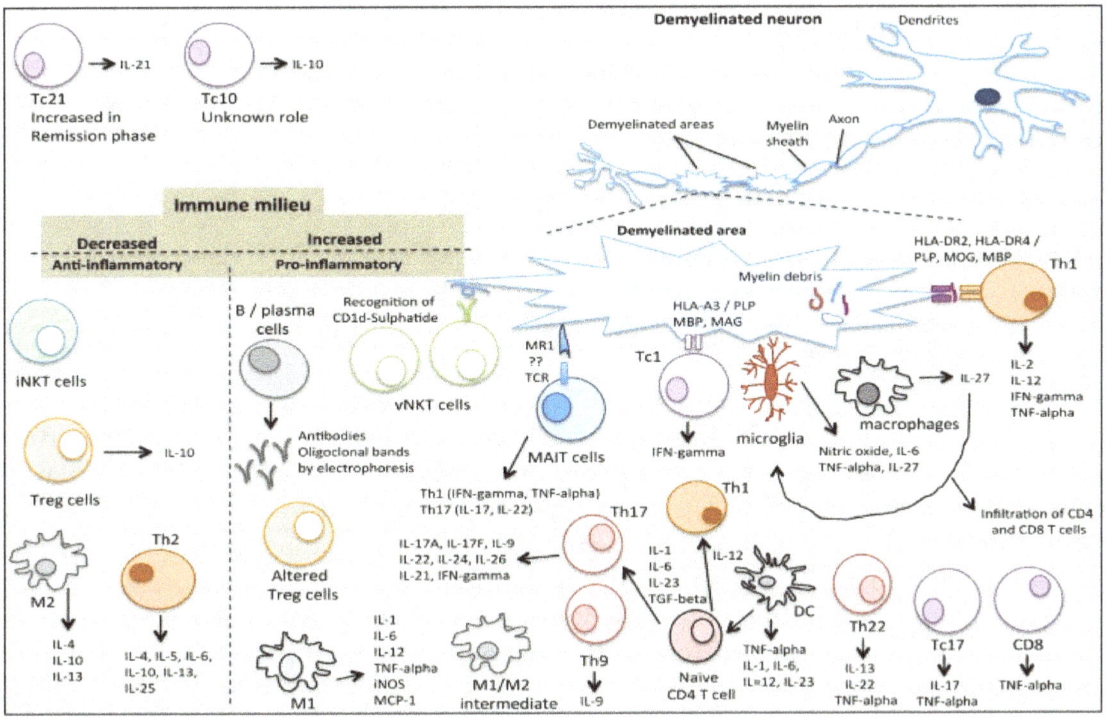

Figure 1. The immunological complexity of the immune/cytokine network in multiple sclerosis (MS). Adapted from Dargahi et al. [25].

Traditionally, the etiology of MS was based on an "outside-in" autoimmune hypothesis, whereby dysregulated auto-reactive T cells in the periphery cross into the CNS parenchyma and, together with macrophages and B cells, proceed to attack myelin. Contrariwise, the "inside-out" hypothesis argues that MS is a primary degenerative disease, where the initial malfunction occurs within the CNS and is accompanied by varying degrees of inflammation, as a secondary response, leading to the release of various antigenic cell components. According to the "inside-out" hypothesis, the primary degeneration is present from the start (probably years before the first overt clinical symptoms) and continues throughout the entire course of the disease. Whether early neurodegeneration drives autoimmune injury, or whether ongoing inflammation reaches a threshold to trigger neurodegeneration is still unclear, while another question is whether neurodegeneration is independent or not of chronic inflammation. The lack of understanding with regard to mechanisms of progression phase, when the most irreversible disability takes place, is responsible for the extremely limited treatment options that are currently available to patients with progressive MS. Until now, many different treatment approaches for progressive MS were proposed including mitochondrion-protective strategies, anti-inflammatory strategies, strategies targeting microglia and astrocytes, inhibitors of microglial activity, remyelination therapies, and strategies targeting lymphocytes [20,23,40].

2.2. Current Therapeutics of MS

Until now, the Food and Drug Administration (FDA) approved over a dozen therapeutic agents to reduce the number of attacks and delay MS progression in terms of available DMTs. Disease-modifying agents are commonly shown to reduce the rate of relapses, reduce magnetic resonance imaging (MRI) lesions, and stabilize or delay MS disability. However, MS remains incurable. Interferon beta (IFN-β) and glatiramer acetate (GA), being the first two introduced drugs, are able to alter T-cell responses, are injectable, and still remain the "first line" therapies for MS, owing to their relative safety and proven efficacy. Oral DMTs available for RRMS include immunosuppressives, which inhibit lymphocyte trafficking, namely, fingolimod and the teriflunomide (TFM) that inhibit activated T and B cells, as well as the immunomodulatory/immunosuppressive dimethyl fumarate (DMF) that alters T-cell responses. The above are characterized as long-term treatments. In addition, a number of humanized monoclonal antibody-based therapeutics for RRMS were developed, including natalizumab, alemtuzumab, and ocrelizumab. Unfortunately, their disadvantage is the high risk of side effects, including progressive multifocal leukoencephalopathy (PML) and the development of secondary autoimmune diseases [4,12,25,26,39,41–45].

2.3. Experimental Autoimmune Encephalomyelitis (EAE) as an Animal Model for MS

Experimental autoimmune encephalomyelitis (EAE) is a widely used animal model of MS because it shares several features with the human disease, including neurological dysfunction and perivascular inflammation in the CNS. It is considered to be the most frequently used model to study the demyelinating and immune pathology of MS. EAE can be induced in several mammalian species by directly immunizing animals with CNS homogenate or myelin proteins, such as myelin oligodendrocyte glycoprotein (MOG), myelin basic protein (MBP), and proteolipid protein (PLP), or using small peptides derived from these proteins; alternatively, the transfer of isolated activated CD4+ T cells or less commonly CD8+ T cells, may be introduced to a naïve animal. The fact that demyelination and lesion formation occur predominantly in the spinal cord rather than the CNS is a disadvantage indicating that EAE does not fully recapitulate human MS pathology [46–50]. However, there is no other model representing better the pathophysiology of MS. EAE extensively contributed toward the knowledge and understanding of the pathophysiology of the MS, as well as contributed to the discovery and the understanding of the mechanism of action of some of the current approved therapies [39,51–53].

3. Nanotechnology and MS

Drug delivery nanosystems are considered as innovative technological platforms that are able to transport bioactive molecules to target tissues, modifying their solubility and improving their bioavailability, by altering their pharmacokinetic profile [54]. The existence of physiological barriers, such as the BBB and the blood–cerebrospinal fluid barrier (BCSFB), limits the access of several therapeutic agents to the CNS and downgrades their therapeutic activity. In this regard, nanotechnology is considered to be a promising strategy to improve drug targeting to the brain, as well as increase bioavailability. There is great research attention toward the employment of nanotechnology, as well as the development of new therapies and improvement of the therapeutic efficacy for MS [55]. Taking advantage of their size, nanoparticles are easily internalized by the cells, being suitable carriers for drugs, immunomodulatory molecules, or antigens. Nanosystems are able to improve the drug solubility, provide targeted delivery, diminish potential side effects from high doses, and establish controlled drug release. Moreover, nanoparticles can be administrated through various routes apart from systemic administration, such as intranasally, for example, in cases where nose-to-brain delivery is desired.

In the following paragraphs, different literature cases on nanoparticles and MS are examined. There are referred nanoparticles that are used as drug delivery systems, in order to improve the pharmacokinetics and bioavailability, while enhancing the therapeutic efficacy when compared to the free administered drugs; furthermore, nanoparticles can be used as vectors for antigen-specific immunomodulation. Through antigen-specific immunomodulation, the immune system is repeatedly exposed to a specific antigen, which results in immunomodulation from the disease to the tolerance state. Antigen-loaded nanoparticles provide several advantages for antigen-specific immunomodulation, such as sustained antigen release, the co-delivery of antigens and adjuvants, the formation of antigen depots at the injection site, the effective presentation of B-cell epitopes, and an increase in the uptake and stimulation of cell-mediated immune responses against acellular antigens. These nanoparticles are coupled with specific antigens related to the autoimmune response in MS and their epitopes. These nanoparticles are able to regulate T-cell function, as well as induce Treg cell and dendritic cell differentiation, restoring immunological tolerance [56]. More details are analytically described throughout the paragraphs below.

Another subject of great scientific interest regarding MS, which is also correlated with the development of new therapeutics, is remyelination. While some patients suffer from progressive neurological deficits, other patients occasionally display improved neurological function. The mechanism via which some patients experience neurological improvement remains unclear. However, increasing evidence shows that remyelination occurs in the MS/EAE [57–60]. In addition, recent studies showed that activated neural stem/progenitor cells around region sites contribute to remyelination [61,62]. Promoting remyelination, therefore, provides an additional line of defense against the axonal damage that follows the loss of myelin. Several potential drugs that target CNS inflammation and the different aspects and stages of remyelination (for example, by inducing oligodendrocyte precursor cell (OPC) differentiation) are being identified [9,63]. Nanoparticles themselves can also act as remyelinating agents. Most recently, Robinson et al. [64] reported a new nanocatalytic therapeutic candidate for remyelination, consisting of a suspension of clean-surfaced, faceted nanocrystals of gold, which was found to demonstrate robust remyelinating activity in response to demyelinating agents, in both chronic cuprizone and acute lysolecithin rodent animal models. More analytically, the administrated nanoparticles induced differentiation of OPCs and enhanced activities of neurons and oligodendrocytes through enhancement of bioenergetic processes of key indicators of aerobic glycolysis. According to the in vivo results, the oral delivery of gold nanocrystals improved the motor functions of cuprizone-treated mice in both open-field and kinematic gait studies. Additional in vitro data indicated an upregulation of myelin synthesis-related genes, collectively resulting in functional myelin generation.

However, there is still no available treatment to regenerate myelin, and several strategies are being scrutinized, while there are difficulties in translating these potential drug targets into practical therapies for patients, as these must cross the BBB to reach OPCs in the CNS, and ideally should be delivered directly to OPCs, to avoid off-target effects. Once again, nanotechnology may solve these problems, with nanoparticles crossing the BBB and facilitating targeting to specific cells, as highlighted in the below-described literature examples.

3.1. Lipid-Based Nanosystems

Lipid nanocarriers such as liposomes, solid lipid nanoparticles (SLNs), nanostructured lipid carriers (NLCs), and nanoemulsions (Figure 2) are considered an ideal strategy for effective delivery of the therapeutic agents against MS at the CNS, enhancing brain transport. They possess the ability to cross the BBB by naturally entering the brain capillary endothelial cells, reducing the peripheral side effects. Furthermore, through suitable surface decoration, lipid nanocarriers can be engineered to interact with particular types of molecules or cell receptors presented in the BBB, even delivering drugs which normally cannot cross the BBB [65,66].

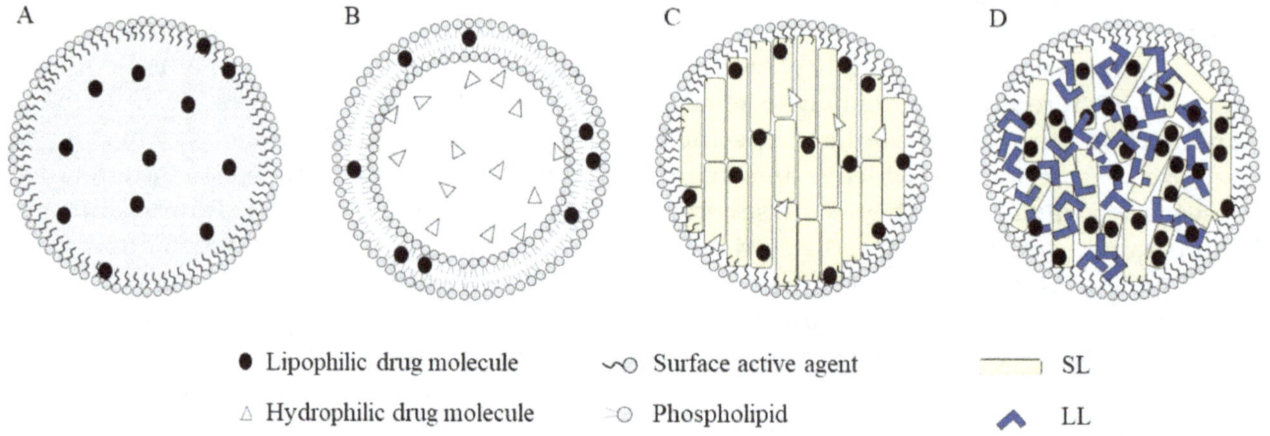

Figure 2. Different types of lipid-based nanoparticles: (**A**) nanoemulsions; (**B**) liposomes; (**C**) solid lipid nanoparticles (SLNs); (**D**) nanostructured lipid carriers (NLCs). Adapted from Haider et al. [67].

3.1.1. Nanolipid Carriers (NLCs) and Solid Lipid Nanoparticles (SLNs)

The lipid-based nanoparticulate system with a solid matrix primarily originated from an oil-in-water type emulsion, by replacing the oil phase or liquid lipids with solid lipids to make it solid at body temperature. Solid lipid nanoparticles (SLNs) are usually considered as the first-generation lipid nanoparticle developed from solid lipid, while nanolipid carriers (NLCs) are known as second-generation lipid nanoparticles, comprising a solid and liquid lipid blend, as well as a surfactant (Figure 2C,D) [68,69]. Although the formulation contains a liquid lipid, NLCs remain in the solid state at body and room temperatures, by adjusting the levels of the liquid lipid. SLNs are colloidal particles with increased physical stability derived from oil-in-water (O/W) emulsions, by replacing liquid lipids with a lipid matrix that is solid at both room and body temperature. The lipid core of SLNs typically consists of fatty acids, monoglycerides, diglycerides, triglycerides, waxes, or steroids and is stabilized by surfactants [70,71]. SLNs and NLCs differ in the composition and organization of the lipids of the matrix, which causes different morphological structures. Commonly used solid lipids for NLC formulation are stearic acid, stearyl alcohol, glycerol monostearate, mono-stearin, etc., while common examples of liquid lipids involve the use of olive oil, sesame oil, almond oil, peanut oil, soyabean oil, oleic acid, corn oil, soy lecithin, phosphatidyl choline, vitamin E, etc. [69].

Recently, Gadhave et al. [72] formulated intranasal nanolipid carriers loaded with TFM, an inhibitor of dihydroorotate dehydrogenase, exhibiting anti-inflammatory activity. The TFM-loaded NLCs were prepared via the melt emulsification ultrasonication method, while the Box–Behnken statistical design was applied to optimize the formulation. The lipid nanocarriers were composed of Compritol® 888 ATO (solid lipid), maisine 35–1 (liquid lipid), gelucire 44/14 (stabilizer) (all by Gattefosse, Mumbai, India), and its aqueous phase from water and Tween-20 (surfactant) (S.D. Fine Chemicals, Pune, India). They were evaluated regarding their particle size, entrapment efficiency (%), in vitro and ex vivo permeation, and their pharmacological and toxicological properties. According to the results, the optimized formulation exhibited particle size, surface charge, and entrapment efficiency of 99.82 nm, −22.29 mV, and 83.39%, respectively. The formulation was enriched with mucoadhesive and gelling agents. The ex vivo drug permeation study and the permeation flux of the prepared mucoadhesive nanosystem was higher than the plain one. From the therapeutic point of view, the intranasal administration of the prepared nanostructures facilitates the rapid remyelination of damaged neurons in the cuprizone-treated rat model, without any significant change in hepatic biomarkers and sub-acute toxicity of the drug; thus, it can be considered as effective and safe delivery for brain disorders.

Kumar et al. [73] developed nanolipid carriers for the delivery of DMF and tocopherol acetate, in an effort to enhance the brain permeability of DMF, improve its gastric tolerance, and reduce its side effects. They used stearic acid (M/s Central Drug House, New Delhi, India) as the solid-phase lipid, tocopherol acetate as the liquid-phase lipid, and Tween 80 (M/s Fisher Scientific India Pvt. Limited, Mumbai, India) as an emulsifier, while the hot microemulsion technique was utilized as the preparation method. The prepared formulation was then evaluated by physicochemical, Caco-2 cellular permeability, in vitro drug release, in vivo pharmacokinetics, and biodistribution studies. The physicochemical study revealed characteristics suitable for brain drug delivery, namely, an average size of 69.70 nm, polydispersity index (PDI) of 0.317, and zeta potential of −9.71 mV. At the same time, the loading efficiency and entrapment efficiency of the formulation were observed as 20.13% and 90.12%, respectively. The obtained controlled release profile, in both gastric and intestinal pH (up to 68% of drug in 24 h), was attributed to the better encapsulation of DMF within the NLC. The drug release was found to best fit the Higuchi equation of release kinetics. Cellular uptake studies on Caco-2 and SH-SY5Y monolayers confirmed better intestinal absorption, due to its biodegradable, lipidic formulation and small size, as well as higher neuronal uptake of the developed system. Furthermore, the in vivo pharmacokinetic data showed a significant improvement in C_{max} and $t_{1/2}$, three times higher drug absorption, and a reduction in the drug clearance, volume of distribution, T_{max}, and drug elimination. The findings are promising and offer preclinical evidence for better brain bioavailability of DMF, which can improve the clinical therapy of MS through reduction of the dosing frequency.

Ghasemian et al. [74] developed baclofen-loaded nanolipid carriers for effective brain drug delivery, in order to reach the site of baclofen action in the CNS. Although baclofen is not an MS-specific therapy, it is used in the treatment of multiple sclerosis, in order to eliminate the spasticity that usually appears in MS. However, the effect of oral baclofen is limited due to its hydrophilic nature, which creates insufficient concentrations in the brain and CSF. The proposed lipid nanocarrier was prepared via the double emulsification solvent evaporation technique and was composed of glyceryl monostearate, glyceryl distearate, glyceryl trioleate (all by Gattefossè, France), and an aqueous phase containing Tween 80 (Sigma-Aldrich, Darmstadt, Germany), as a surface acting agent. Taking into account the obtained physicochemical results, the formulation gave suitable ranges of particle size, size distribution, and zeta potential, while encapsulation efficiencies ranged between 39% and 42%. Glyceryl trioleate lipid gave the minimum particle size. The obtained sustained release profile (up to 74.6% of drug in 28 h) was found to best fit the Higuchi equation of release kinetics and to take place via Fickian diffusion. The formulation of baclofen in nanolipid carriers increased the half-life of drug in plasma and brain by up to 10 and 1.5 times, respectively, and provided a prolonged effect compared to the solution formulation.

Most recently, Kumar et al. [75] loaded methylthioadenosine in SLNs for oral delivery to the brain for the management of MS. The SLNs were prepared via the well-reported microencapsulation technique and were composed of stearic acid (M/s Central Drug House, New Delhi, India), phospholipid 90 G (IPCA Laboratories, Mumbai, India), and Tween-80. The obtained SLNs exhibited sizes below 100 nm, being well within the range to offer a promise of enhanced BBB permeability and bypassing the reticuloendothelial system, with almost neutral zeta potential; they also offered higher drug entrapment and drug loading. Cuprizone-induced demyelination model in mice was employed to mimic the MS-like conditions of demyelination. We should mention that the cuprizone model does not accurately capture the MS disease state, but it is useful for pro-remyelination investigations. It is mainly neurodegenerative-based, exhibiting toxin-based demyelination, rather than immune-mediated demyelination [9]. The symptoms were monitored to some level by plain methylthioadenosine and to a major extent by the SLN version of this nucleoside. According to the pharmacokinetic studies, the methylthioadenosine was better absorbed from SLNs vis-à-vis plain methylthioadenosine, and the biological residence was substantially enhanced so as to reach the target site, thus improving bioavailability and enhancing bioresidence. Methylthioadenosine-loaded SLNs were able to maintain the normal metabolism, locomotor activity, motor coordination, balancing, and grip strength of the rodents compared to plain MTA. The pharmacokinetics corroborated the pharmacodynamic findings, indicating that the orally administrated SLNs can be substantially delivered to the brain and can effectively remyelinate the neurons.

In another case of SLNs, Gandomi et al. [76] developed polyethylene glycol (PEG)ylated SLNs in order to efficiently deliver the glycocorticosteroid methylprednisolone to the brain. The corticosteroids, including the glucocorticosteroids, which are mentioned in many literature cases of drug delivery nanosystems described in the present review article, are used in pulse curses, in order to clinically treat significant relapses in MS patients, in an attempt to hasten recovery. Although they are one of the most common clinically prescribed drugs for reducing MS symptoms, due to their anti-inflammatory and immunosuppressive effects, we should note that they are not a specific treatment of MS. The SLNs were surface-modified by using two targeting moieties and, more specifically, glycoprotein antigens, either anti-Contactin2 or anti-Neurofascin, which are two axo-glial-glycoprotein antigens located in the node of Ranvier and are considered to be the main targets of autoimmune reaction in MS. Myelin-based SLNs were prepared via the solvent evaporation method and were composed of myelin lipids including cholesterol, sphingosine, phosphatidylethanolamine, phosphatidylcholine, sphingomyelin, and phosphatidylserine (all by Sigma Aldrich, St. Louis, MO, USA). In order to obtain targeted SLNs, the antibody, either anti-Contactin2 or anti-Neurofascin, was conjugated to the drug-loaded polyethylene glycol (PEG)-covered SLNs (PEGylated SLNs). The prepared SLNs were physicochemically characterized, while their in vitro release profile, cell viability, and cell uptake were studied. Their brain uptakes were also probed following injections into MS-induced mice. The formulation differentiated the particle size; for example, smaller particle sizes following the antibody bindings were observed, due to the lesser hydration of polymer after the antibody conjugation. The SLNs presented good release profiles, where variations in the lipid type slightly affected the drug release profile, while the PEG and/or antibody coating provided a sink boundary condition for the drug diffusion within the lipoid matrix. It was found that the targeted PEGylated SLNs had no significant cytotoxicity on U87MG-cells, although their cellular uptake was increased four- and eight-fold when surface-modified with anti-Contactin2 or anti-Neurofascin, respectively, compared to control. However, the non-surface-modified SLNs exhibited better penetration ability of the BBB compared to the PEGylated and antibody-functionalized SLNs. The authors suggested that the antibodies may facilitate the adsorption of the SLNs to myelin due to binding to the related antigens, i.e., Contactin2 or Neurofascin, on the CNS axon, and the above information would help toward the development of more efficient nanocarriers for the treatment of MS.

3.1.2. Liposomes

Liposomes (Figure 2B) are considered to be one of the most well-investigated drug delivery nanosystems, presenting major advantages, such as biocompatibility and biodegradability, while also exhibiting great versatility, because they can be easily surface-modified with functional biomaterials, in order to acquire advanced properties, such as escaping rapid clearance in circulation and presenting increased targeting to pathological tissues [54,77].

In addition to lipid nanoparticles, liposomes and especially the PEGylated ones were also reported as potential drug carriers for MS and specially for the delivery of glycosteroids. Schmidt et al. [78] developed a novel formulation of PEG-coated long-circulating liposomes, prepared from dipalmitoyl phosphatidylcholine (Lipoid GmbH, Ludwigshafen, Germany), encapsulating prednisolone that was administrated to the CNS of rats exhibiting EAE. The authors tried to achieve ultra-high tissue concentrations of glucocorticosteroids in the inflamed target organ as compared to an equivalent dose given as free drug, along with a much lower systemic concentration with a reduction of unwanted side effects. Radioactive labeling showed the accumulation of liposomes in the inflamed target organ. More specifically, ^{3}H-labeled prednisolone liposomes showed selective targeting to the inflamed CNS, where up to 4.5-fold higher radioactivity was achieved compared to healthy control animals. Moreover, much higher and more persistent levels of prednisolone in the spinal cord were detected by liposomal administration than in the case of free administrated drug. Gold-labeled liposomes were used, while they could be detected in the spinal cord within the vascular endothelium, as well as in inflammatory macrophages, microglial cells, and astrocytes. The BBB disruption, the T-cell and macrophage infiltration, and the percentage of tumor necrosis factor-α (TNF-α) in these cells were monitored, indicating superior performance by the liposomal administration of prednisolone. It was also reported that a single injection of the liposomes clearly ameliorated the course of adoptive transfer EAE and EAE induced by immunization. The authors finally stated that the liposomal prednisolone was found to be highly effective in the treatment of EAE, being superior to a five-fold higher dose of free methylprednisolone, possibly due to liposomal targeting.

Later, Gailard et al. [79] used PEGylated liposomes conjugated to the brain-targeting ligand glutathione (GSH-PEG), in order to optimally improve the therapeutic window of methylprednisolone, composed of hydro soy phosphatidylcholine lipid (Lipoid, Cham, Switzerland). The authors chose the GSH-PEG liposomes because they include the safety of the liposomal constituents, the ability to encapsulate compounds without modification, the prolonged plasma exposure, and the possibility to enhance drug delivery to the brain. The prepared liposomes were administrated to rats with acute EAE. Apart from the prolonged plasma circulation and increased brain uptake as revealed by the pharmacokinetic analysis, the treatment with GSH-PEG liposomes was found to be significantly more effective in EAE as compared to PEG liposomes, while the same dose level of free methylprednisolone even worsened disease outcome. The rats received intravenous treatment, before disease onset, at disease onset, or at the peak of disease. Free methylprednisolone and non-targeted pegylated (PEG) liposomal methylprednisolone served as control treatments. It was reported that, when the treatment was initiated at disease onset, free methylprednisolone showed no effect, while GSH-PEG liposomal methylprednisolone significantly reduced the clinical signs to 42% ± 6.4% of the saline control, confirming that GSH-PEG liposomes improve the therapeutic availability of methylprednisolone and, therefore, a lower dose and lower dosing frequency can be used to obtain an effective brain concentration.

Lee et al. [80] further exploited the efficacy of the GSH-PEG liposomes carrying methylprednisolone, by using mice exhibiting murine myelin oligodendrocyte-induced EAE (MOG-EAE). This animal model mimics many neurodegenerative features of MS, including axonal damage. The experimental protocol was as follows: after the disease onset, mice were randomized to receive saline, three injections of free drug (high dose methylprednisolone), two injections of free drug (low dose methylprednisolone), or two injections of liposomes. The infiltration of T cells and macrophage/microglia, the amount of astrocyte activation, the extent of axonal loss, and the demyelination in spinal cord lesions were also monitored, indicating good performance of liposomes compared to a low dose of the free drug. Treatment with a low dose of liposomes significantly reduced the severity of EAE, similar to treatment with high-dose free drug but at one-tenth of the dosage, while a low dose of free methylprednisolone was not effective. The proposed liposomes were clinically and histologically effective as a high dose of free drug, thus allowing treatment by liposomal administration at a lower application frequency.

More recently, sterically stabilized liposomes were designed by Turjeman et al. [81] in order to carry glucocorticosteroids and treat the neuroinflammation presented in MS. More specifically, the authors investigated the remote loading of the "water-soluble", amphipathic weak acid glucocorticosteroid prodrug methylprednisolone hemisuccinate (MPS) or the amphipathic weak base nitroxide tempamine (TMN) and compared the effect of passive targeting alone and of active targeting based on short peptide fragments of ApoE or of β-amyloid. The stealthiness of the liposomes was achieved by incorporating the PEG-DSPE-2000 lipid (Genzyme Pharmaceuticals, Liestal, Switzerland). The peptide-conjugated sterically stabilized liposomes (actively targeted) were prepared via the covalent attachment of either ApoE or β-amyloid to dioleoyl (DO)-succinate, in order to form the lipidated peptides. These two peptides can be transported through the BBB. In addition to the physicochemical and thermotropic characterization of the fabricated liposomes, the EAE mice model was used, in order to monitor their therapeutic efficacy, while its mechanism of action in both the acute and the adoptive transfer EAE models was investigated. According to the results, for the liposomes carrying

MPS, active targeting is not superior to passive targeting. For both groups of liposomes, carrying MPS or TMN, it was demonstrated that these nano-drugs ameliorated the clinical signs and the pathology of EAE. The authors concluded that the highly efficacious anti-inflammatory therapeutic feature of these two nano-drugs meets the criteria of disease-modifying drugs and supports further development and evaluation of these nano-drugs as potential therapeutic agents for diseases with an inflammatory component.

The prevalence of autoimmunity is on the rise, and there is no cure for any autoimmune disease, caused by the loss of tolerance to self. Apart from delivering drugs, liposomes were applied as immunotherapy, due to their ability of apoptosis to induce immunological tolerance. One of the mechanisms to maintain self-tolerance is the efficient removal of apoptotic cells. For example, liposomes were generated mimicking apoptotic β-cells, where they arrest autoimmunity in type 1 diabetes, through specific and definitive re-establishment of tolerance. This type of liposome was also investigated to be applied in other autoimmune diseases, such as MS. More analytically, phosphatidylserine-rich liposomes were prepared and loaded with MS-specific autoantigen and, more specifically, the myelin-oligodendrocyte glycoprotein peptide 40–55 (MOG_{40-55}), in order to co-deliver a double signal of tolerance and specificity to arrest autoimmunity in a synergistic, effective, and safe manner. Phosphatidylserine is considered to be the main "eat me" and "tolerate me" signal of the apoptotic cell membrane, which allows recognition and phagocytosis by antigen-presenting cells, such as dendritic cells. According to the results, the prepared liposomes induced a tolerogenic phenotype in dendritic cells and arrested autoimmunity, while they were efficiently phagocytosed by dendritic cells and induced tolerogenic features in dendritic cells. Moreover, after immunization administration, the MOG-loaded phosphatidylserine liposomes reduced the incidence and severity of EAE, as well as delayed the onset of the disease, correlating with an increase in the regulatory CD25+ FoxP3− CD4+ T-cell subset. The authors concluded that the proposed nanosystems exhibit high potential to operate as a platform for MS and autoimmune diseases [82].

3.1.3. Other Lipid-Based Nanocarriers

Binyamin et al. [83] developed a nanodroplet formulation of pomegranate seed oil (PSO), denominated as nano-PSO, which was an oil-in-water (O/W) nanoemulsion (Figure 2A) administrated in an EAE model. PSO comprises high levels of punicic acid, a unique poly-unsaturated fatty acid considered as one of the strongest natural antioxidants. Nano-PSO was supposed to enhance the bioavailability and activity of PSO. According to the results, the beneficial effect of PSO was increased significantly when EAE mice were treated with nano-PSO of specific size nanodroplets (200 nm) size and much lower concentrations of the oil. Nano-PSO was also beneficial to the EAE mice when treatment commenced close to disease manifestation (day 7) and not only when administered concomitant with disease induction, highlighting its potential to abrogate the disease progression and not only prevent it. Pathological examinations revealed that nano-PSO administration dramatically reduced demyelination and oxidation of lipids in the brains of the affected animals, even in the existence of immune infiltrates in the CNS. Nano-PSO may be a good choice for individuals at the initial stages of MS, as well as at later stages, where it may be used in combination with advanced MS treatments such as natalizumab or antioxidant formulations. Last but not least, nano-PSO was also beneficial in the prevention and treatment of genetic prion disease model, indicating that reagents that can prevent lipid oxidation may be beneficial for an array of neurodegenerative diseases.

Most recently, Lu et al. [84] tried to take advantage of the significant role of the monocytes in the process of MS and, thus, developed a targeting immunomodulatory carrier from high-density lipoprotein-mimicking peptide–phospholipid scaffold (HPPS), which can target monocytes, in order to improve the bioavailability of curcumin. Monocytes are considered to be mediators and immunomodulation targets because they are considered to be similar to most of the amplified inflammatory monocytes crossing the BBB, to promote neuron injury and recruit more immune cells to infiltrate the CNS. More specifically, peripheral monocytes were chosen as the immunomodulation targets and curcumin as the anti-inflammatory agent, which was delivered by HPPS nanoparticles. The nanoparticles were taken up efficiently, specifically by monocytes through the scavenger receptor class B type I (SR-B1) receptor, which is a receptor of high-density lipoprotein (HDL) that is highly expressed in the peripheral monocytes; thus, the proposed nanoparticles could be used for early detection of CNS inflammation in EAE. The nanoparticle distribution in monocytes was confirmed in vivo by using optical imaging, while the nanoparticles were loaded with a fluorescent dye. According to the results, the delivery of curcumin by HPPS nanoparticles hindered inflammatory monocytes across the BBB in EAE mice, owing to the downregulation of intercellular adhesion molecules 1 (ICAM-1) and macrophage-1 antigen (MAC-1) expression in the monocytes by inhibiting the activation of the nuclear factor-κB (NF-κB). Moreover, the proposed nanoparticles inhibited the proliferation of microglia and restricted the infiltration of other effect or immune cells, such as TH1, TH17, and myeloid cells, due to the blockade of inflammatory monocyte infiltration, resulting in the reduction of EAE morbidity from 100% (10 of 10 mice exhibited EAE pathology in the phosphate-buffered saline (PBS) group) to 30% (three of 10 mice showed mild clinical signs). The authors concluded that the targeted modulation of monocytes with such HPPS nanoparticles, carrying therapeutic and/or imaging agents, offers a novel strategy for MS diagnosis and treatment.

MicroRNAs were postulated as a promising tool to induce OPC differentiation and, therefore, remyelination, albeit exhibiting significant limitations in terms of the administration of microRNAs to the CNS. Osorio-Querejeta et al. [85] utilized three different categories of nanosystems for miR-219a-5p encapsulation, release, and remyelination promotion, namely, liposomes from 1,2-dioctadecanoyl-sn-glycero-3-phosphocholine (DSPC) lipid (Avanti Polar Lipids, Alabaster, AL, USA), poly(lactic-*co*-glycolic) acid polymeric nanoparticles, and finally biologically engineered extracellular vesicles overexpressing miR-219a-5p, which are also lipid-based, due to their biological origin. Extracellular vesicles are biological delivery systems that contain other proteins, lipids, and genetic material, apart from RNA, which can be integrated into the cell in several ways, and which contain microRNA-processing molecules. The three nanosystem categories were compared by assessing their ability to induce OPC differentiation in a primary oligodendrocyte precursor cell culture and cross the BBB. According to the results, on the one hand, the liposomes and the polymeric nanoparticles were able to entrap higher amounts of miR-219a-5p and showed higher uptake levels than extracellular vesicles. On the other hand, the extracellular vesicles, due to their biological complexity, were surprisingly the only delivery system that was able to induce a significant OPC differentiation, while they also showed the highest BBB permeability levels. Finally, the EAE animal model was used to study the remyelination potential of the extracellular vesicles. The intranasally administered miR-219a-5p-enriched extracellular vesicles successfully decreased clinical scores in the EAE model, without affecting the tested anti-inflammatory pathways. As the authors concluded, the significant differences in clinical score observed after the disease peak indicate that extracellular vesicles might be increasing the myelin production.

3.2. *Polymer-Based Nanosystems*

Several types of polymers and their respective nanoparticles were studied for efficient BBB crossing, the delivery of therapeutic agents to the CNS, and their contribution to the treatment of neurodegenaration diseases, such as MS. Polymer nanoparticles can be prepared using various synthetic and natural monomers/polymers and via different preparation methods. Their surface can also be functionalized for specific brain targeting. It is crucial for the used polymers in manufacturing these nanocarriers to be biocompatible and biodegradable. The mechanisms for brain uptake and drug release to the CNS of the polymeric nanoparticles involve endocytosis or transcytosis through the endothelial cells, as well as accumulation in the brain capillaries, resulting in transfer to the brain parenchyma, owing to the high concentration gradient, and membrane fluidization through lipid solubilization, due to the surfactant effect and tight junctions opening. One of their most significant advantage is their potential to be easily surface-functionalized by the conjugation of targeting peptides or cell-penetrating ligands, in order to improve their targeting ability and crossing through the BBB [86].

3.2.1. Poly(Lactic-*co*-Glycolic Acid) (PLGA) Polymeric Nanoparticles

Polymeric poly(lactic-*co*-glycolic acid) (PLGA) or poly(lactide-*co*-glycolide) (PLG) nanoparticles are attractive carriers due to their biodegradability, bio-compatibility, and approval by the FDA. One of the key advantages of using PGLA nanoparticles is that they can be easily loaded with a wide variety of molecules. The degradation kinetics of nanoparticles and the release rate of the encapsulated molecules can be easily monitored by controlling the PGLA physicochemical properties, such as the lactide-to-glycolide ratio, molecular weight, crystal profile, storage temperature, and surface coating materials [87–91].

"Inverse vaccination" includes antigen-specific tolerogenic immunization treatments that are capable of inhibiting autoimmune responses, exhibiting great therapeutic potential in MS. Antigen-specific treatments are highly desirable for autoimmune diseases in contrast to treatments which induce systemic immunosuppression. Several myelin proteins, such as MBP, PLP, and MOG, were implicated as targets of autoreactive T cells in MS and EAE [92]. The use of protein-based inverse vaccines in the EAE model, loaded in polymeric biodegradable PLGA nanoparticles, in order to obtain the sustained release of antigens and regulatory adjuvants, can be an alternative strategy to overcome the main obstacles of the administration of free myelin antigens, which exhibit rapid clearance, or of the DNA-based vaccines encoding for myelin autoantigens, whose potential risks limit their use in humans. These data suggest that subcutaneous PLGA nanoparticle-based inverse vaccination maybe an effective tool to treat autoimmune diseases (Figure 3), such as MS, and reduce the significant toxicity, as well as the high costs, caused by the chronic therapies [93,94].

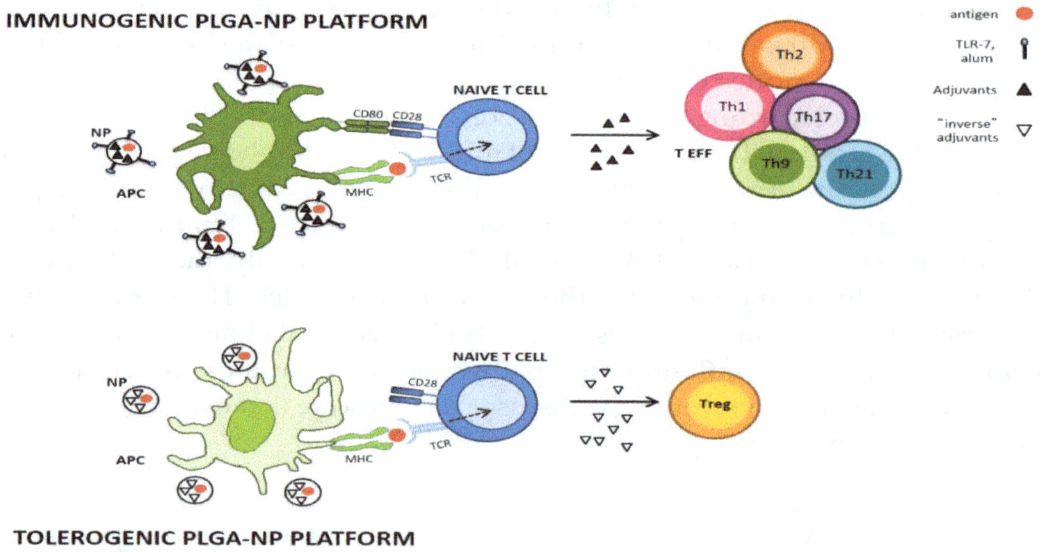

Figure 3. Immunogenic and tolerogenic poly(lactic-*co*-glycolic acid) (PLGA) NP (nanoparticle) platforms. Immunogenic PLGA-NPs may include standard adjuvants such as alum or Toll-like receptor 7 (TLR-7) agonists, capable of activating APCs (antigen-presenting cells) and promoting naïve T-cell differentiation into effector T cells (TEFFs); on the contrary, in the absence of costimulatory signals, tolerogenic PLGA-NPs by employing "inverse adjuvants" induce tolerogenic APCs that lead to the expansion of antigen-specific regulatory T cells (Tregs). The dotted arrow indicates activation of naïve T cells, and the solid arrow indicates its differentiation into TEFFs or Tregs. Adapted from Cappellano et al. [94].

Cappellano et al. [93] developed PLGA nanoparticles loaded with either the immunodominant 35–55 epitope of MOG (MOG_{35-55}) in C57BL/6 mice or the recombinant interleukin-10 (IL-10), used as an inverse adjuvant, for prophylactic and therapeutic treatment of a chronic progressive model of EAE.

The authors prepared 65:35 PLGA nanoparticles because they slowly release the loaded molecule for several weeks, which was also confirmed in vitro, and they display minimal cell toxicity along with low intrinsic adjuvant activity. More specifically, the prepared nanoparticles did not display cytotoxic or proinflammatory activity and were partially endocytosed by phagocytes. The prepared nanoparticles loaded with IL-10 completely lost their ability to induce secretion of TNF-α in vitro in peripheral blood mononuclear cells, while the in vivo subcutaneous injection of the prepared nanoparticles in C57BL/6 mice, loaded with either MOG_{35-55} or IL-10, being both simultaneously injected, ameliorated the course of EAE in both prophylactic and therapeutic vaccination. The EAE onset was earlier in the prophylactic vaccination than in the therapeutic vaccination, which suggests that pre-treatment with the PLGA nanoparticles may precondition the induction of EAE by stimulating the innate immunity. Contrariwise, immunization with only one type of nanoparticle, loaded with either MOG_{35-55} or IL-10, did not have any effect. Moreover, they decreased the histopathological lesions in the central nervous tissue, the inflammation, and the T-cell infiltration in the CNS, as well as the secretion of proinflammatory cytokines IL-17 and interferon (IFN)-γ induced by MOG_{35-55} in splenic T cells in vitro.

Maldonaldo et al. [95] developed synthetic, biodegradable PLGA nanoparticles loaded with the immunodominant 139–151 epitope of myelin proteolipid protein ($PLP_{139-151}$) together with the tolerogenic immunomodulator rapamycin, used as an inverse adjuvant, in order to induce durable and antigen-specific immune tolerance, even in the presence of potent Toll-like receptor agonists and control both cellular and humoral immune responses. The nanoparticles were administrated in a relapse remitting model of EAE in mice. According to the results, the treatment, by either subcutaneous or intravenous administration, with tolerogenic nanoparticles results in the inhibition of the activation of the antigen-specific CD4+ and CD8+ T cell, an increase in regulatory cells, durable B-cell tolerance with resistance to multiple immunogenic challenges, and the inhibition of antigen-specific hypersensitivity reactions at relapsing EAE. More specifically, when Swiss Jack Lambert (SJL) mice were immunized with the $PLP_{139-151}$ peptide in complete Freud's adjuvant ($PLP_{139-151}$/CFA) and treated therapeutically with a single dose of tolerogenic nanoparticles at the peak of disease, the mice were completely protected from developing relapsing paralysis. Prophylactic treatment using these nanoparticles inhibited the onset of EAE, whereas the therapeutic treatment inhibited relapse. Moreover, an inhibition of the neutralizing antibody responses against coagulation factor VIII in hemophilia A mice, was observed, even in animals previously sensitized to antigen. Only the encapsulated rapamycin and not the free form in solution could induce immunological tolerance, preventing both cellular and humoral immunity. The authors concluded that therapy with tolerogenic nanoparticles can be applied against allergies and autoimmune diseases, such as MS, as well as for the prevention of antidrug antibodies against biologic therapies.

Cho et al. [96] developed a formulation of dual-sized, polymeric microparticles from PLGA, referred as dMPs, which were loaded with multiple immunomodulatory factors, namely, specific antigen and tolerizing factors, targeting both intra- and extracellular tolerogenic receptors, in order to block the autoimmunity. The epitope MOG_{35-55}, along with vitamin D, was encapsulated in the phagocytosable small particles, while transforming growth factor beta 1 (TGF-β1) and granulocyte-macrophage colony-stimulating factor (GM-CSF) were encapsulated in the large non-phagocytosable particles. According to the results, the administration of the dMPs resulted in a reduction of infiltrating CD4+ T cells, inflammatory cytokine-producing pathogenic CD4+ T cells, activated macrophages, and microglia in the CNS, as well as reduced frequency of $CD86^{hi}MHCII^{hi}$ dendritic cells in draining lymph nodes of EAE mice. Thus, the formulation was successfully recruited and modulated the dendritic cells toward a tolerogenic phenotype, while also exhibiting a local controlled release and achieving robust durable antigen-specific autoimmune protection.

Tolerogenic PLGA nanoparticles can also function as on-target and direct modulators of myelin-autoreactive T cells without eliciting the intervention of tolerogenic dendritic cells. Pei et al. [97] developed PLGA nanoparticles for the encapsulation of multiple regulatory molecules. More specifically, the TGF-β was encapsulated in nanoparticles that were surface-decorated by multimers of MHC class I and II molecules loaded with myelin peptides to target autoreactive T cells (MOG_{40-54}/H-2D^b-Ig dimer, MOG_{35-55}/I-A^b multimer), by the regulatory molecules (anti-Fas, PD-L1-Fc), being capable of inducing apoptosis or dysfunction of the autoreactive T cells bound to the MHC multimers, or by the "self-marker" CD47-Fc, being able to inhibit nanoparticle phagocytosis. The suggested nanoparticles exhibited a size of 217 nm and were administrated by intravenous infusion, where they were capable of durably ameliorating EAE, with a marked reduction of clinical score, neuroinflammation, and demyelination. Their mechanism of action was based on the inhibition of the myelin-autoreactive T-cell surface presentation of multiple ligands and the paracrine release of cytokine. According to the results, the MOG_{35-55}-reactive Th1 and Th17 cells, as well as the MOG_{40-55}-reactive Tc1 and Tc17 cells, were decreased, and the regulatory T cells were increased, while inhibited T-cell proliferation and elevated T-cell apoptosis in the spleen took place.

Another report on inducing peripheral, antigen-specific T-cell tolerance for treatment of MS describes the use of biodegradable PLG tolerogenic nanoparticles, being loaded with myelin antigens ($PLP_{139-151}$ and $OVA_{323-339}$ (ovalbumin)) and administrated in mice with relapsing/remitting EAE. PLG particles were fabricated on-site via an emulsion process with modifications using poly(ethylene-*co*-maleic acid) as a surfactant (PLG-PEMA), in order to increase their ability to couple with peptides and to prevent disease induction. In addition to the characterization of the physical properties of the particles, their safety and their therapeutic efficacy for EAE were evaluated by clinical score, histology, and flow cytometric assessment of CNS inflammatory cell infiltration. Their intravenous infusion yielded a significant improvement in the ongoing disease and subsequent relapses when administered at onset or at peak of acute disease, as well as a minimization of epitope spreading when administered during disease remission, resulting in complete long-term protection from disease with superior effects to the already existing commercial PLG nanoparticles. The tolerance was induced by the combined effects of T-cell anergy and the activation of Treg. According to the results, there were reduced CNS infiltration of encephalitogenic Th1 (IFN-γ) and Th17 (IL-17a) cells, as well as inflammatory monocytes/macrophages and demyelination in the CNS of the treated animals [98].

Casey et al. [99] compared the differences between the intravenous and subcutaneous administration of PLG nanoparticles containing disease-relevant antigens (denoted as silver nanoparticles (Ag-NPs)), being surface decorated with TGF-β. The purpose of Ag-NP therapies is to treat autoimmunity. Although the Ag-NPs being intravenously administrated exhibit antigen (Ag)-specific immune tolerance in models of autoimmunity, there is a lower efficacy with subcutaneous administration. Thus, the authors tried to investigate whether the co-delivery of the immunomodulatory cytokine TGF-β using the Ag-NPs would modulate the immune response to Ag-NPs and improve the efficiency of tolerance induction. The selected antigen was $PLP_{139-151}$. An in vitro co-culture system of bone marrow-derived dendritic cells (BMDCs) and naive T cells was used to evaluate the bioactivity and the immunomodulatory effects of the Ag-NPs with TGF-β, by monitoring the surface costimulatory markers and inflammatory cytokine production. According to the results, the Ag-NPs with TGF-β provided Ag-specific T-cell stimulation, decreased co-stimulatory molecule presentation, and suppressed inflammatory cytokine secretions. The in vivo Treg frequency and number were measured following the injection of particles into OT-II mice that expressed $OVA_{323-339}$-restricted T-cell receptors, resulting in the surface binding of TGF-β to PLGA-NPs loaded with OVA being required to efficiently induce tolerance to OVA in an antigen-specific manner. Finally, the ability of surface-bound TGF-β to enhance the tolerogenicity of Ag-NPs was evaluated using the EAE mouse model in the context of intravenous and subcutaneous administration routes, revealing improved efficacy at lower doses by intravenous administration and significantly reduced disease severity by subcutaneous administration. Thus, subcutaneous inverse vaccination needs inverse adjuvants in order to be effective.

Getts et al. [100] used either polystyrene or biodegradable PLG microparticles bearing encephalitogenic peptides, being administrated by intravenous infusion, in order to prevent the onset and modify the course of the disease. These antigen-decorated microparticles, exhibiting an approximate 500-nm diameter induced a long-term T-cell tolerance in mice with relapsing EAE. The chosen antigen for the nanoparticle decoration was MOG_{35-55}, being covalently linked to the surface of the nanoparticle. This treatment reduced the inflammatory cell infiltration and the damage of the CNS. The authors stated that the beneficial effect of these antigen-linked particles requires the scavenger receptor MARCO, being expressed at the marginal zone macrophages. Moreover, the results of the treatment were also monitored by the activity of regulatory T cells, the abortive T-cell activation, and the T-cell anergy. The obtained results highlighted the potential for using microparticles in order to target natural apoptotic clearance pathways, to inactivate pathogenic T cells, to stop the disease process in autoimmunity, and to treat T-cell-based autoimmune disorders, by inducing T-cell tolerance.

Kuo et al. [101] investigated the effect of the amount of antigen conjugated to PLG nanoparticles, as well as of the nanoparticle dose for the induction of immune tolerance, during the treatment of MS with disease-relevant antigens. More specifically, different amounts of the $PLP_{139-151}$ antigen were loaded in PLG nanoparticles that were intravenously administrated in vivo, in different doses to mice with EAE. As a result, the amounts of antigen conjugation and nanoparticle dose were correlated with the severity of EAE. More specifically, the high dose of PLG nanoparticles carrying high amounts of $PLP_{139-151}$ significantly decreased the severity of the EAE with a more durable immune tolerance, also preventing relapses, while a low dose of the nanoparticles carrying high amounts of the antigen or a high dose of the nanoparticles carrying low antigen amounts were not so efficient, as indicated by the observed relapses. The increase of nanoparticle dose and antigen amount was also correlated with the suppression of inflammatory signaling pathways in vitro. Through the analysis of the cells expressing MHC-restricted antigen, significant decreases in positive co-stimulatory molecules (CD86, CD80, and CD40) and a high expression of a negative co-stimulatory molecule (PD-L1) were found in high doses of both nanoparticles and with high antigen conjugation. Tolerance induction was evaluated by co-culturing cells administrated with the nanoparticles and autoreactive T cells isolated from mice immunized against $PLP_{139-151}$. According to the results, reduced T-cell proliferation, increased T-cell apoptosis, and a stronger anti-inflammatory response were observed.

More recently, Saito et al. [102] investigated whether the use of multiple nanoparticle formulations and the extent of antigen loading at the carrier could impact the immune cell internalization and polarization of the immune cells that get associated with the particles and the subsequent disease progression. The nanoparticles were administrated for antigen-specific immunotherapy for the efficient induction of tolerance in the EAE disease model. More specifically, the formulation was composed of three polymeric carriers, 50:50 poly (DL-lactide-*co*-glycolide) with inherent viscosity (IV) = 0.17 dL/g and 0.66 dL/g (termed agPLG-L and agPLG-H, respectively), and poly(DL-lactide) (PLA) particles with IV = 0.21 dL/g (termed agPLA) loaded with the disease-specific antigen myelin protein ($PLP_{139-151}$), being administrated in a single injection for mice with EAE. According to the results, at a low particle dose, mice treated with PLA-based particles had significantly lower clinical scores at the chronic stage, while neither PLG-based particles nor OVA control particles reduced the clinical scores. Moreover, the higher antigen loading PLA-based particles helped to reduce inflammation during the acute stage of the disease, as well as completely ameliorate EAE over 200 days, along with the inhibition of Th1 and Th17 polarization, allowing a smaller particle dosage and, thus, fewer potential adverse effects. PLA, which was correlated with a more tolerogenic polarization of the antigen-presenting cells, was found to be a more efficacious platform relative to PLG. Fluorescently labeled particles were employed to examine the biodistributions among the organs, the interaction with specific antigen-presenting cells within the organs, and the resulting phenotypes. Compared to PLG-based particles, PLA-based particles, interacting with antigen-presenting cells, were largely associated with Kupffer cells and liver sinusoidal endothelial cells, reducing the CD4+ T-cell populations that were activated locally and not trafficked in the CNS.

In addition to antigen-specific tolerogenic immunization, the PLGA nanoparticles were also employed in the remyelination strategy. Rittchen et al. [103] developed a PLGA nanoparticle-based strategy for the targeted delivery of leukemia inhibitory factor (LIF) to OPCs, in order to promote their differentiation into mature oligodendrocytes that are able to repair myelin. Among the potential therapeutics that promote remyelination is the LIF, a cytokine known to play a key regulatory role in self-tolerant immunity and recently identified as a promyelination factor. However, LIF is rapidly degraded in vivo, and high doses may have unwanted off-target effects; therefore, a nanotechnology strategy could help toward its targeted delivery to OPCs. In detail, PLGA-based nanoparticles of ~120 nm diameter were prepared, loaded with LIF (LIF-NP), and functionalized with surface antibodies against NG-2 chondroitin sulfate proteoglycan, expressed on OPCs. The nanoparticle platform used in this study previously featured in clinical trials (e.g., Clinicaltrials.gov NCT01812746, NCT01792479). According to the in vitro results, the NG2-targeted LIF-NPs bound to OPCs activated pSTAT-3 signaling and induced OPC differentiation into mature oligodendrocytes. As per the in vivo results, where a model of focal CNS demyelination was used, the NG2-targeted LIF-NP increased myelin repair, at the level of both increased number of myelinated axons and increased thickness (maturity of sheath) of myelin per axon. The authors also noted that the potency was high, because even a single dose of nanoparticles delivering picomolar quantities of LIF was sufficient to increase remyelination. The nanoparticles were added intralesionally, as a proof of concept, confirming the powerful potential of this delivery system as a targeted approach to deliver bioactive molecules for in situ myelin repair. The authors concluded that, for translation into clinical use, it is notable that the intravenously delivered nanoparticles should be able to cross the BBB, at least in rodents, or they can be delivered intranasally directly to the CNS, bypassing the BBB.

3.2.2. Other Polymeric Nanoparticles

Führmann et al. [104] tried to exploit the physiopathology of MS, regarding the presence of leaky permeable blood vessels, where fibrinogen and nidogen are progressively upregulated after disease onset. Peptide-modified polymeric nanoparticles that are able to target the blood clots and the extracellular matrix (ECM) molecules, such as nidogen, can be used for the targeted drug delivery and the reduction of "off-target" effects. More specifically, poly(ethylene glycol)-*block*-poly(caprolactone) (PEG-*b*-PCL) nanoparticles, functionalized with fibrin peptides, were developed. The prepared nanoparticles were administrated in rats that exhibited EAE along with upregulation of fibrin and nidogen/entactin-1. The administrated nanoparticles showed enhanced binding to these targets and to lesion sites ex vivo and in vivo, compared to non-functionalized or scrambled-peptide control nanoparticles. By using a minimally invasive technique, the active targeting of leaky blood vessels in the diseased spinal cord of animals with EAE can be achieved after the systemic injection of fibrin-targeting nanoparticles. Thus, increased drug concentrations at the site of injury, reduction of undesirable side effects of systemic delivery, and enhanced efficacy of hydrophobic drugs can be achieved in MS conditions.

In another study [105] employing PCL nanoparticles, the recombinant human myelin basic protein (rhMBP) was purified from the milk of transgenic cows, by using a vacuum-driven cation exchanger, and it was formulated into PCL nanoparticles in order to achieve an rhMBP controlled release kinetic, fabricating a therapeutic vaccine for protection against EAE symptoms in mice. RhMBP-loaded PCL nanoparticles were prepared and characterized in terms of entrapment efficiency, size, morphology, charge, and release pattern. The nanoparticles were optimized, until discrete spherical, rough-surfaced rhMBP nanoparticles with small particle size, high surface charge, lower concentration of stabilizer, and intermediate concentration of polymer were obtained, in order to achieve high entrapment efficiency and a controlled release pattern. According to the in vivo results, after the subcutaneous administration of free or rhMBP nanoparticles before EAE induction, the average behavioral score in EAE mice was reduced, and only mild histological alterations and preservation of myelin sheath were observed, indicating increased protection and enhanced efficacy of rhMBP as a therapeutic vaccine due to the nanoformulation. Being hydrophobic, the PCL nanoparticles provided an improved drug delivery system for rhMBP, enabling it to cross the BBB and deliver rhMBP into the mice brains, while the differences in activity between the immediate release and sustained release of the nanoparticle formulations were highlighted. Moreover, the analysis of inflammatory cytokines (IFN-γ and IL-10) in mice brains revealed that the pre-treatment with free or rhMBP nanoparticles significantly protected against EAE-induced behavioral, histopathological, and inflammatory changes.

Lunin et al. [106] developed poly(butylcyanoacrylate) (PBCA) nanoparticles, in order to deliver the thymic peptide thymulin and prolong its presence in the blood of mice with relapsing/remitting EAE (rEAE). The increase in the blood content of thymulin, which is depleted with age, and the prolongation of its blood half-life, alone or in combination with other treatments, may be a prospective strategy for treatment of chronic inflammatory conditions, such as MS. More analytically, as revealed by the results, thymulin significantly decreased symptoms of rEAE and lowered plasma cytokine levels, both in early and in later stages of rEAE, as well as decreased the NF-κB and stress-activated protein kinase/Jun amino-terminal kinase (SAPK/JNK) cascade activation, as confirmed by ELISA measurements of cytokine levels in the blood. In terms of the cytokine response in rEAE, it was multi-staged, where an early phase was accompanied by an increase in plasma IFN-γ, while the IL-17 response was markedly increased at a later stage. According to the results, the nanoparticle-bound thymulin had enhanced efficacy in comparison to the effect of free thymulin.

Kondiah et al. [107] synthesized a pH-sensitive copolymer (TMC-PEGDMA-MAA) from trimethyl-chitosan (TMC), poly(ethylene glycol)dimethacrylate (PEGDMA), and methacrylic acid (MAA), via free radical suspension polymerization, in order to produce microparticles for the oral delivery of IFN-β. The polymer was designed to possess pH-sensitive, mucoadhesive, and hydrophilic properties. A Box–Behnken experimental design was used for optimization of the formulation, where varying concentrations of TMC and percentage crosslinker (polyethylene glycol diacrylate) were investigated. The prepared copolymeric microparticulate system was characterized for its morphological, porositometric, and mucoadhesive properties. The optimized microparticles with 0.5 g/100 mL TMC and 3% crosslinker had an IFN-β loading efficiency of 53.25%. The microparticles were subsequently compressed into a suitable oral tablet formulation. The in vitro release of IFN-β had a pH-sensitive pattern, being increased in intestinal (pH 6.8) and decreased in gastric (pH 1.2) environments. Regarding the in vivo results, the tablets were orally administrated in the New Zealand White rabbit, and the plasma concentration of IFN-β was compared to a known subcutaneous formulation during a 24-h blood sampling procedure. The IFN-β-loaded particulate system demonstrated a remarkable drug release in vivo, greater than the subcutaneous commercial formulation (Rebif®) over a 24-h duration, with a larger bioavailable IFN-β concentration after 2 h.

Youssef et al. [108] investigated the effect of intranasal administration of LINGO-1-directed small interfering RNA (siRNA)-loaded chitosan nanoparticles on demyelination and remyelination processes in a rat model of demyelination. Chitosan nanoparticles are one of the most studied polymers in non-viral siRNA delivery, due to their polycationic nature and biocompatibility. Suppression of LINGO-1 by different strategies, such as LINGO-1 gene knockout or infusion of LINGO-1 antagonists, was associated with enhancement of remyelination in different animal models of CNS demyelination. The RNA interference is a new strategy to block LINGO-1 expression in the target lesions with low doses and fewer systemic side effects, provided that there are efficient gene delivery carriers. In detail, the authors studied whether the nasal administration of LINGO-1-directed siRNA-loaded chitosan nanoparticles in rats could inhibit pontine LINGO-1 expression and enhance the remyelination in a model of demyelination induced by ethidium bromide (EB). The chitosan nanoparticle dose was given alone after the induction of EB in rats that were categorized into demyelination and remyelination groups. According to the results, following the LINGO-1-directed siRNA–chitosan nanoparticle treatment, the animals performed better than controls. Specifically, the remyelination-treated group showed better motor performance than the demyelination group. LINGO-1 downregulation was associated with signs of repair in histopathological sections, higher expression of pontine myelin basic protein (MBP) messenger RNA (mRNA) and protein, and lower levels of caspase-3 activity, indicating neuroprotection and remyelination enhancement.

4. Conclusions

Drug delivery into the CNS is one of the most inhibitory points in the treatment of MS. Nanotechnology opened a new window for the treatment of MS and created promising opportunities by providing drug delivery nanosystems, as well as tolerance-inducing nanocarriers. On the one hand, several novel promising drug delivery systems are being developed for the targeted delivery of MS therapeutics and remyelinating agents into the CNS, in order to increase their therapeutic efficiency and decrease the unwanted side effects that are caused by the high doses. On the other hand, tolerance-inducing nanocarriers can be used as promising vaccines for antigen-specific immunotherapy. Currently, numerous studies describe the successful administration and the promising results of various nanoparticles, both lipidic and polymeric, in the EAE animal model at the preclinical stage, although there is a lack of clinical data in MS patients. Finally, the great potential in the improvement of nanotechnological formulations via the proper monitoring of their physical characteristics or the right choice and functionalization of their biomaterials continually creates future perspectives for the upgrade of current MS therapies.

Author Contributions: Writing—original draft preparation, M.C.; writing—review and editing, C.D.; visualization, M.C.; supervision, C.D. All authors read and agreed to the published version of the manuscript.

References

1. Compston, A.; Coles, A. Multiple sclerosis. *Lancet* **2002**, *359*, 1221–1231. [CrossRef]
2. Passos, G.R.D.; Sato, D.K.; Becker, J.; Fujihara, K. Th17Cells pathways in multiple sclerosis and neuromyelitis optica spectrum disorders: Pathophysiological and therapeutic implications. *Mediat. Inflamm.* **2016**, *2016*, 5314541. [CrossRef]
3. Koch, M.W.; Metz, L.M.; Kovalchuk, O. Epigenetic changes in patients with multiple sclerosis. *Nat. Rev. Neurol.* **2013**, *9*, 35–43. [CrossRef] [PubMed]
4. Tillery, E.E.; Clements, J.N.; Howard, Z. What's new in multiple sclerosis? *Ment. Health Clin.* **2018**, *7*, 213–220. [CrossRef] [PubMed]
5. Boissy, A.R.; Cohen, J.A. Multiple sclerosis symptom management. *Expert Rev. Neurother.* **2007**, *7*, 1213–1222. [CrossRef] [PubMed]
6. Pugliatti, M.; Rosati, G.; Carton, H.; Riise, T.; Drulovic, J.; Vecsei, L.; Milanov, I. The Epidemiology of Multiple Sclerosis in Europe. *Eur. J. Neurol.* **2006**, *13*, 700–722. [CrossRef]
7. Dendrou, C.A.; Fugger, L.; Friese, M.A. Immunopathology of multiple sclerosis. *Nat. Rev. Immunol.* **2015**, *15*, 545–558. [CrossRef]
8. Diebold, M. Immunological treatment of multiple sclerosis. *Semin Hematol.* **2016**, *53*, 54–57. [CrossRef]
9. Melchor, G.S.; Khan, T.; Reger, J.F.; Huang, J.K. Remyelination Pharmacotherapy Investigations Highlight Diverse Mechanisms Underlying Multiple Sclerosis Progression. *ACS Pharmacol. Transl. Sci.* **2019**, *2*, 372–386. [CrossRef]
10. Ghalamfarsa, G.; Hojjat-Farsangi, M.; Mohammadnia-Afrouzi, M.; Anvari, E.; Farhadi, S.; Yousefi, M.; Jadidi-Niaragh, F. Application of nanomedicine for crossing the blood–brain barrier: Theranostic opportunities in multiple sclerosis. *J. Immunotoxicol.* **2016**, *13*, 603–619. [CrossRef]
11. Ballerini, C.; Baldi, G.; Aldinucci, A.; Maggi, P. Nanomaterial applications in multiple sclerosis inflamed brain. *J. Neuroimmune Pharmacol.* **2015**, *10*, 1–13. [CrossRef] [PubMed]
12. Gironi, M.; Arno, C.; Comi, G.; Penton-Rol, G.; Furlan, R. Chapter 4—Multiple Sclerosis and Neurodegenerative Diseases. In *Immune Rebalancing: The Future of Immunosuppression*; Elsevier Inc.: Amsterdam, The Netherlands, 2016; pp. 63–84.
13. Leray, E.; Moreau, T.; Fromont, A.; Edan, G. Epidemiology of multiple sclerosis. *Rev. Neurol.* **2016**, *172*, 3–13. [CrossRef] [PubMed]
14. Beecham, A.H.; Patsopoulos, N.A.; Xifara, D.K.; Davis, M.F.; Kemppinen, A.; Cotsapas, C.; Shah, T.S.; Spencer, C.; Booth, D.; Goris, A.; et al. Analysis of Immune-Related Loci Identifies 48 New Susceptibility Variants for Multiple Sclerosis. *Nat. Genet.* **2013**, *45*, 1353–1360.

15. Belbasis, L.; Bellou, V.; Evangelou, E.; Ioannidis, J.P.A.; Tzoulaki, I. Environmental Risk Factors and Multiple Sclerosis: An Umbrella Review of Systematic Reviews and Meta-Analyses. *Lancet Neurol.* **2015**, *14*, 263–273. [CrossRef]
16. Hedström, A.K.; Åkerstedt, T.; Hillert, J.; Olsson, T.; Alfredsson, L. Shift Work at Young Age Is Associated with Increased Risk for Multiple Sclerosis. *Ann. Neurol.* **2011**, *70*, 733–741. [CrossRef]
17. Sadovnick, A.D.; Ebers, G.C.; Dyment, D.A.; Risch, N.J. Evidence for genetic basis of multiple sclerosis. *Lancet* **1996**, *347*, 1728–1730. [CrossRef]
18. Hemmer, B.; Nessler, S.; Zhou, D.; Kieseier, B.; Hartung, H.P. Immunopathogenesis and immunotherapy of multiple sclerosis. *Nat. Clin. Pract. Neurol.* **2006**, *2*, 201–211. [CrossRef]
19. Lublin, F.D.; Reingold, S.C.; Cohen, J.A.; Cutter, G.R.; Sørensen, P.S.; Thompson, A.J.; Wolinsky, J.S.; Balcer, L.J.; Banwell, B.; Barkhof, F.; et al. Defining the clinical course of multiple sclerosis: The 2013 revisions. *Neurology* **2014**, *83*, 278–286. [CrossRef]
20. Faissner, S.; Plemel, J.R.; Gold, R.; Yong, V.W. Progressive multiple sclerosis: From pathophysiology to therapeutic strategies. *Nat. Rev. Drug Discov.* **2019**, *18*, 905–922. [CrossRef]
21. Eckstein, C.; Bhatti, M.T. Currently approved and emerging oral therapies in multiple sclerosis: An update for the ophthalmologist. *Surv. Ophthalmol.* **2016**, *61*, 318–332. [CrossRef]
22. Ian Douglas, J.K.C.; Rompani, P.; Singhal, B.S.; Thompson, A. Multiple sclerosis. In *Neurological Disorders: Public Health Challenges*; Saraceno, B., Ed.; WHO (World Health Organization): Geneva, Switzerland, 2005; pp. 85–94.
23. Correale, J.; Gaitan, M.I.; Ysrraelit, M.C.; Fiol, M.P. Progressive multiple sclerosis: From pathogenic mechanisms to treatment. *Brain J. Neurol.* **2017**, *140*, 527–546. [CrossRef]
24. Baecher-Allan, C.; Kaskow, B.J.; Weiner, H.L. Multiple Sclerosis: Mechanisms and Immunotherapy. *Neuron* **2018**, *97*, 742–768. [CrossRef]
25. Dargahi, N.; Katsara, M.; Tselios, T.; Androutsou, M.E.; de Courten, M.; Matsoukas, J.; Apostolopoulos, V. Multiple sclerosis: Immunopathology and treatment update. *Brain Sci.* **2017**, *7*, 78. [CrossRef] [PubMed]
26. Reich, D.S.; Lucchinetti, C.F.; Calabresi, P.A. Multiple sclerosis. *N. Engl. J. Med.* **2018**, *378*, 169–180. [CrossRef] [PubMed]
27. Kallaur, A.P.; Lopes, J.; Oliveira, S.R.; Simão, A.N.; Reiche, E.M.; de Almeida, E.R.; Morimoto, H.K.; de Pereira, W.L. Immune-Inflammatory and oxidative and nitrosative stress biomarkers of depression symptoms in subjects with multiple sclerosis: Increased peripheral inflammation but less acute neuroinflammation. *Mol. Neurobiol.* **2015**, *53*, 5191–5202. [CrossRef] [PubMed]
28. McFarland, H.F.; Martin, R. Multiple Sclerosis: A Complicated Picture of Autoimmunity. *Nat. Immunol.* **2007**, *8*, 913–919. [CrossRef] [PubMed]
29. Fletcher, J.M.; Lalor, S.J.; Sweeney, C.M.; Tubridy, N.; Mills, K.H.G. T Cells in Multiple Sclerosis and Experimental Autoimmune Encephalomyelitis. *Clin. Exp. Immunol.* **2010**, *162*, 1–11. [CrossRef] [PubMed]
30. Kaskow, B.J.; Baecher-Allan, C. Effector T Cells in Multiple Sclerosis. *Cold Spring Harb. Perspect. Med.* **2018**, *8*, 029025. [CrossRef]
31. Farjam, M.; Zhang, G.X.; Ciric, B.; Rostami, A. Emerging immunopharmacological targets in multiple sclerosis. *J. Neurol. Sci.* **2015**, *358*, 22–30. [CrossRef]
32. Xie, Z.X.; Zhang, H.L.; Wu, X.J.; Zhu, J.; Ma, D.H.; Jin, T. Role of the immunogenic and tolerogenic subsets of dendritic cells in multiple sclerosis. *Mediators Inflamm.* **2015**, *2015*, 513295. [CrossRef]
33. Hemmer, B.; Kerschensteiner, M.; Korn, T. Role of the innate and adaptive immune responses in the course of multiple sclerosis. *Lancet Neurol.* **2015**, *14*, 406–419. [CrossRef]
34. Jadidi-Niaragh, F.; Shegarfi, H.; Naddafi, F.; Mirshafiey, A. The role of natural killer cells in Alzheimer's disease. *Scand. J. Immunol.* **2012**, *76*, 451–456. [CrossRef]
35. Jadidi-Niaragh, F.; Mirshafiey, A. Regulatory T-cell as orchestra leader in immunosuppression process of multiple sclerosis. *Immunopharmacol. Immunotoxicol.* **2011**, *33*, 545–567. [CrossRef] [PubMed]
36. Jadidi-Niaragh, F.; Mirshafiey, A. Th17 cell, the new player of neuroinflammatory process in multiple sclerosis. *Scand. J. Immunol.* **2011**, *74*, 1–13. [CrossRef] [PubMed]
37. Ghalamfarsa, G.; Hadinia, A.; Yousefi, M.; Jadidi-Niaragh, F. The role of natural killer T cells in B cell malignancies. *Tumor Biol.* **2013**, *34*, 1349–1360. [CrossRef]

38. Mishra, M.K.; Yong, V.W. Myeloid Cells—Targets of Medication in Multiple Sclerosis. *Nat. Rev. Neurol.* **2016**, *12*, 539–551. [CrossRef]
39. Nally, F.K.; De Santi, C.; McCoy, C.E. Nanomodulation of Macrophages in Multiple Sclerosis. *Cells* **2019**, *8*, 543. [CrossRef] [PubMed]
40. Stys, P.K.; Tsutsui, S. Recent advances in understanding multiple sclerosis. *F1000Res* **2019**, *8*, F1000 Faculty Rev-2100. [CrossRef] [PubMed]
41. Wingerchuk, D.M.; Carter, J.L. Multiple Sclerosis: Current and Emerging Disease-Modifying Therapies and Treatment Strategies. *Mayo Clin. Proc.* **2014**, *89*, 225–240. [CrossRef]
42. Cross, A.H.; Naismith, R.T. Established and Novel Disease-Modifying Treatments in Multiple Sclerosis. *J. Intern. Med.* **2014**, *275*, 350–363. [CrossRef]
43. Polman, C.H.; O'Connor, P.W.; Havrdova, E.; Hutchinson, M.; Kappos, L.; Miller, D.H.; Phillips, J.T.; Lublin, F.D.; Giovannoni, G.; Wajgt, A.; et al. A Randomized, Placebo-Controlled Trial of Natalizumab for Relapsing Multiple Sclerosis. *N. Engl. J. Med.* **2006**, *354*, 899–910. [CrossRef]
44. Coles, A.J.; Twyman, C.L.; Arnold, D.L.; Cohen, J.A.; Confavreux, C.; Fox, E.J.; Hartung, H.-P.; Havrdova, E.; Selmaj, K.W.; Weiner, H.L.; et al. Alemtuzumab for Patients with Relapsing Multiple Sclerosis after Disease-Modifying Therapy: A Randomised Controlled Phase 3 Trial. *Lancet* **2012**, *380*, 1829–1839. [CrossRef]
45. Katsara, M.; Matsoukas, J.; Deraos, G.; Apostolopoulos, V. Towards immunotherapeutic drugs and vaccines against multiple sclerosis. *Acta Biochim. Biophys. Sin.* **2008**, *40*, 636–642. [CrossRef] [PubMed]
46. Bettelli, E. Building different mouse models for human MS. *Ann. N. Y. Acad. Sci.* **2007**, *1103*, 11–18. [CrossRef]
47. Burt, R.K.; Testori, A.; Craig, R.; Cohen, B.; Suffit, R.; Barr, W. Hematopoietic stem cell transplantation for autoimmune diseases: What have we learned? *J. Autoimmun.* **2008**, *30*, 116–120. [CrossRef]
48. Lassmann, H.; Bradl, M. Multiple Sclerosis: Experimental Models and Reality. *Acta Neuropathol.* **2017**, *133*, 223–244. [CrossRef] [PubMed]
49. Terry, R.L.; Ifergan, I.; Miller, S.D. Experimental Autoimmune Encephalomyelitis in Mice. *Methods Mol. Biol.* **2016**, *1304*, 145–160. [PubMed]
50. Sun, D.; Whitaker, J.N.; Huang, Z.; Liu, D.; Coleclough, C.; Wekerle, H.; Raine, C.S. Myelin Antigen-Specific CD8+ T Cells Are Encephalitogenic and Produce Severe Disease in C57BL/6 Mice. *J. Immunol.* **2001**, *166*, 7579–7587. [CrossRef] [PubMed]
51. Bjelobaba, I.; Begovic-Kupresanin, V.; Pekovic, S.; Lavrnja, I. Animal Models of Multiple Sclerosis: Focus on Experimental Autoimmune Encephalomyelitis. *J. Neurosci. Res.* **2018**, *96*, 1021–1042. [CrossRef]
52. Robinson, A.P.; Harp, C.T.; Noronha, A.; Miller, S.D. The Experimental Autoimmune Encephalomyelitis (EAE) Model of MS. In *Handbook of Clinical Neurology*; Elsevier: Amsterdam, The Netherlands, 2014; Volume 122, pp. 173–189.
53. Kipp, M.; Nyamoya, S.; Hochstrasser, T.; Amor, S. Multiple Sclerosis Animal Models: A Clinical and Histopathological Perspective. *Brain Pathol.* **2017**, *27*, 123–137. [CrossRef]
54. Demetzos, C.; Pippa, N. Advanced drug delivery nanosystems (aDDnSs): A mini-review. *Drug Deliv.* **2014**, *21*, 250–257. [CrossRef] [PubMed]
55. Ortiz, G.G.; Pacheco-Moisés, F.P.; Macías-Islas, M.Á.; Flores-Alvarado, L.J.; Mireles-Ramírez, M.A.; González-Renovato, E.D.; Hernández-Navarro, V.E.; Sánchez-López, A.L.; Alatorre-Jiménez, M.A. Role of the blood-brain barrier in multiple sclerosis. *Arch. Med. Res.* **2014**, *45*, 687–697. [CrossRef]
56. Shakya, A.K.; Nandakumar, K.S. Antigen-Specific Tolerization and Targeted Delivery as Therapeutic Strategies for Autoimmune Diseases. *Trends Biotechnol.* **2018**, *36*, 686–699. [CrossRef]
57. Prinz, J.; Karacivi, A.; Stormanns, E.R.; Recks, M.S.; Kuerten, S. Time-Dependent Progression of Demyelination and Axonal Pathology in MP4-Induced Experimental Autoimmune Encephalomyelitis. *PLoS ONE* **2015**, *10*, e0144847. [CrossRef] [PubMed]
58. Keough, M.B.; Yong, V.W. Remyelination therapy for multiple sclerosis. *Neurotherapeutics* **2013**, *10*, 44–54. [CrossRef] [PubMed]
59. Aharoni, R.; Herschkovitz, A.; Eilam, R.; Blumberg-Hazan, M.; Sela, M.; Bruck, W.; Arnon, R. Demyelination arrest and remyelination induced by glatiramer acetate treatment of experimental autoimmune encephalomyelitis. *Proc. Natl. Acad. Sci. USA* **2008**, *105*, 11358–11363. [CrossRef] [PubMed]

60. Deshmukh, V.A.; Tardif, V.; Lyssiotis, C.A.; Green, C.C.; Kerman, B.; Kim, H.J.; Padmanabhan, K.; Swoboda, J.G.; Ahmad, I.; Kondo, T.; et al. A regenerative approach to the treatment of multiple sclerosis. *Nature* **2013**, *502*, 327–332. [CrossRef]
61. Maeda, Y.; Nakagomi, N.; Nakano-Doi, A.; Ishikawa, H.; Tatsumi, Y.; Bando, Y.; Yoshikawa, H.; Matsuyama, T.; Gomi, F.; Nakagomi, T. Potential of Adult Endogenous Neural Stem/Progenitor Cells in the Spinal Cord to Contribute to Remyelination in Experimental Autoimmune Encephalomyelitis. *Cells* **2019**, *8*, 1025. [CrossRef]
62. Arvidsson, L.; Covacu, R.; Estrada, C.P.; Sankavaram, S.R.; Svensson, M.; Brundin, L. Long-distance effects of inflammation on differentiation of adult spinal cord neural stem/progenitor cells. *J. Neuroimmunol.* **2015**, *288*, 47–55. [CrossRef]
63. Münzel, E.J.; Williams, A. Promoting remyelination in multiple sclerosis—Recent advances. *Drugs* **2013**, *73*, 2017–2029. [CrossRef] [PubMed]
64. Robinson, A.P.; Zhang, J.Z.; Titus, H.E.; Karl, M.; Merzliakov, M.; Dorfman, A.R.; Karlik, S.; Stewart, M.G.; Watt, R.K.; Facer, B.D.; et al. Nanocatalytic activity of cleansurfaced, faceted nanocrystalline gold enhances remyelination in animal models of multiple sclerosis. *Sci. Rep.* **2020**, *10*, 1936. [CrossRef] [PubMed]
65. Zhang, T.T.; Li, W.; Meng, G.; Wang, P.; Liao, W. Strategies for transporting nanoparticles across the blood-brain barrier. *Biomater. Sci.* **2016**, *4*, 219–229. [CrossRef] [PubMed]
66. Niu, X.; Chen, J.; Gao, J. Nanocarriers as a powerful vehicle to overcome bloodbrain barrier in treating neurodegenerative diseases: Focus on recent advances. *Asian J. Pharm. Sci.* **2019**, *14*, 480–496. [CrossRef]
67. Haider, M.; Abdin, S.M.; Kamal, L.; Orive, G. Nanostructured Lipid Carriers for Delivery of Chemotherapeutics: A Review. *Pharmaceutics* **2020**, *12*, 288. [CrossRef]
68. Puri, A.; Loomis, K.; Smith, B.; Lee, J.H.; Yavlovich, A.; Heldman, E.; Blumenthal, R. Lipid-based nanoparticles as pharmaceutical drug carriers: From concepts to clinic. *Crit. Rev. Ther. Drug Carrier Syst.* **2009**, *26*, 523–580. [CrossRef]
69. Agrawal, M.; Saraf, S.; Saraf, S.; Dubey, S.K.; Puri, A.; Patel, R.J.; Ajazuddin; Ravichandiran, V.; Murty, U.S.; Amit, A. Recent strategies and advances in the fabrication of nano lipid carriers and their application towards brain targeting. *J. Control. Release* **2020**, *321*, 372–415. [CrossRef] [PubMed]
70. Shah, R.; Eldridge, D.; Palombo, E.; Harding, I. Composition and structure. In *Lipid Nanoparticles: Production, Characterization and Stability*; Shah, R., Eldridge, D., Palombo, E., Harding, I., Eds.; Springer International Publishing: Cham, Switzerland, 2014; pp. 11–22.
71. Ganesan, P.; Narayanasamy, D. Lipid nanoparticles: Different preparation techniques, characterization, hurdles, and strategies for the production of solid lipid nanoparticles and nanostructured lipid carriers for oral drug delivery. *Sustain. Chem. Pharm.* **2017**, *6*, 37–56. [CrossRef]
72. Gadhave, D.G.; Kokare, C.R. Nanostructured lipid carriers engineered for intranasal delivery of teriflunomide in multiple sclerosis: Optimization and in vivo studies. *Drug Dev. Ind. Pharm.* **2019**, *45*, 839–851. [CrossRef]
73. Kumar, P.; Sharma, G.; Kumar, R.; Malik, R.; Singh, B.; Katare, O.P.; Raza, K. Enhanced brain delivery of dimethyl fumarate employing tocopherol-acetate-based nanolipidic carriers: Evidence from pharmacokinetic, biodistribution, and cellular uptake studies. *ACS Chem. Neurosci.* **2017**, *8*, 860–865. [CrossRef]
74. Ghasemian, E.; Vatanara, A.; Navidi, N.; Rouini, M.R. Brain delivery of baclofen as a hydrophilic drug by nanolipid carriers: Characteristics and pharmacokinetics evaluation. *J. Drug Deliv. Sci. Technol.* **2017**, *37*, 67–73. [CrossRef]
75. Kumar, P.; Sharma, G.; Gupta, V.; Kaur, R.; Thakur, K.; Malik, R.; Kumar, A.; Kaushal, N.; Katare, O.P.; Raza, K. Oral Delivery of Methylthioadenosine to the Brain Employing Solid Lipid Nanoparticles: Pharmacokinetic, Behavioral, and Histopathological Evidences. *AAPS PharmSciTech.* **2019**, *20*, 74. [CrossRef]
76. Gandomi, N.; Varshochian, R.; Atyabi, F.; Ghahremani, M.H.; Sharifzadeh, M.; Amini, M.; Dinarvand, R. Solid lipid nanoparticles surface modified with anti-Contactin-2 or anti-Neurofascin for brain-targeted delivery of medicines. *Pharm. Dev. Technol.* **2017**, *22*, 426–435. [CrossRef]
77. Chountoulesi, M.; Naziris, N.; Pippa, N.; Pispas, S.; Demetzos, C. Differential scanning calorimetry (DSC): An invaluable tool for the thermal evaluation of advanced chimeric liposomal drug delivery nanosystems. In *Thermodynamics and Biophysics of Biomedical Nanosystems. Applications and Practical Considerations. Series: Series in BioEngineering*; Demetzos, C., Pippa, N., Eds.; Springer: Berlin/Heidelberg, Germany, 2019; pp. 297–337.
78. Schmidt, J.; Metselaar, J.M.; Wauben, M.H.M.; Toyka, K.V.; Storm, G.; Gold, R. Drug targeting by long-circulating liposomal glucocorticosteroids increases therapeutic efficacy in a model of multiple sclerosis. *Brain* **2003**, *126*, 1895–1904. [CrossRef]

79. Gaillard, P.J.; Appeldoorn, C.C.; Rip, J.; Dorland, R.; van der Pol, S.M.; Kooij, G.; de Vries, H.E.; Reijerkerk, A. Enhanced brain delivery of liposomal methylprednisolone improved therapeutic efficacy in a model of neuroinflammation. *J. Control. Release* **2012**, *164*, 364–369. [CrossRef]
80. Lee, D.H.; Rötger, C.; Appeldoorn, C.C.; Reijerkerk, A.; Gladdines, W.; Gaillard, P.J.; Linker, R.A. Glutathione PEGylated liposomal methylprednisolone (2B3-201) attenuates CNS inflammation and degeneration in murine myelin oligodendrocyte glycoprotein induced experimental autoimmune encephalomyelitis. *J. Neuroimmunol.* **2014**, *274*, 96–101. [CrossRef]
81. Turjeman, K.; Bavli, Y.; Kizelsztein, P.; Schilt, Y.; Allon, N.; Katzir, T.B.; Sasson, E.; Raviv, U.; Ovadia, H.; Barenholz, Y. Nano-Drugs Based on Nano Sterically Stabilized Liposomes for the Treatment of Inflammatory Neurodegenerative Diseases. *PLoS ONE* **2015**, *10*, e0130442. [CrossRef]
82. Pujol-Autonell, I.; Mansilla, M.J.; Rodriguez-Fernandez, S.; Cano-Sarabia, M.; Navarro-Barriuso, J.; Ampudia, R.M.; Rius, A.; Garcia-Jimeno, S.; Perna-Barrull, D.; Martinez-Caceres, E.; et al. Liposome-based immunotherapy against autoimmune diseases: Therapeutic effect on multiple sclerosis. *Nanomedicine* **2017**, *12*, 1231–1242. [CrossRef]
83. Binyamin, O.; Larush, L.; Frid, K.; Keller, G.; Friedman-Levi, Y.; Ovadia, H.; Abramsky, O.; Magdassi, S.; Gabizon, R. Treatment of a multiple sclerosis animal model by a novel nanodrop formulation of a natural antioxidant. *Int. J. Nanomed.* **2015**, *10*, 7165–7174. [CrossRef]
84. Lu, L.; Qi, S.; Chen, Y.; Luo, H.; Huang, S.; Yu, X.; Luo, Q.; Zhang, Z. Targeted immunomodulation of inflammatory monocytes across the blood-brain barrier by curcumin-loaded nanoparticles delays the progression of experimental autoimmune encephalomyelitis. *Biomaterials* **2020**, *245*, 119987. [CrossRef]
85. Osorio-Querejeta, I.; Carregal-Romero, S.; Ayerdi-Izquierdo, A.; Mäger, I.; Nash, L.A.; Wood, M.; Egimendia, A.; Betanzos, M.; Alberro, A.; Iparraguirre, L.; et al. MiR-219a-5p Enriched Extracellular Vesicles Induce OPC Differentiation and EAE Improvement More Efficiently Than Liposomes and Polymeric Nanoparticles. *Pharmaceutics* **2020**, *12*, 186. [CrossRef]
86. El-Say, K.M.; El-Sawy, H.S. Polymeric nanoparticles: Promising platform for drug delivery. *Int. J. Pharm.* **2017**, *528*, 675–691. [CrossRef]
87. Houchin, M.L.; Topp, E.M. Chemical degradation of peptides and proteins in PLGA:a review of reactions and mechanisms. *J. Pharm. Sci.* **2008**, *97*, 2395–2404. [CrossRef]
88. Makadia, H.K.; Siegel, S.J. Poly Lactic-co-Glycolic Acid (PLGA) as Biodegradable Controlled Drug Delivery Carrier. *Polymers* **2011**, *3*, 1377–1397. [CrossRef]
89. Gentile, P.; Chiono, V.; Carmagnola, I.; Hatton, P.V. An overview of poly(lactic-co-glycolic) acid (PLGA)-based biomaterials for bone tissue engineering. *Int. J. Mol. Sci.* **2014**, *15*, 3640–3659. [CrossRef]
90. Samavedi, S.; Poindexter, L.K.; Van Dyke, M.; Goldstein, A.S. Synthetic biomaterials for regenerative medicine applications. *Regen. Med. Appl. Organ. Transpl.* **2014**, 81–99. [CrossRef]
91. Houchin, M.L.; Topp, E.M. Physical properties of PLGA films during polymer degradation. *J. Appl. Polym. Sci.* **2009**, *114*, 2848–2854. [CrossRef]
92. Johnson, D.; Hafler, D.A.; Fallis, R.J.; Lees, M.B.; Brady, R.O.; Quarles, R.H.; Weiner, H.L. Cell-mediated immunity to myelin-associated glycoprotein, proteolipid pro-tein, and myelin basic protein in multiple sclerosis. *J. Neuroimmunol.* **1986**, *13*, 99–108. [CrossRef]
93. Cappellano, G.; Woldetsadik, A.D.; Orilieri, E.; Shivakumar, Y.; Rizzi, M.; Carniato, F.; Gigliotti, C.L.; Boggio, E.; Clemente, N.; Comi, C.; et al. Subcutaneous inverse vaccination with PLGA particles loaded with a MOG peptide and IL-10 decreases the severity of experimental autoimmune encephalomyelitis. *Vaccine* **2014**, *32*, 5681–5689. [CrossRef]
94. Cappellano, G.; Comi, C.; Chiocchetti, A.; Dianzani, U. Exploiting PLGA-Based Biocompatible Nanoparticles for Next-Generation Tolerogenic Vaccines against Autoimmune Disease. *Int. J. Mol. Sci.* **2019**, *20*, 204. [CrossRef]
95. Maldonado, R.A.; LaMothe, R.A.; Ferrari, J.D.; Zhang, A.H.; Rossi, R.J.; Kolte, P.N.; Griset, A.P.; O'Neil, C.; Altreuter, D.H.; Browning, E.; et al. Polymeric synthetic nanoparticles for the induction of antigen-specific immunological tolerance. *Proc. Natl. Acad. Sci. USA* **2015**, *112*, 156–165. [CrossRef]
96. Cho, J.J.; Stewart, J.M.; Drashansky, T.T.; Brusko, M.A.; Zuniga, A.N.; Lorentsen, K.J.; Keselowsky, B.G.; Avram, D. An antigen-specific semi-therapeutic treatment with local delivery of tolerogenic factors through a dual-sized microparticle system blocks experimental autoimmune encephalomyelitis. *Biomaterials* **2017**, *143*, 79–92. [CrossRef]

97. Pei, W.; Wan, X.; Shahzad, K.A.; Zhang, L.; Song, S.; Jin, X.; Wang, L.; Zhao, C.; Shen, C. Direct modulation of myelin-autoreactive CD4(+) and CD8(+) T cells in EAE mice by a tolerogenic nanoparticle co-carrying myelin peptide-loaded major histocompatibility complexes, CD47 and multiple regulatory molecules. *Int. J. Nanomed.* **2018**, *13*, 3731–3750. [CrossRef]
98. Hunter, Z.; McCarthy, D.P.; Yap, W.T.; Harp, C.T.; Getts, D.R.; Shea, L.D.; Miller, S.D. A biodegradable nanoparticle platform for the induction of antigen-specific immune tolerance for treatment of autoimmune disease. *ACS Nano* **2014**, *8*, 2148–2160. [CrossRef]
99. Casey, L.M.; Pearson, R.M.; Hughes, K.R.; Liu, J.M.H.; Rose, J.A.; North, M.G.; Wang, L.Z.; Lei, M.; Miller, S.D.; Shea, L.D. Conjugation of Transforming Growth Factor Beta to Antigen-Loaded Poly(lactideco-glycolide) Nanoparticles Enhances Efficiency of Antigen-Specific Tolerance. *Bioconjug. Chem.* **2018**, *29*, 813–823. [CrossRef]
100. Getts, D.R.; Martin, A.J.; McCarthy, D.P.; Terry, R.L.; Hunter, Z.N.; Yap, W.T.; Getts, M.T.; Pleiss, M.; Luo, X.; King, N.J.; et al. Microparticles bearing encephalitogenic peptides induce T-cell toleranceand ameliorate experimental autoimmune encephalomyelitis. *Nat. Biotechnol.* **2012**, *30*, 1217–1224. [CrossRef]
101. Kuo, R.; Saito, E.; Miller, S.D.; Shea, L.D. Peptide-Conjugated Nanoparticles Reduce Positive Co-stimulatory Expression and T Cell Activity to Induce Tolerance. *Mol. Ther.* **2017**, *25*, 1676–1685. [CrossRef]
102. Saito, E.; Kuo, R.; Kramer, K.R.; Gohel, N.; Giles, D.A.; Moore, B.B.; Miller, S.D.; Shea, L.D. Design of biodegradable nanoparticles to modulate phenotypes of antigen-presenting cells for antigen-specific treatment of autoimmune disease. *Biomaterials* **2019**, *222*, 119432. [CrossRef]
103. Rittchen, S.; Boyd, A.; Burns, A.; Park, J.; Fahmy, T.M.; Metcalfe, S.; Williams, A. Myelin repair in vivo is increased by targeting oligodendrocyte precursor cells with nanoparticles encapsulating leukaemia inhibitory factor (LIF). *Biomaterials* **2015**, *56*, 78–85. [CrossRef]
104. Führmann, T.; Ghosh, M.; Otero, A.; Goss, B.; Dargaville, T.R.; Pearse, D.D.; Dalton, P.D. Peptide-functionalized polymeric nanoparticles for active targeting of damaged tissue in animals with experimental autoimmune encephalomyelitis. *Neurosci. Lett.* **2015**, *602*, 126–132. [CrossRef]
105. Al-Ghobashy, M.A.; El Meshad, A.N.; Abdelsalam, R.M.; Nooh, M.M.; Al-Shorbagy, M.; Laible, G. Development and Pre-Clinical Evaluation of Recombinant Human Myelin Basic Protein Nano Therapeutic Vaccine in Experimental Autoimmune Encephalomyelitis Mice Animal Model. *Sci. Rep.* **2017**, *7*, 46468. [CrossRef]
106. Lunin, S.M.; Khrenov, M.O.; Glushkova, O.V.; Parfenyuk, S.B.; Novoselova, T.V.; Novoselova, E.G. Protective Effect of PBCA Nanoparticles Loaded with Thymulin Against the Relapsing-Remitting Form of Experimental Autoimmune Encephalomyelitis in Mice. *Int. J. Mol. Sci.* **2019**, *20*, 5374. [CrossRef]
107. Kondiah, P.P.; Tomar, L.K.; Tyagi, C.; Choonara, Y.E.; Modi, G.; du Toit, L.C.; Kumar, P.; Pillay, V. A novel pH-sensitive interferon-β (INF-β) oral delivery system for application in multiple sclerosis. *Int. J. Pharm.* **2013**, *456*, 459–472. [CrossRef]
108. Youssef, A.E.H.; Dief, A.E.; El Azhary, N.M.; Abdelmonsif, D.A.; El-fetiany, O.S. LINGO-1 siRNA nanoparticles promote central remyelination in ethidium bromide-induced demyelination in rats. *J. Physiol. Biochem.* **2019**, *75*, 89–99. [CrossRef]

11

Genetic Association and Altered Gene Expression of *CYBB* in Multiple Sclerosis Patients

Giulia Cardamone [1], Elvezia Maria Paraboschi [1], Giulia Soldà [1,2], Stefano Duga [1,2], Janna Saarela [3] and Rosanna Asselta [1,2,*]

1 Department of Biomedical Sciences, Humanitas University, Via Rita Levi Montalcini 4, 20090 Pieve Emanuele, Milan, Italy; giulia.cardamone@st.hunimed.eu (G.C.); elvezia_maria.paraboschi@hunimed.eu (E.M.P.); giulia.solda@hunimed.eu (G.S.); stefano.duga@hunimed.eu (S.D.)
2 Humanitas Clinical and Research Center, Via Manzoni 56, 20089 Rozzano, Milan, Italy
3 Institute for Molecular Medicine Finland, Helsinki Institute of Life Science (HiLIFE), University of Helsinki, 00290 Helsinki, Finland; janna.saarela@helsinki.fi
* Correspondence: rosanna.asselta@hunimed.eu;

Abstract: Multiple sclerosis (MS) is a chronic neurological disorder characterized by inflammation, demyelination, and axonal damage. Increased levels of reactive oxygen species (ROS), produced by macrophages and leading to oxidative stress, have been implicated as mediators of demyelination and axonal injury in both MS and experimental autoimmune encephalomyelitis, the murine model of the disease. On the other hand, reduced ROS levels can increase susceptibility to autoimmunity. In this work, we screened for association with MS 11 single nucleotide polymorphisms (SNPs) and two microsatellite markers in the five genes (*NCF1*, *NCF2*, *NCF4*, *CYBA*, and *CYBB*) of the nicotinamide adenine dinucleotide phosphate (NADPH) oxidase (NOX2) system, the enzymatic pathway producing ROS in the brain and neural tissues, in 347 Finnish patients with MS and 714 unaffected family members. This analysis showed suggestive association signals for *NCF1* and *CYBB* (lowest $p = 0.038$ and $p = 0.013$, respectively). Functional relevance for disease predisposition was further supported for the *CYBB* gene, by microarray analysis in $CD4^{+/-}$ mononuclear cells of 21 individuals from five Finnish multiplex MS families, as well as by real-time RT-PCRs performed on RNA extracted from peripheral blood mononuclear cells of an Italian replication cohort of 21 MS cases and 21 controls. Our results showed a sex-specific differential expression of *CYBB*, suggesting that this gene, and more in general the NOX2 system, deserve to be further investigated for their possible role in MS.

Keywords: multiple sclerosis; association study; reactive oxygen species; NADPH oxidase; *CYBB*

1. Introduction

Multiple sclerosis (MS) (Online Mendelian Inheritance in Men, OMIM #126200) is a chronic disease of the central nervous system (CNS) characterized by multifocal inflammation, plaques of myelin degeneration, axonal damage, and by a high degree of individual variability in the severity and progression of symptoms [1–3]. Among neurological disorders of young adults, MS is the most common: in Europe, where a latitude-correlated distribution of prevalence and incidence rates can be observed, prevalence ranges from 70 to 100 per 100,000, whereas incidence varies between 2 and 4 per 100,000 person/year; the highest prevalence and incidence rates have been reported in Finland [4]. Here, incidence and prevalence reach the exceptional rate of 11.6 and 200 per 100,000 in the Southern Ostrobothnian region (western coast of Finland), reflecting several centuries of genetic drift in a small and isolated population [5].

In agreement with the multigenic character of MS, genome-wide linkage scans, genome-wide association studies (GWAS), as well as meta-analyses performed in large cohorts disclosed more than 200 non-HLA (human leukocyte antigen) single nucleotide polymorphisms (SNPs) associated with MS, each having a small effect size on MS predisposition [6–10]. Typically, the identified association signals point to genes belonging to innate and adaptive pathways [9,10]. The deep involvement of a dysregulated immune system in MS is also supported by the efficacy of drugs targeting T- and B-cell functions in the treatment of the disease, as well as by the numerous studies indicating $CD4^+$ and $CD8^+$ T cells as strong contributors to the pathogenic process [11–14].

Apart from immune-mediated mechanisms, a growing body of evidence indicates that oxidative stress (OS) may play a role in the etiology of MS [15–17]. Increased levels of oxygen-free radicals (collectively called reactive oxygen species, ROS), produced by macrophages and leading to OS, have been implicated as mediators of demyelination and axonal injury in both MS and experimental autoimmune encephalomyelitis, the murine model of the disease [18–20]. Moreover, ROS: (i) activate specific transcription factors, such as the nuclear transcription factor kappa B, which in turn upregulates the expression of genes associated with MS or its progression (e.g., tumor necrosis factor α) [21,22]; (ii) mediate the activity of matrix metalloproteinases, which are involved in T-cell activation and trafficking into the CNS and hence probably involved in some of the early pro-inflammatory events in MS [23–25]; (iii) are produced in increased amount by activated mononuclear cells of patients, resulting in oxygen damage to DNA, lipids, and proteins—these molecules are frequently found in active MS lesions and are associated with apoptotic oligodendrocytes and neurodegeneration in the brains of patients with MS [16,26–28].

Besides reactions involving the electron-transport chain of mitochondria or those related to the metabolism of amino acids and neurotransmitters, in the brain and neural tissue ROS are also produced by enzymatic pathways, such as xanthine oxidase, lipoxygenase, and cyclooxygenase, as well as by the nicotinamide adenine dinucleotide phosphate (NADPH) oxidase (NOX) systems [29,30]. Specifically, the NOX2 system is a complex that, in resting cells, is compartmentalized between cytosol and plasma membrane: the core enzyme is composed of three cytoplasmic polypeptides (p47phox, p67phox, and p40phox, encoded by *NCF1*, *NCF2*, and *NCF4* genes, respectively), and a membrane-bound flavo-hemo-cytochrome, b558, constituted by two components, the p22phox and gp91phox subunits (encoded by *CYBA* and *CYBB*, respectively) [29,30]. When the resting cell is exposed to stimuli (i.e., chemotactic reactants or particulate stimuli, such as bacteria and fungi), p47phox becomes heavily phosphorylated, inducing all cytoplasmic components to translocate to the membrane-bound cytochrome in order to form the active enzyme complex [29,30].

Given the proposed role of OS in MS, its contribution to the pathogenesis of the disease was here investigated by genetic association and expression analyses of the five genes coding for the main components of the NOX2 complex.

2. Results

2.1. *NCF1* and *CYBB* Are Associated with MS in the Finnish Population

For investigating the potential role of OS genes in the pathogenesis of MS, we performed an association analysis on a Finnish cohort of 63 MS families (547 individuals) with two microsatellite markers and 11 SNPs mapping in or located close to the five genes coding for the main components of the NOX2 complex (the soluble factors *NCF1*, *NCF2*, and *NCF4*, and the membrane-bound redox core proteins of the complex, *CYBA* and *CYBB*) (see Table S1 in the Supplementary Materials). No significant deviation from Hardy-Weinberg equilibrium (HWE) and no Mendelian inheritance errors were observed for any of the markers included in this study. The overall average genotype call rate was 96.5%, and the accuracy was >99.5% according to duplicated genotyping (5%) of all samples.

Table 1 shows the results of the allelic association analysis for each of the 11 variants for the whole study cohort. Two polymorphisms, D7S1870 in *NCF1* and rs5963310 in *CYBB*, showed suggestive evidence of association with MS in the transmission/disequilibrium (TDT) test ($p = 0.038$ and $p = 0.027$ for *NCF1* and *CYBB*, respectively; not corrected for multiple testing). By using the more powerful approach based on the TDT statistic implemented with the parental discordance test (see the Materials and Methods section), we confirmed the association signal for the rs5963310 polymorphism in *CYBB* ($p = 0.013$), which confers a protective effect against MS (the minor allele A is untransmitted in MS cases). No significant allelic association between MS and the other NADPH variants could be detected (Table 1).

2.2. CYBB Is Differentially Expressed in MS Cases

To verify the possible functional relevance of NADPH genes for MS predisposition, we performed a genome-wide microarray-based gene expression analysis. We extracted total RNA from $CD4^+$ and $CD4^-$ samples isolated from peripheral blood mononuclear cells (PBMCs) of 21 individuals from five Finnish multiplex MS families. An adequate amount of high-quality total RNA was obtained from nine MS cases (four males, five females) and ten controls (four males, six females) for the $CD4^-$ cells, and from nine cases (five males, four females) and 11 controls (six males, five females) for the $CD4^+$ cells. All patients had a relapsing-remitting (RR) subtype, i.e., the most common form of MS (~80% of cases), which is characterized by periods of acute intensification of symptoms followed by phases of almost complete remission [31].

To screen for differential expression of the genes of interest in MS, we specifically searched for probe sets corresponding to *NCF1*, *NCF2*, *NCF4*, *CYBA*, and *CYBB* in the NetAffx annotation site (http://www.affymetrix.com/analysis/index.affx). The 11 identified probes were individually searched in the University of California Santa Cruz (UCSC) Genome Browser (hg19; Blat search) to identify the correct target gene (http://genome.ucsc.edu/cgi-bin/hgGateway). Probe sets recognizing only intronic sequences or mapping to several loci were excluded: in this way expression data were available for seven probes mapping in the five genes.

As for the *NCF1* gene, none of the probes were mapping correctly/specifically. As for *NCF2*, it did not show appreciable expression signals in any of the $CD4^+/CD4^-$ samples. We hence monitored for potential differential expression of these two genes by using the more sensitive semi-quantitative real-time reverse transcription-PCR (RT-PCR) approach. Figure 1 shows the results of RT-PCR assays: no significant difference between cases and controls in the expression levels of either genes was evidenced (no significant difference between cases and controls was seen even stratifying individuals on the basis of the D7S1870 genotype in *NCF1*; data not shown).

Table 1. NADPH polymorphisms: Results of family-based association TDT and haplotype relative risk (HRR) tests.

Gene	Marker	ANALYZE Analyses [1]		PLINK Analyses						
		HRR p Value	TDT p Value	Minor Allele [2]	MAF	Transmitted/Untransmitted [3]	TDT p Value	OR [95% CI]	p Par [4]	p Comb [4]
NCF1	D7S1870	**0.0491**	**0.0383**	20 repeats	0.4533	Untransmitted	0.330	0.727 [0.38–1.385]	0.157	0.206
	D7S2518	0.376	0.431	7 repeats	0.3986	/	1	1 [0.351–2.851]	0.414	0.655
NCF2	rs796860	0.895	0.500	C	0.06548	/	1	1 [0.250–3.998]	1	1
	rs2296164	0.568	0.399	T	0.4861	Untransmitted	0.297	0.643 [0.278–1.485]	0.564	0.239
	rs3818364	0.604	0.500	T	0.4688	Transmitted	0.847	1.0770 [0.506–2.291]	0.564	0.715
	rs789192	0.183	0.253	G	0.4268	Transmitted	0.144	1.727 [0.822–3.630]	0.317	0.423
	rs2274065	0.293	0.500	C	0.0974	Transmitted	0.180	4 [0.447–35.790]	0.317	0.414
NCF4	rs1883112	0.991	0.500	A	0.3861	Transmitted	0.353	1.417 [0.677–2.966]	0.257	0.182
	rs741999	0.680	0.444	A	0.4444	Transmitted	0.336	1.455 [0.675–3.134]	0.479	0.237
CYBA	rs4673	0.319	0.199	T	0.1795	Untransmitted	0.317	0.600 [0.218–1.651]	0.564	0.251
	rs2306422	0.661	0.500	T	0.494	Transmitted	0.739	1.118 [0.581–2.150]	0.655	0.876
CYBB	rs5963310	0.239	**0.0274**	A	0.09848	Untransmitted	0.0578	0.250 [0.0531–1.177]	0.0833	**0.0126**
	rs9330580	0.663	0.206	A	0.1203	Untransmitted	0.366	0.571 [0.167–1.952]	0.0833	0.109

Suggestive p values ($p < 0.05$) are indicated in bold. Results are presented not corrected for multiple testing (total number of performed analyses for each test: 11; Bonferroni threshold for significance: $p < 0.0045$). [1] Analyses were run both considering MS frequency of 0.01 and penetrance of 0.05, as well as considering MS frequency of 0.0006 and penetrance of 0.76 (identical results). [2] In the case of multiallelic markers (D7S1870, D7S2518), the minor allele corresponds to the most frequent repeat, which was analyzed against all the others clumped together. [3] Indication referred to the minor allele. [4] p par (p values for parents) and p comb (combined p value, deriving from the asymptotic TDT p value and the p par value). NADPH, nicotinamide adenine dinucleotide phosphate; CI, confidence interval; HRR, haplotype relative risk; MAF, minor allele frequency; OR, odds ratio; TDT, transmission disequilibrium test.

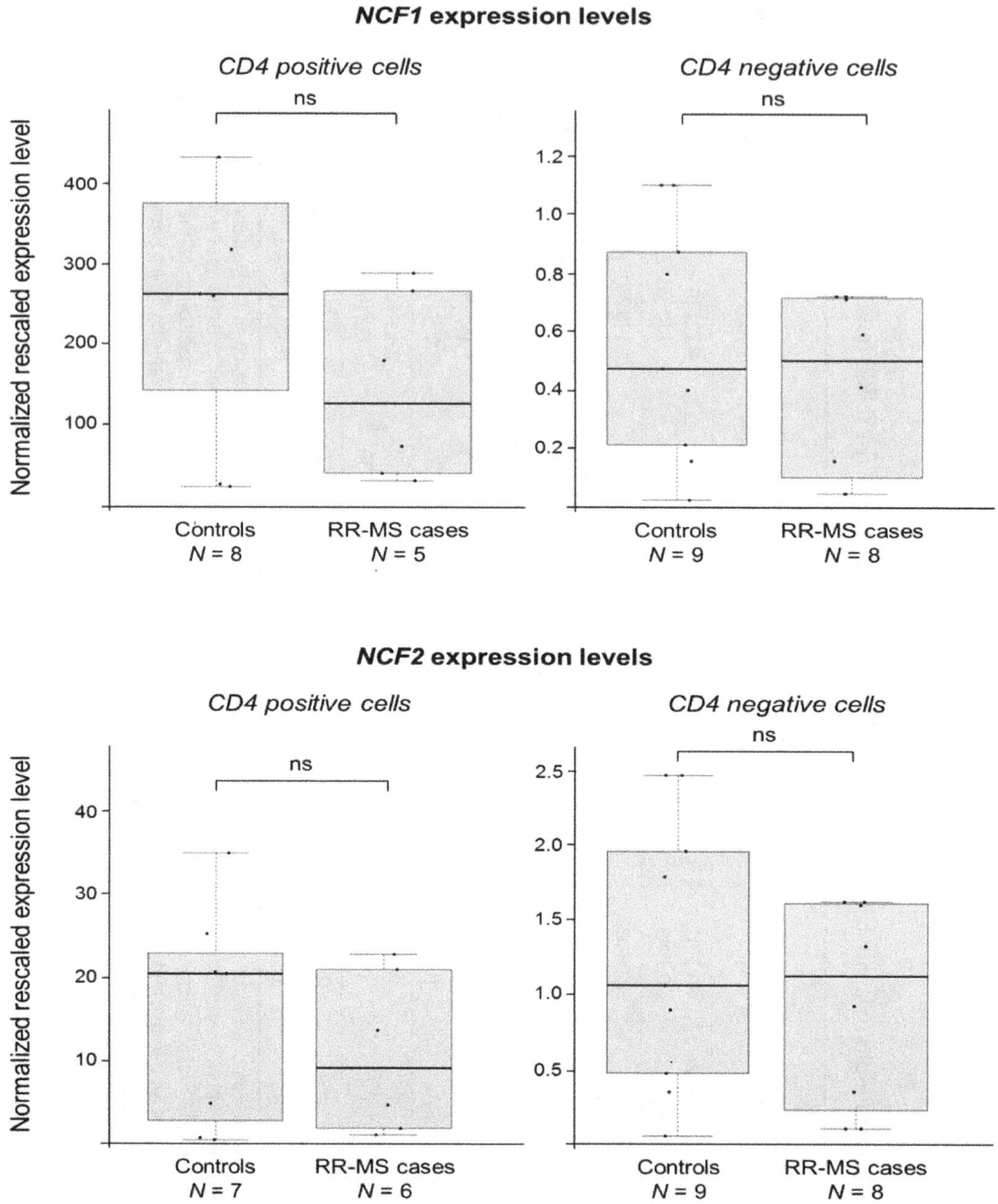

Figure 1. *NCF1* and *NCF2* do not show any significant difference between MS cases and controls. Boxplots show the expression levels of the *NCF1* and *NCF2* genes measured by semi-quantitative real-time RT-PCR in $CD4^+$ and $CD4^-$ cells (prepared from peripheral blood mononuclear cells, PBMCs). MS cases and controls belong to five multiplex Finnish families (comprising both male and female individuals). Boxes define the interquartile range; the thick line refers to the median. Results were normalized to expression levels of the *HMBS* and *ACTB* housekeeping genes and are presented as rescaled values. The number of subjects belonging to each group is indicated (*N*). The significance level of *t*-tests was in all cases not significant (ns).

Concerning *NCF4, CYBA,* and *CYBB,* probes were correctly mapping on the corresponding transcripts and gave appreciable signals. In Figure 2a, differential expression analysis for MS cases and controls is shown for both $CD4^-$ and $CD4^+$ cells, again indicating no differences between the two groups. However, considering that the *CYBB* gene is located on chromosome X, we stratified patients according to gender. Interestingly, this analysis allowed us to highlight an opposite molecular signature not only between males and females, but also between $CD4^-$ and $CD4^+$ cells (Figure 2b). In particular, we found a 1.76-fold significant up-regulation ($p = 0.021$) of *CYBB* in RR-MS male patients in $CD4^-$ cells (with females showing an opposite, though not significant, trend; 0.80-fold decrease). Conversely, in $CD4^+$ cells, we noticed the opposite situation, with a 1.75-fold significant *CYBB* increased expression in RR-MS females patients ($p = 0.014$) and a 0.74-fold decrease (not significant) in MS male cases compared to healthy controls.

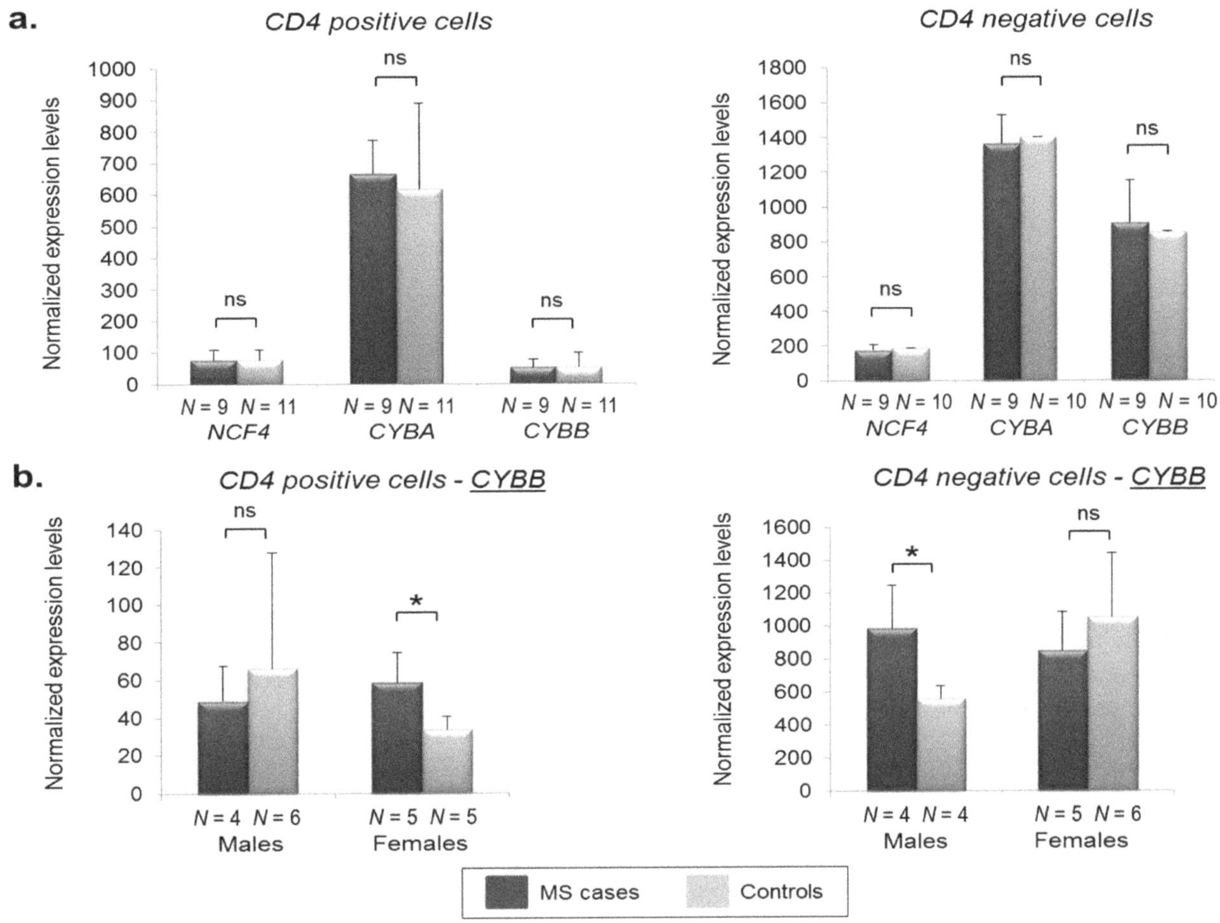

Figure 2. *CYBB* shows sex-related and cell-specific differential expression in MS cases and controls. *NCF4*, *CYBA*, and *CYBB* expression levels (shown by histograms) were measured by means of microarray-based experiments (see the "Materials and Methods" section). The number of subjects belonging to each group is indicated (*N*). Error bars represent means + SD (standard deviation). Significance levels of *t*-tests are shown. *: $p < 0.05$.

To validate the most interesting result obtained from the microarray profiling, expression of *CYBB* was quantitated by real-time RT-PCR assays, performed on RNA extracted from PBMCs of an independent cohort of 21 RR-MS Italian cases and an equal number of age-matched controls. Only females were included in this analysis. We found a 1.43-fold significant up-regulation ($p = 0.032$) of *CYBB* in RR-MS patients (Figure 3), which is consistent with the high abundance of $CD4^+$ cells in the heterogeneous pool of PBMCs (25–60% of PBMC is composed of $CD4^+$ cells) [32].

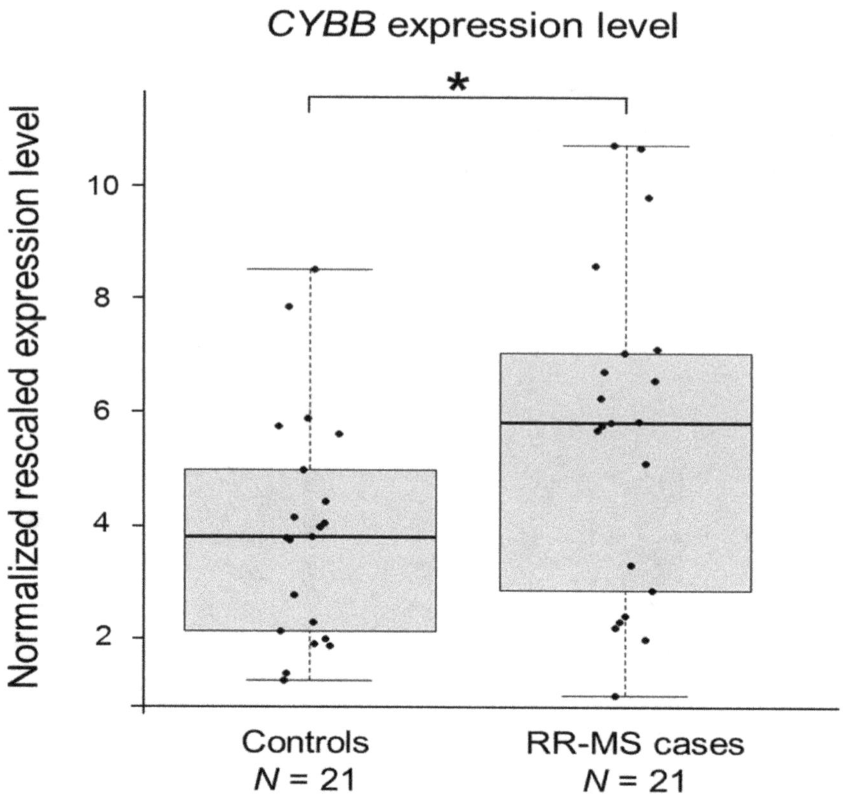

Figure 3. *CYBB* is upregulated in MS patients. Boxplots show the expression levels of the *CYBB* gene measured by semi-quantitative real-time RT-PCR in PBMCs of an Italian case-control cohort (only female individuals). Boxes define the interquartile range; the thick line refers to the median. Results were normalized to expression levels of the *HMBS* and *ACTB* housekeeping genes and are presented as rescaled values. The number of subjects belonging to each group is indicated (*N*). Significance levels of *t*-tests are shown. * $p < 0.05$.

3. Discussion

Apart from the well-known implication of mutations affecting the NOX2 complex in the pathogenesis of chronic granulomatous disease (CGD) [33], some information is currently available in the literature on the possible predisposing role of polymorphisms in *NCF1*, *NCF2*, *NCF4*, *CYBA*, and *CYBB* genes in other immune disorders. Among others, missense variants in the *NCF1* gene have been associated with systemic lupus erythematosus (SLE), Sjögren's syndrome, and rheumatoid arthritis (RA) [34]; two missense polymorphisms in *NCF2* were described as predisposing to SLE [35]; and common polymorphisms in *NCF4* were associated both with RA and Crohn's disease [36,37]. In our exploratory study, we aimed at investigating the possible genetic association between MS and all of the five genes coding for the NADPH oxidase complex. We found suggestive association signals for the *NCF1* and *CYBB* genes (lowest $p = 0.038$ and $p = 0.013$, respectively), which were paralleled, in the case of *CYBB*, by a gender-specific differential gene expression between MS cases and controls.

However, we acknowledge the limited size of our study material, and a lack of a replication step confirming the association of *CYBB* with MS. No significant association between the *CYBB* locus and MS was reported in the previous GWAS analyses, which, however, excluded the X chromosome harboring the *CYBB* gene from the genome-wide analysis. The role of the X chromosome in MS—a pathology characterized by higher susceptibility in females than males—remains still largely unknown. For instance, in the largest MS-related meta-analysis so far published, genome-wide, a total of 233 loci were found to be significantly associated with the disease, and only one maps to chromosome X [10]. The case-control analysis did not take gender into account, while the study presented here was utilizing family-based transmission analysis. Overall, the lack of association signals on chromosome X is indeed a common feature of complex traits: the X chromosome accounts for 5% of the nuclear genome and underlies almost 10% of Mendelian disorders [38]. Nonetheless, only 114 associations (0.8%) at $p \leq 5 \times 10^{-8}$ have been reported on the X chromosome, on a total of more than 14,700 signals identified by GWAS for ~300 traits [39]. These data could potentially be explained by the fact that the vast majority of GWAS have not included chromosome X in their analyses and have not considered gender. There is also a lack of specific bioinformatics pipelines to adopt in the analytic steps [40].

To overcome the limitation of the lack of a replication cohort in the association study, we focused on the investigation of an "intermediate phenotype", i.e., the gene expression profile of NOX2 components in $CD4^+$ and $CD4^-$ cells. We used a two-tiered approach, based on both microarray and real-time RT-PCR experiments. The most striking result was the differential gene expression for the *CYBB* gene in MS cases, with opposite molecular signatures not only between males and females, but also between $CD4^-$ and $CD4^+$ cells. Indeed, sex-differential expression has recently emerged as a common feature of many genes. For instance, by comprehensively analyzing the Genotype-Tissue Expression (GTEx) data across 53 tissues (publicly available at https://www.gtexportal.org/home/), Gershoni and Pietrokovski were able to demonstrate that more than 6500 protein-coding genes showed significant sex-differential expression in one or more tissues [41]. In most of the cases, these genes are differentially expressed according to gender in just one or a few tissues. The *CYBB* gene seems to conform to this rule, showing a certain degree of sex-differential expression in kidney cortex, bladder, and thyroid (see Figure S1 in the Supplementary Materials); similar observations can be made for *NCF1*, *NCF2*, *NCF4*, and *CYBA*. Of note, data relative to blood cell sub-populations are missing in the GTEx portal.

The differential gene expression evidenced by stratifying patients and controls on the basis of the gender and, above all, according to the cell type, could contribute to explaining—if confirmed in other immune disorders—some of the puzzling observations that have accumulated over the years on CGD, SLE, or RA. For instance, RA patients show in blood a marked increase in ROS formation, protein oxidation, as well as lipid peroxidation [42]. In addition, they also present a synovial tissue that is invaded by inflammatory cells, a large proportion of which are activated $CD4^+$ T cells [43]. Both these phenomena can collectively account for tissue damage and for the chronicity of the disease. However, the development of RA has been associated with a lower copy number of the *NCF1* gene [44], and this association was supported by *ncf1* mutant rodents [45,46]. In this regard, it could be speculated that lower expression levels of the NOX2 complex could be protective against the chronic inflammation in RA relevant tissues; on the other hand, a lower oxidative burst response in antigen-presenting cells, especially in the thymus during priming, could change the antigen-presentation capacity of the cells, thus inducing autoimmunity [46]. Besides RA and SLE, previously shown examples of immune pathology characterized by inappropriate over-activation or down-regulation of ROS also include psoriasis, Hashimoto thyroiditis, vitiligo, and inflammatory bowel disease [47,48].

Concerning specifically MS, our results well fit with the observations of Fischer and colleagues [16], who described a global NOX2 over-expression in microglia and infiltrating macrophages of MS patients' autopsy brain tissues. These data also suggest that an inflammation-associated oxidative burst could play a fundamental role in the demyelination process typical of MS.

In conclusion, our work adds another piece of information on the possible involvement of NOX2 in the pathogenesis of MS, suggesting that this particular topic deserves to be further investigated, especially in the light of potential therapies based on decreasing/enhancing the oxidative burst.

4. Materials and Methods

4.1. Materials

All oligonucleotides for SNP genotyping and quantitative real-time RT-PCRs were purchased from Proligo (Paris, France). Primer couples for microsatellite analysis were from Applied Biosystems (Foster City, CA, USA). All sequences can be provided on request. The AmpliTaq Gold, DynaZyme, and HotStar Taq DNA polymerases were from Applied Biosystems, Finnzymes (Espoo, Finland), and Qiagen (Hilden, Germany), respectively.

4.2. MS Pedigrees

The study was approved by the ethical committee of the Helsinki and Uusimaa hospital district (Decision 46/2002, #192/E9/02), and all individuals included in the study gave their informed consent. The study material consisted of a total of 63 families: 22 of them were multiplex MS families, having two to six affected cases per pedigree, whereas the remaining 41 families were composed of MS patients with their parents and unaffected siblings. These families were previously described [49] and they all originate from the high-risk region for MS in Southern Ostrobothnia, Finland. In total, the cohort consisted of 547 individuals, 116 being MS cases. Patient selection was hospital-based; only definite cases were included (clinically or laboratory-supported definite). Diagnosis of MS in affected individuals strictly followed Poser's diagnostic criteria [50].

4.3. Genotyping

Genomic DNA was extracted from peripheral blood cells following standard procedures.

Two non-chimeric microsatellite markers (D7S1870 and D7S2518) were selected from databases for the association analysis of the *NCF1* gene, avoiding the highly duplicated regions characterizing this chromosomal locus (7q11.23). Microsatellite markers were PCR amplified in two-plex format in 10-μL reaction mixtures under standard conditions, using VIC (D7S1870) or PET (D7S2518) labeled primers, the AmpliTaq Gold DNA polymerase, a MJ Tetrad thermal cycler (MJ Research INC, Waltham, MA, USA), and a touch-down thermal profile. PCR products were run on an ABI-3730 Genetic Analyzer (Applied Biosystems) and analyzed using the Genotyper software (Applied Biosystems).

For the association analysis of the other genes, we selected 21 SNPs, having heterozygosity >10%. Primers flanking the putative SNPs were designed for multiplex PCR amplification using the web-based program MPprimer (https://omictools.com/mpprimer-tool?t=tab-tool-variant-0). SNPs were first tested for polymorphic content by direct sequencing the relevant PCR-amplified fragment in 32 healthy Finnish individuals. Nine SNPs were monomorphic in the Finnish population, whereas one was tri-allelic; those ten SNPs were not further investigated. The remaining 11 SNPs were typed in MS samples using an in-house developed microarray, based on allele-specific primer extension [51]. In particular, two allele-specific detection oligonucleotides were designed for each SNP: these primers were characterized by the presence of a 5′ aminolinker and a stretch of 9T (poly-T), followed by the SNP-specific sequence. The 5′ aminolinker and the poly-T served to spot and anchor detection oligonucleotides onto silane/isothiocyanate-coated chrome mirror microscope slides (Evaporated Coatings, Willow Grove, PA, USA). Spotting was performed in duplicate using an OmniGrid 100 arrayer (Discovery Scientific, Vancouver, BC, Canada). Regions containing the SNPs were PCR amplified with a touch-down protocol from genomic DNA in two multiplex reactions, using SNP-specific primers with a T3 (forward) or a T7 (reverse) tail. Multiplex reactions were in-vitro transcribed using the AmpliScribe T7 or T3 High Yield Transcription Kit (Epicentre Technologies, Madison, WI, USA). The DNAseI-treated T3 or T7 RNA pools were hybridized to the arrays in a hybridization buffer (1.67 M NaCl) at 42 °C for 20 min. Arrays were washed twice in a washing buffer (0.3 M NaCl, 0.5× TE, 0.1% TritonX-100) and subsequently rinsed in ice-cold water. The allele-specific extension was performed using the MMLV Reverse Transcriptase (Epicentre Technologies) in a 20-μL reaction containing 50 mM Tris-HCl (pH 8.3), 10 mM $MgCl_2$, 75 mM KCl, 10 mM DTT, 0.5 μM dATP, 0.5 μM dGTP, 0.5 μM ddATP, 0.5 μM ddGTP, 1 μM Cy5-labeled dCTP, 1 μM Cy5-labeled dUTP (Cy5-labeled nucleotides were from Amersham Pharmacia Biotech, Uppsala, Sweden), 15% glycerol, and 0.24 M trehalose. Reverse transcription was carried out at 52 °C for 20 min. Finally, arrays were put in washing buffer under mild agitation for 15 min, dipped quickly in 50 mM NaOH, washed again in washing buffer, rinsed in ice-cold water, air dried, and scanned using a ScanArray 4000 instrument (Packard Biochip Technologies, Perkin Elmer Life Sciences, Boston, MA, USA). The image was analyzed using the ScanArray software (Packard Biochip Technologies, Perkin Elmer Life Sciences). Genotypes were called using an in-house developed software (W. Wong and C. Li, unpublished data).

The list of selected polymorphisms is presented in the Supplementary Materials (Table S1).

Important note: the entire analysis was performed a while ago, i.e., before the genomic databases became available with all the associated information on allele frequencies in different ethnicities.

4.4. Statistical Analyses

All genotypes were checked for Mendelian errors using PedCheck [52]. The check for the HWE was performed using the Genepop program (option 1), which also admits multiallelic markers [53]; only genotypes of women were considered for X-linked SNPs.

TDT [54] and HRR (a modified TDT test that uses siblings as "pseudo-controls") [55] analyses, both implemented in the ANALYZE package [55], were used in the association study. Since the inheritance pattern of MS is unknown, analyses were performed using two different modes of inheritance, i.e., dominant with reduced penetrance of $f = 0.05$ (with disease allele-frequency estimate of 0.01) or $f = 0.76$ (with disease allele-frequency estimate of 0.0006) [56].

Analyses were repeated using the PLINK software v.1.07 [57] by applying a more powerful method based on the TDT statistic implemented with the parental discordance test. This test is based on counting the number of alleles in affected versus unaffected parents (using each nuclear-family parental pair as a matched pair). These counts are then combined with the transmitted and untransmitted counts of the basic TDT to give a combined test statistic [58]. In this analysis, multiallelic markers were analyzed as biallelic, considering from one hand the most common allele, and from the other all the remaining ones clumped together as they were a unique alternative allele. In the text, p values, ORs, and 95% CIs always referred to the minor allele.

Considering the exploratory hypothesis-generating nature of the present study and the limited sample size as compared to the number of investigated genetic variants, we did not adjust for multiple testing, and p values < 0.05 were considered to be statistically significant. However, the total number of performed tests as well as the threshold of significance based on the over-conservative Bonferroni correction has been indicated in the footnote of the relevant table.

4.5. RNA Samples

Fresh blood samples from 25 members (both male and female subjects) belonging to five of the above-mentioned multiplex MS families were collected. PBMCs were separated using a Ficoll-Paque (Amersham Pharmacia Biotech) density gradient centrifugation, and hence stratified to $CD4^+$ and $CD4^-$ cell populations by negative selection using the $CD4^+$ T-cell isolation kit (Miltenyi Biotec, Auburn, CA, USA) and an autoMACS instrument (Miltenyi Biotec). Total RNA was extracted from $CD4^+$ and $CD4^-$ samples using the Trizol reagent (Ambion, Austin, TX, USA), treated with DNAse-I, and further purified with RNeasy Mini Kit columns (Qiagen, Valencia, CA, USA) according to the manufacturers' instruction. RNA quality was assessed using the RNA 6000 Nano assay in a Bioanalyzer (Agilent Technologies, Foster City, CA, USA).

As for the replication cohort, we collected PBMCs from 21 unrelated RR-MS patients and 21 healthy subjects, all females and Caucasians (coming from Northern Italy). Controls were age-matched with cases. To avoid possible confounding effects, we focused only on RR-MS cases in remitting phase, who had not received any immune-modulatory therapy within the month prior to blood withdrawal. PBMCs were isolated from heparinized blood immediately after phlebotomy by centrifugation on a Lympholyte Cell separation media (Cederlane Laboratories Limited, Hornby, ON, Canada) gradient. Total RNA was isolated using the Eurozol kit (Euroclone, Wetherby, UK).

4.6. Sample Preparation, Microarray Processing, and Data Analysis

RNA samples were prepared for hybridization on the Affymetrix GeneChip Human Genome U133 Plus 2.0 Array (Affymetrix, Santa Clara, CA, USA) according to the manufacturer's recommendations.

In brief, 1 μg of total RNA was converted to biotin-labelled cRNA using the Affymetrix HT One-Cycle cDNA Synthesis Kit and the HT IVT Labelling Kit. Fifteen μg of cRNA were then fragmented and hybridized for 16 hours at 45 °C, washed in Affymetrix Fluidics Station 450, and then scanned with Affymetrix GeneChip Scanner 3000. Hybridization, washing, staining, and scanning were conducted using the same instruments for all samples.

Raw intensity data files were imported to GeneSpring 7.3 (Agilent Technologies) and GC Robust Multi-array Average (GC-RMA) normalized. We then excluded probe sets with low signal intensity (GC-RMA normalized signal < 50). Probe sets with a $p \leq 0.05$ were considered to be differentially expressed.

4.7. Semi-Quantitative Real-Time RT-PCRs

Random hexamers and the TaqMan Gold RT-PCR kit (Applied Biosystems) were used to perform first-strand cDNA synthesis starting from 1 μg of total RNA from $CD4^{+/-}$ cells, according to the manufacturer's instructions. From a total of 20 μL of the RT reaction, 4 μL were used as template for semi-quantitative real-time RT-PCRs for the quantitation of the *NCF1* and *NCF2* mRNAs. Assays were carried out using the SYBR-Green Kit (Applied Biosystems) and a standard PCR thermal protocol on the ABI Prism 7900 HT Sequence Detection System. Data were analyzed with the Sequence Detector version 2.0 software (Applied Biosystems).

As for *CYBB* evaluation, random hexamers and the Superscript-III Reverse Transcriptase (Invitrogen, Carlsbad, CA, USA) were used in the RT step starting from 1 μg of RNA extracted from PBMCs of MS patients and controls. From a total of 20 μL of the RT reaction, 1 μL was used as a template for amplifications, using the FastStart SYBR Green Master Mix (Roche, Basel, Switzerland) on a LightCycler 480 (Roche), following a touch-down thermal protocol. Data were analyzed by the GeNorm software [59].

In all cases, RT-PCRs were performed at least in triplicate. Expression levels were normalized using *HMBS* (hydroxymethylbilane synthase gene) and *ACTB* (β-actin) as housekeeping genes. Primer sequences can be provided on request.

Author Contributions: R.A. and J.S. conceived and designed the experiments; R.A., G.C., and E.M.P. performed the experiments; R.A., G.S., S.D., and J.S. analyzed the data; R.A. wrote the paper; J.S. and R.A. supervised the entire study.

Acknowledgments: The European Science foundation is acknowledged for the support to R.A. (Grant program GENOMICS/2003/19).

Abbreviations

ACTB	β-actin
$CD4^+$	Cluster of differentiation 4 positive
$CD4^-$	Cluster of differentiation 4 negative
CGD	Chronic granulomatous disease
CI	Confidence interval
CNS	Central nervous system
CYBA	Cytochrome B-245 alpha chain, coding for the p22phox subunit of the NOX2 system
CYBB	Cytochrome B-245 beta chain, coding for the gp91phox subunit of the NOX2 system
GC-RMA	GC Robust Multi-array Average
GWAS	Genome-wide association study
HLA	Human leukocyte antigen
HMBS	Hydroxymethylbilane synthase gene
HRR	Haplotype relative risk
HWE	Hardy-Weinberg equilibrium

MMLV	Moloney Murine Leukemia Virus
MS	Multiple sclerosis
NADPH	nicotinamide adenine dinucleotide phosphate
NCF1	Neutrophil cytosolic factor 1, coding for the p47phox subunit of the NOX2 system
NCF2	Neutrophil cytosolic factor 2, coding for the p67phox subunit of the NOX2 system
NCF4	Neutrophil cytosolic factor 4, coding for the p40phox subunit of the NOX2 system
NOX	NADPH oxidase system
NOX2	NADPH oxidase system 2 (isoform 2 of the complex)
OMIM	Online Mendelian Inheritance in Men
OR	Odds ratio
OS	Oxidative stress
PBMCs	Peripheral blood mononuclear cells
RA	Rheumatoid arthritis
ROS	Reactive oxygen species
RR	Relapsing-remitting
RT-PCR	Reverse-transcription polymerase chain reactions
SD	Standard deviation
SLE	Systemic lupus erythematosus
SNP	Single nucleotide polymorphism
TDT	Transmission/disequilibrium test

References

1. Trapp, B.D.; Peterson, J.; Ransohoff, R.M.; Rudick, R.; Mörk, S.; Bö, L. Axonal transection in the lesions of multiple sclerosis. *N. Engl. J. Med.* **1998**, *338*, 278–285. [CrossRef] [PubMed]
2. Hauser, S.L.; Oksenberg, J.R. The neurobiology of multiple sclerosis: Genes, inflammation, and neurodegeneration. *Neuron* **2006**, *52*, 61–76. [CrossRef] [PubMed]
3. Thompson, A.J. Multiple sclerosis—A global disorder and still poorly managed. *Lancet Neurol.* **2008**, *7*, 1078–1079. [CrossRef]
4. Kingwell, E.; Marriott, J.J.; Jetté, N.; Pringsheim, T.; Makhani, N.; Morrow, S.A.; Fisk, J.D.; Evans, C.; Béland, S.G.; Kulaga, S.; et al. Incidence and prevalence of multiple sclerosis in Europe: A systematic review. *BMC Neurol.* **2013**, *13*, 128. [CrossRef] [PubMed]
5. Sumelahti, M.L.; Tienari, P.J.; Wikström, J.; Palo, J.; Hakama, M. Regional and temporal variation in the incidence of multiple sclerosis in Finland 1979–1993. *Neuroepidemiology* **2000**, *19*, 67–75. [CrossRef] [PubMed]
6. International Multiple Sclerosis Genetics Consortium; Hafler, D.A.; Compston, A.; Sawcer, S.; Lander, E.S.; Daly, M.J.; De Jager, P.L.; de Bakker, P.I.; Gabriel, S.B.; Mirel, D.B.; et al. Risk alleles for multiple sclerosis identified by a genomewide study. *N. Engl. J. Med.* **2007**, *357*, 851–862. [CrossRef] [PubMed]
7. Sawcer, S.; Hellenthal, G.; Pirinen, M.; Spencer, C.C.; Patsopoulos, N.A.; Moutsianas, L.; Dilthey, A.; Su, Z.; Freeman, C.; Hunt, S.E.; et al. Genetic risk and a primary role for cell-mediated immune mechanisms in multiple sclerosis. *Nature* **2011**, *476*, 214–219. [CrossRef] [PubMed]
8. International Multiple Sclerosis Genetics Consortium (IMSGC); Beecham, A.H.; Patsopoulos, N.A.; Xifara, D.K.; Davis, M.F.; Kemppinen, A.; Cotsapas, C.; Shah, T.S.; Spencer, C.; Booth, D.; et al. Analysis of immune-related loci identifies 48 new susceptibility variants for multiple sclerosis. *Nat. Genet.* **2013**, *45*, 1353–1360. [CrossRef] [PubMed]
9. Bos, S.D.; Berge, T.; Celius, E.G.; Harbo, H.F. From genetic associations to functional studies in multiple sclerosis. *Eur. J. Neurol.* **2016**, *23*, 847–853. [CrossRef] [PubMed]
10. Patsopoulos, N.; Baranzini, S.E.; Santaniello, A.; Shoostari, P.; Cotsapas, C.; Wong, G.; Beecham, A.H.; James, T.; Replogle, J.; Vlachos, I.; et al. The Multiple Sclerosis Genomic Map: Role of peripheral immune cells and resident microglia in susceptibility. *bioRxiv* **2017**. [CrossRef]
11. Linker, R.A.; Kieseier, B.C.; Gold, R. Identification and development of new therapeutics for multiple sclerosis. *Trends Pharm. Sci.* **2008**, *29*, 558–565. [CrossRef] [PubMed]

12. Broux, B.; Stinissen, P.; Hellings, N. Which immune cells matter? The immunopathogenesis of multiple sclerosis. *Crit. Rev. Immunol.* **2013**, *33*, 283–306. [CrossRef] [PubMed]
13. Salou, M.; Nicol, B.; Garcia, A.; Laplaud, D.A. Involvement of CD8(+) T Cells in Multiple Sclerosis. *Front. Immunol.* **2015**, *6*, 604. [CrossRef] [PubMed]
14. Jones, A.P.; Kermode, A.G.; Lucas, R.M.; Carroll, W.M.; Nolan, D.; Hart, P.H. Circulating immune cells in multiple sclerosis. *Clin. Exp. Immunol.* **2017**, *187*, 193–203. [CrossRef] [PubMed]
15. Gilgun-Sherki, Y.; Melamed, E.; Offen, D. The role of oxidative stress in the pathogenesis of multiple sclerosis: The need for effective antioxidant therapy. *J. Neurol.* **2004**, *251*, 261–268. [CrossRef] [PubMed]
16. Fischer, M.T.; Sharma, R.; Lim, J.L.; Haider, L.; Frischer, J.M.; Drexhage, J.; Mahad, D.; Bradl, M.; van Horssen, J.; Lassmann, H. NADPH oxidase expression in active multiple sclerosis lesions in relation to oxidative tissue damage and mitochondrial injury. *Brain* **2012**, *135*, 886–899. [CrossRef] [PubMed]
17. Adamczyk, B.; Adamczyk-Sowa, M. New Insights into the Role of Oxidative Stress Mechanisms in the Pathophysiology and Treatment of Multiple Sclerosis. *Oxidative Med. Cell. Longev.* **2016**, *2016*, 1973834. [CrossRef] [PubMed]
18. Van der Goes, A.; Brouwer, J.; Hoekstra, K.; Roos, D.; van den Berg, T.K.; Dijkstra, C.D. Reactive oxygen species are required for the phagocytosis of myelin by macrophages. *J. Neuroimmunol.* **1998**, *92*, 67–75. [CrossRef]
19. Nikić, I.; Merkler, D.; Sorbara, C.; Brinkoetter, M.; Kreutzfeldt, M.; Bareyre, F.M.; Brück, W.; Bishop, D.; Misgeld, T.; Kerschensteiner, M. A reversible form of axon damage in experimental autoimmune encephalomyelitis and multiple sclerosis. *Nat. Med.* **2011**, *17*, 495–499. [CrossRef] [PubMed]
20. Friese, M.A.; Schattling, B.; Fugger, L. Mechanisms of neurodegeneration and axonal dysfunction in multiple sclerosis. *Nat. Rev. Neurol.* **2014**, *10*, 225–238. [CrossRef] [PubMed]
21. Barnes, P.J.; Karin, M. Nuclear factor-kappaB: A pivotal transcription factor in chronic inflammatory diseases. *N. Engl. J. Med.* **1997**, *336*, 1066–1071. [CrossRef] [PubMed]
22. Srinivasan, M.; Lahiri, D.K. Significance of NF-κB as a pivotal therapeutic target in the neurodegenerative pathologies of Alzheimer's disease and multiple sclerosis. *Expert Opin. Ther. Targets* **2015**, *19*, 471–487. [CrossRef] [PubMed]
23. Romanic, A.M.; Madri, J.A. Extracellular matrix-degrading proteinases in the nervous system. *Brain Pathol.* **1994**, *4*, 145–156. [CrossRef] [PubMed]
24. Merrill, J.E.; Murphy, S.P. Inflammatory events at the blood brain barrier: Regulation of adhesion molecules, cytokines, and chemokines by reactive nitrogen and oxygen species. *Brain Behav. Immun.* **1997**, *11*, 245–263. [CrossRef] [PubMed]
25. Chiurchiù, V.; Orlacchio, A.; Maccarrone, M. Is Modulation of Oxidative Stress an Answer? The State of the Art of Redox Therapeutic Actions in Neurodegenerative Diseases. *Oxidative Med. Cell. Longev.* **2016**, *2016*, 7909380. [CrossRef] [PubMed]
26. Vladimirova, O.; Lu, F.M.; Shawver, L.; Kalman, B. The activation of protein kinase C induces higher production of reactive oxygen species by mononuclear cells in patients with multiple sclerosis than in controls. *Inflamm. Res.* **1999**, *48*, 412–416. [CrossRef] [PubMed]
27. Lu, F.; Selak, M.; O'Connor, J.; Croul, S.; Lorenzana, C.; Butunoi, C.; Kalman, B. Oxidative damage to mitochondrial DNA and activity of mitochondrial enzymes in chronic active lesions of multiple sclerosis. *J. Neurol. Sci.* **2000**, *177*, 95–103. [CrossRef]
28. Van Horssen, J.; Witte, M.E.; Schreibelt, G.; de Vries, H.E. Radical changes in multiple sclerosis pathogenesis. *Biochim. Biophys. Acta* **2011**, *1812*, 141–150. [CrossRef] [PubMed]
29. Babior, B.M. NADPH Oxidase: An update. *Blood* **1999**, *93*, 1464–1476. [PubMed]
30. Vignais, P.V. The superoxide-generating NADPH oxidase: Structural aspects and activation mechanism. *Cell. Mol. Life Sci.* **2002**, *59*, 1428–1459. [CrossRef] [PubMed]
31. Trapp, B.D.; Nave, K.A. Multiple sclerosis: An immune or neurodegenerative disorder? *Annu. Rev. Neurosci.* **2008**, *31*, 247–269. [CrossRef] [PubMed]
32. Kleiveland, C.R. Peripheral Blood Mononuclear Cells. In *The Impact of Food Bioactives on Health*; Verhoeckx, K., Cotter, P., López-Expósito, I., Kleiveland, C., Lea, T., Mackie, A., Requena, T., Swiateck, D., Wicher, H., Eds.; Springer: Cham, Switzerland, 2015. [CrossRef]

33. Wu, J.; Wang, W.F.; Zhang, Y.D.; Chen, T.X. Clinical Features and Genetic Analysis of 48 Patients with Chronic Granulomatous Disease in a Single Center Study from Shanghai, China (2005–2015): New Studies and a Literature Review. *J. Immunol. Res.* **2017**, *2017*, 8745254. [CrossRef] [PubMed]
34. Zhao, J.; Ma, J.; Deng, Y.; Kelly, J.A.; Kim, K.; Bang, S.Y.; Lee, H.S.; Li, Q.Z.; Wakeland, E.K.; Qiu, R.; et al. A missense variant in NCF1 is associated with susceptibility to multiple autoimmune diseases. *Nat. Genet.* **2017**, *49*, 433–437. [CrossRef] [PubMed]
35. Armstrong, D.L.; Eisenstein, M.; Zidovetzki, R.; Jacob, C.O. Systemic lupus erythematosus-associated neutrophil cytosolic factor 2 mutation affects the structure of NADPH oxidase complex. *J. Biol. Chem.* **2015**, *290*, 12595–12602. [CrossRef] [PubMed]
36. Olsson, L.M.; Lindqvist, A.K.; Källberg, H.; Padyukov, L.; Burkhardt, H.; Alfredsson, L.; Klareskog, L.; Holmdahl, R. A case-control study of rheumatoid arthritis identifies an associated single nucleotide polymorphism in the NCF4 gene, supporting a role for the NADPH-oxidase complex in autoimmunity. *Arthritis Res. Ther.* **2007**, *9*, R98. [CrossRef] [PubMed]
37. Rioux, J.D.; Xavier, R.J.; Taylor, K.D.; Silverberg, M.S.; Goyette, P.; Huett, A.; Green, T.; Kuballa, P.; Barmada, M.M.; Datta, L.W.; et al. Genome-wide association study identifies new susceptibility loci for Crohn disease and implicates autophagy in disease pathogenesis. *Nat. Genet.* **2007**, *39*, 596–604. [CrossRef] [PubMed]
38. Amberger, J.; Bocchini, C.A.; Scott, A.F.; Hamosh, A. McKusick's Online Mendelian Inheritance in Man (OMIM). *Nucleic Acids Res.* **2009**, *37*, D793–D796. [CrossRef] [PubMed]
39. MacArthur, J.; Bowler, E.; Cerezo, M.; Gil, L.; Hall, P.; Hastings, E.; Junkins, H.; McMahon, A.; Milano, A.; Morales, J.; et al. The new NHGRI-EBI Catalog of published genome-wide association studies (GWAS Catalog). *Nucleic Acids Res.* **2017**, *45*, D896–D901. [CrossRef] [PubMed]
40. Wise, A.L.; Gyi, L.; Manolio, T.A. eXclusion: Toward integrating the X chromosome in genome-wide association analyses. *Am. J. Hum. Genet.* **2013**, *92*, 643–647. [CrossRef] [PubMed]
41. Gershoni, M.; Pietrokovski, S. The landscape of sex-differential transcriptome and its consequent selection in human adults. *BMC Biol.* **2017**, *15*, 7. [CrossRef] [PubMed]
42. Mateen, S.; Moin, S.; Khan, A.Q.; Zafar, A.; Fatima, N. Increased Reactive Oxygen Species Formation and Oxidative Stress in Rheumatoid Arthritis. *PLoS ONE* **2016**, *11*, e0152925. [CrossRef] [PubMed]
43. Kondo, Y.; Yokosawa, M.; Kaneko, S.; Furuyama, K.; Segawa, S.; Tsuboi, H.; Matsumoto, I.; Sumida, T. Review: Transcriptional Regulation of CD4+ T Cell Differentiation in Experimentally Induced Arthritis and Rheumatoid Arthritis. *Arthritis Rheumatol.* **2018**, *70*, 653–661. [CrossRef] [PubMed]
44. Olsson, L.M.; Nerstedt, A.; Lindqvist, A.K.; Johansson, S.C.; Medstrand, P.; Olofsson, P.; Holmdahl, R. Copy number variation of the gene NCF1 is associated with rheumatoid arthritis. *Antioxid Redox Signal* **2012**, *16*, 71–78. [CrossRef] [PubMed]
45. Olofsson, P.; Holmberg, J.; Tordsson, J.; Lu, S.; Akerström, B.; Holmdahl, R. Positional identification of Ncf1 as a gene that regulates arthritis severity in rats. *Nat. Genet.* **2003**, *33*, 25–32. [CrossRef] [PubMed]
46. Hultqvist, M.; Olofsson, P.; Holmberg, J.; Bäckström, B.T.; Tordsson, J.; Holmdahl, R. Enhanced autoimmunity, arthritis, and encephalomyelitis in mice with a reduced oxidative burst due to a mutation in the Ncf1 gene. *Proc. Natl. Acad. Sci. USA* **2004**, *101*, 12646–12651. [CrossRef] [PubMed]
47. Kienhöfer, D.; Boeltz, S.; Hoffmann, M.H. Reactive oxygen homeostasis—The balance for preventing autoimmunity. *Lupus* **2016**, *25*, 943–954. [CrossRef] [PubMed]
48. Di Dalmazi, G.; Hirshberg, J.; Lyle, D.; Freij, J.B.; Caturegli, P. Reactive oxygen species in organ-specific autoimmunity. *Autoimmun. Highlights* **2016**, *7*, 11. [CrossRef] [PubMed]
49. Saarela, J.; Kallio, S.P.; Chen, D.; Montpetit, A.; Jokiaho, A.; Choi, E.; Asselta, R.; Bronnikov, D.; Lincoln, M.R.; Sadovnick, A.D.; et al. PRKCA and multiple sclerosis: Association in two independent populations. *PLoS Genet.* **2006**, *2*, e42. [CrossRef] [PubMed]
50. Poser, C.M.; Paty, D.W.; Scheinberg, L.; McDonald, W.I.; Davis, F.A.; Ebers, G.C.; Johnson, K.P.; Sibley, W.A.; Silberberg, D.H.; Tourtellotte, W.W. New diagnostic criteria for multiple sclerosis: Guidelines for research protocols. *Ann. Neurol.* **1983**, *13*, 227–231. [CrossRef] [PubMed]
51. Pastinen, T.; Raitio, M.; Lindroos, K.; Tainola, P.; Peltonen, L.; Syvänen, A.C. A system for specific, high-throughput genotyping by allele-specific primer extension on microarrays. *Genome Res.* **2000**, *10*, 1031–1042. [CrossRef] [PubMed]

52. O'Connell, J.R.; Weeks, D.E. PedCheck: A program for identification of genotype incompatibilities in linkage analysis. *Am. J. Hum. Genet.* **1998**, *63*, 259–266. [CrossRef] [PubMed]
53. Raymond, M.; Rousset, F. GENEPOP (version 1.2): Population genetics software for exact tests and ecumenicism. *J. Hered.* **1995**, *86*, 248–249. [CrossRef]
54. Spielman, R.S.; McGinnis, R.E.; Ewens, W.J. Transmission test for linkage disequilibrium: The insulin gene region and insulin-dependent diabetes mellitus (IDDM). *Am. J. Hum. Genet.* **1993**, *52*, 506–516. [PubMed]
55. Terwilliger, J.D.; Ott, J. A haplotype-based 'haplotype relative risk' approach to detecting allelic associations. *Hum. Hered.* **1992**, *42*, 337–346. [CrossRef] [PubMed]
56. Kuokkanen, S.; Sundvall, M.; Terwilliger, J.D.; Tienari, P.J.; Wikström, J.; Holmdahl, R.; Pettersson, U.; Peltonen, L. A putative vulnerability locus to multiple sclerosis maps to 5p14-p12 in a region syntenic to the murine locus Eae2. *Nat. Genet.* **1996**, *13*, 477–480. [CrossRef] [PubMed]
57. Purcell, S.; Neale, B.; Todd-Brown, K.; Thomas, L.; Ferreira, M.A.; Bender, D.; Maller, J.; Sklar, P.; de Bakker, P.I.; Daly, M.J.; et al. PLINK: A tool set for whole-genome association and population-based linkage analyses. *Am. J. Hum. Genet.* **2007**, *8*, 559–575. [CrossRef] [PubMed]
58. Purcell, S.; Sham, P.; Daly, M.J. Parental phenotypes in family-based association analysis. *Am. J. Hum. Genet.* **2005**, *76*, 249–259. [CrossRef] [PubMed]
59. Vandesompele, J.; De Preter, K.; Pattyn, F.; Poppe, B.; Van Roy, N.; De Paepe, A.; Speleman, F. Accurate normalization of real-time quantitative RT-PCR data by geometric averaging of multiple internal control genes. *Genome Biol.* **2002**, *3*, RESEARCH0034. [CrossRef] [PubMed]

12

Autoimmune Encephalitis and CSF Anti-GluR3 Antibodies in an MS Patient after Alemtuzumab Treatment

Maria Chiara Buscarinu [1], Arianna Fornasiero [1], Giulia Pellicciari [2], Roberta Reniè [2], Anna Chiara Landi [2], Alessandro Bozzao [1], Cristina Cappelletti [3], Pia Bernasconi [3], Giovanni Ristori [1,*] and Marco Salvetti [1,4,*]

1 Department of Neurosciences, Mental Health and Sensory Organs, Centre for Experimental Neurological Therapies (CENTERS), Faculty of Medicine and Psychology, Sapienza University, 00189 Rome, Italy; mchiara.buscarinu@gmail.com (M.C.B.); ari.fornasiero@gmail.com (A.F.); alessandro.bozzao@uniroma1.it (A.B.)

2 Faculty of Medicine and Psychology, Sapienza University, 00189 Rome, Italy; giuliapellicciari11@gmail.com (G.P.); roberta.renie@gmail.com (R.R.); landiannachiara@gmail.com (A.C.L.)

3 Neurology IV–Neuroimmunology and Neuromuscular Diseases Unit, Fondazione IRCCS Istituto Neurologico Carlo Besta, 20133 Milan, Italy; cristina.cappelletti@istituto-besta.it (C.C.); pia.bernasconi@istituto-besta.it (P.B.)

4 IRCCS Istituto Neurologico Mediterraneo (INM) Neuromed, 86077 Pozzilli, Italy

* Correspondence: giovanni.ristori@uniroma1.it (G.R.); marco.salvetti@uniroma1.it (M.S.);

Abstract: A 45-year-old Italian woman, affected by relapsing–remitting multiple sclerosis (RR-MS) starting from 2011, started treatment with alemtuzumab in July 2016. Nine months after the second infusion, she had an immune thrombocytopenic purpura (ITP) with complete recovery after steroid treatment. Three months after the ITP, the patient presented with transient aphasia, cognitive deficits, and focal epilepsy. Serial brain magnetic resonance imaging showed a pattern compatible with encephalitis. Autoantibodies to glutamate receptor 3 peptide A and B were detected in cerebrospinal fluid and serum, in the absence of any other diagnostic cues. After three courses of intravenous immunoglobulin (0.4 mg/kg/day for 5 days, 1 month apart), followed by boosters (0.4 mg/kg/day) every 4–6 weeks, her neurological status improved and is currently comparable with that preceding the encephalitis. Autoimmune complications of the central nervous system during alemtuzumab therapy are relatively rare: only one previous case of autoimmune encephalitis following alemtuzumab treatment has been reported to date.

Keywords: multiple sclerosis; autoimmune diseases; immune thrombocytopenic purpura; autoimmune encephalitis; alemtuzumab; antibodies against GluR3 peptide

1. Introduction

Alemtuzumab, a humanized monoclonal antibody indicated for the treatment of patients with relapsing–remitting multiple sclerosis (RR-MS), increases the risk of autoimmune adverse events, including thyroid disorder, renal disease, and immune thrombocytopenic purpura (ITP) [1]. Recently, new complications after alemtuzumab treatment have been described, like stroke, myocardial infarction, diffuse alveolar hemorrhage, and hemophagocytic lymphohistiocytosis (as reported in the European Medicine Agency note EMEA/H/A-20/1483/C/3718/0028).

We here report a case of presumed autoimmune encephalitis (AE) after the second course of alemtuzumab. AE is one of the most common causes of non-infectious encephalitis, with a variety of clinical manifestations, including behavioral and psychiatric symptoms, autonomic disturbances, movement disorders, and seizures. First-line immune therapies in AE consist of corticosteroids (intravenous and oral), sometimes coupled with intravenous immunoglobulin (IVIG) and/or plasma exchange (PE). Second-line treatments, including rituximab, cyclophosphamide, azathioprine, and mycophenolate mofetil, are administered when the first-line therapies fail to produce adequate benefits, when the disease is severe or relapsing, or, even in case of response to first-line treatments, with the goal of decreasing the risk of relapse in AE [2].

2. Case Report

We report the case of a 45-year-old Italian woman affected by RR-MS from 2011, when she had a diplopia and underwent a magnetic resonance imaging (MRI) showing multiple contrast-enhancing lesions in her brain and spinal cord white matter. After a spontaneous recovery, she later had another clinical attack and was treated with high intravenous steroids. Having fulfilled the criteria of definite diseases, a spinal tap was not performed and a disease-modifying therapy was started. After the failure of two first-line therapies (glatiramer acetate and dimethylfumarate) with clinical reactivations and new lesions identified after a new MRI, she started alemtuzumab in July 2016. Other second-line treatments, including natalizumab and fingolimod, were contraindicated for the presence of anti-JC virus antibodies at high titer (stratify index 3.20) and bradycardia. The alemtuzumab schedule (12 mg once daily (QD) for 5 days, followed by 12 mg QD for 3 days after one year) was approved for MS treatment.

In June 2018, 9 months after the second alemtuzumab infusion cycle, she reported a longer and more abundant menstrual period, bleeding from the gums, and scattered red spots on the skin. She was then referred to the emergency department: her platelet level was 1000/μL (normal range: 150,000–450,000/μL), with positive direct and indirect Coombs tests, and a normal bone marrow biopsy. A diagnosis of ITP was made and steroid treatment (methyl-prednisolone 40 mg daily for 7 days, followed by tapering) was promptly started with improvement: her platelet count became normal and the symptoms regressed in approximately 30 days.

In September 2018, 3 months after ITP, the patient presented with progressive aphasia and underwent a brain MRI that showed a pattern compatible with encephalitis (Figure 1a). She was hospitalized and her neurological examinations showed a change in neurological status with anomic aphasia and motor apraxia. Cerebrospinal fluid (CSF) was clear, with a slight increase in glucose (73 mg/dl) and protein (61 mg/dl) and normal cell numbers (4 cells/mmc; normal range: 0–5 cell/mmc). Immunoelectrophocusing showed an IgG index of 1.45 (0.00–0.65) and the presence of 17 oligoclonal bands. The PCR for herpes viruses (HSV (herpes simplex virus), CMV (cytomegalovirus), VZV (varicella-zoster virus), EBV (Epstein-Barr virus), HHV6 (human herpesvirus 6)) and the JC virus (JCV) was negative. Autoimmune screening (anti-gliadin IgG e IgA, anti-transglutaminase, anti-cardiolipin, antibodies to double-stranded DNA, extractable nuclear antigens, and anti-neutrophil cytoplasmic antibodies) was negative. Serology for common and neurotropic infectious agents (Toxoplasma, B. Burgdorferi, HIV), levels of oncotumor markers (CEA (carcino-embryonic antigen), AFP (alpha fetoprotein), CA (cancer antigen) 125, CA 15-3, CA 19-9, and Cyfra (cytokeratin 19 fragment antigen) 21-1 NSE (neuron-specific enolase)), antibodies against onconeural antigens (anti-amphiphysin, anti-MA2, anti-Yo, anti-Ri, anti-Hu, anti-GAD65, anti-titin, anti-recoverin, anti-Sox1, and anti-Zic4), and a total-body computerized tomography were all normal.

Three days after hospitalization, aphasia recovered completely; however, a new brain MRI showed increased edema in the left fronto-temporal subcortical white matter, without diffusion restriction or contrast enhancement (Figure 1b). Five days after hospitalization, a focal epilepsy started with clonic movements in her left upper limb, associated with the worsening of working memory and mood changes. An electroencephalogram showed non-specific electrical alterations in the bilateral temporo-occipital lobes. The patient started therapy with oral levetiracetam (1500 mg daily), with a stop in seizures and improvement of neurological status. We chose not to start steroid or other immunomodulatory therapies, planning strict clinical and neuroradiological follow-up instead.

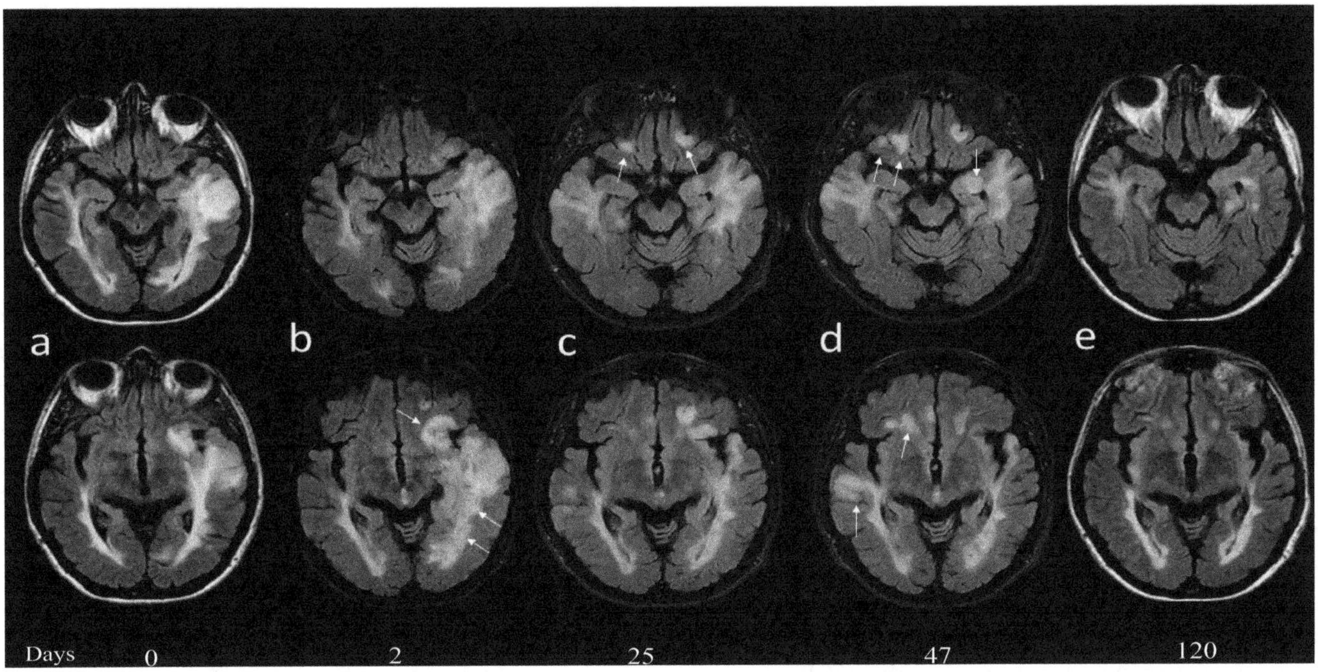

Figure 1. At admission (**a**) showed a large T2 signal alteration involving the left temporal lobe and expanding the superior temporal gyrus. (**b**) Two days later, a new brain magnetic resonance imaging (MRI) showed increased edema also involving the frontal subcortical and periventricular white matter (**b**, arrows); compression of the ventricular system was increased; and no diffusion restriction or contrast enhancement was demonstrated. (**c**) Twenty-five days after admission a new MRI showed reduction of the previously described T2 temporal lobe signal alteration with reduced compression of the temporal horn of the ventricle. Five new lesions were demonstrated and two of these were located in the fronto-orbital regions bilaterally (**c**, arrows). (**d**) Forty-seven days after admission, a new MRI documented a worsening of the T2 signal alterations in the fronto-orbital and in the temporal region on the right, with mild contrast enhancement in the right hippocampus and cingulum cortex (not shown). (**e**) Four months after the beginning of symptomatology all the signal alterations were markedly reduced and no enhancement was evident.

After twenty days, the patient presented with vomiting and mental confusion. A new MRI showed the reduction of a T2 hyperintense lesion previously described, but the appearance of five similar lesions (Figure 1c). Neurological examination showed a worsening of cognitive (especially executive) function and mood status. A second CSF examination was performed that showed 1 cell/mmc, 29 proteins mg/dl, glucose 54 mg/dl, and also included the search for a panel of autoantibodies known to be associated with AE (not investigated in the previous CSF examination). Autoantibodies to glutamate receptor 3 (GluR3) peptide A and B were detected both in the CSF (0.143 and 0.140, respectively, at CSF dilution 1:2) and in the serum (1.074 and 1.155, respectively, at serum dilution 1:200) by an enzyme-linked immunosorbent assay, as described [3,4]. No other findings emerged from the second CSF examination and we therefore started the first course of intravenous immunoglobulin (0.4 mg/kg/day for 5 days).

After a strict follow-up of about 3 weeks, during which the patient showed a partial recovery, a new MRI documented a worsening condition with an extension of signal alterations in the right frontal-orbital and temporal-basal region, with evident contrast enhancements in the hippocampus and cingulum cortex (Figure 1d). The patient underwent another two courses of intravenous immunoglobulin (0.4 mg/kg/day for 5 days), one month apart, with progressive clinical-MRI improvement (Figure 1e).

Her neurological status is currently comparable with that preceding the encephalitis. Given the response to IVIG treatment, we decided to continue that treatment (0.4 g/kg/day, every 4–6 weeks), while we stopped any treatment for MS. The patient is currently on monthly follow-up visits, possibly planning B cell-depleting treatments.

3. Discussion

Autoimmune complications of the central nervous system (CNS) during alemtuzumab therapy are relatively rare: one case of AE was reported to date [5]. The AE case occurred seven months after the second course of alemtuzumab, presenting with a polymorphic epilepsia partialis continua/status epilepticus in a patient with previous autoimmune hypothyroidism and ITP. No autoantibodies were reported in this case.

The clinical-MRI pattern of our patient is comparable with that recently reported. However, the peculiarity of our case was the positivity for anti-GluR3 autoantibodies. This is one of the antibodies directed against ionotropic glutamate receptors. They are present in 25%–30% of patients with different types of epilepsy, underpinning forms of 'autoimmune epilepsy' with frequent cognitive, psychiatric, and behavioral impairments [6]. The finding of anti-GluR3 autoantibodies was also associated with Rasmussen encephalitis, where they cause complement-mediated neuronal damage, irrespective of an excitotoxic effect [7]. A recent case of intractable myoclonus associated with anti-GluR3 antibodies was reported after allogeneic bone marrow transplantation [8].

Overall, our case and that described by Giarola et al. [5] strongly suggest a relationship between AE and previous therapy with alemtuzumab. Especially in patients with other well-known alemtuzumab-associated autoimmune complications (such ITP), monitoring of clinical events that may encompass the AE spectrum is advisable.

Author Contributions: M.C.B., M.S., and G.R. contributed equally to the writing and critical reading of the manuscript; A.B. provided interpretation of MRI imaging; C.C. and P.B. provided interpretation of immunological data; A.F., G.P., R.R., and A.C.L. provided critical reading of the manuscript. All authors read and approved the final manuscript.

References

1. Coles, A.J.; Cohen, J.A.; Fox, E.J.; Giovannoni, G.; Hartung, H.P.; Havrdova, E.; Schippling, S.; Selmaj, K.W.; Traboulsee, A.; Compston, D.A.S.; et al. Alemtuzumab CARE-MS II 5-year follow-up: Efficacy and safety findings. *Neurology* **2017**, *89*, 1117–1126. [CrossRef] [PubMed]
2. Nosadini, M.; Mohammad, S.S.; Ramanathan, S.; Brilot, F.; Dale, R.C. Immune therapy in autoimmune encephalitis: A systematic review. *Expert Rev. Neurother.* **2015**, *15*, 1391–1419. [CrossRef] [PubMed]
3. Mantegazza, R.; Bernasconi, P.; Baggi, F.; Spreafico, R.; Ragona, F.; Antozzi, C.; Bernardi, G.; Granata, T.; Italian Rasmussen's Encephalitis Study Group. Antibodies against GluR3 peptides are nots pecific for Rasmussen's encephalitis but are also present in epilepsy patients with severe, early onset disease and intractable seizures. *J. Neuroimmunol.* **2002**, *131*, 179–185. [CrossRef]
4. Borroni, B.; Stanic, J.; Verpelli, C.; Mellone, M.; Bonomi, E.; Alberici, A.; Bernasconi, P.; Culotta, L.; Zianni, E.; Archetti, S.; et al. Anti-AMPA GluA3 antibodies in frontotemporal dementia: A new molecular target. *Sci. Rep.* **2017**, *7*, 6723. [CrossRef] [PubMed]
5. Giarola, B.; Massey, J.; Barnett, Y.; Rodrigues, M.; Sutton, I. Autoimmune encephalitis following alemtuzumab treatment of multiple sclerosis. *Mult. Scler. Relat. Disord.* **2019**, *28*, 31–33. [CrossRef] [PubMed]
6. Levite, M. Glutamate receptor antibodies in neurological diseases: Anti-AMPA-GluR3 antibodies, Anti-NMDA-NR1 antibodies, Anti-NMDA-NR2A/B antibodies, Anti-mGluR1 antibodies or Anti-mGluR5 antibodies are present in subpopulations of patients with either: Epilepsy, Encephalitis, Cerebellar Ataxia, Systemic Lupus Erythematosus (SLE) and Neuropsychiatric SLE, Sjogren'ssyndrome, Schizophrenia, Mania or Stroke. These autoimmune anti-glutamate receptor antibodies can bind neurons in few brain regions, activate glutamate receptors, decrease glutamate receptor's expression, impair glutamate-induced signaling and function, activate Blood Brain Barrier endothelial cells, kill neurons, damage the brain, induce behavioral/psychiatric/cognitive abnormalities and Ataxia in animal models, and can be removed or silenced in some patients by immunotherapy. *J. Neural. Transm.* **2014**, *121*, 1029–1075. [PubMed]

7. Frassoni, C.; Spreafico, R.; Franceschetti, S.; Aurisano, N.; Bernasconi, P.; Garbelli, R.; Antozzi, C.; Taverna, S.; Granata, T.; Mantegazza, R. Labeling of rat neurons by anti-GluR3 IgG from patients with Rasmussen encephalitis. *Neurology* **2001**, *57*, 324–327. [CrossRef] [PubMed]
8. Solaro, C.; Mantegazza, R.; Bacigalupo, A.; Uccelli, A. Intractable myoclonus associated with anti-GluR3 antibodies after allogeneic bone marrow transplantation. *Haematologica* **2006**, *91*, ECR62. [PubMed]

13

Possible Correlation between Cholinergic System Alterations and Neuro/Inflammation in Multiple Sclerosis

Valentina Gatta [1], Guadalupe Mengod [2], Marcella Reale [3] and Ada Maria Tata [4,5,*]

[1] Department of Psychological, Health and Territorial Sciences, School of Medicine and Health Sciences, "G. d'Annunzio" University, 66100 Chieti, Italy; valentina.gatta@unich.it

[2] IIBB-CSIC, IDIBAPS, CIBERNED, 08036 Barcelona, Spain; guadalupe.mengod@iibb.csic.es

[3] Department of Medical, Oral and Biotechnological Science, University "G. d'Annunzio" Chieti-Pescara, 66100 Chieti, Italy; m.reale@unich.it

[4] Department of Biology and Biotechnologies C. Darwin, "Sapienza" University of Rome, 00185 Rome, Italy

[5] Research Center of Neurobiology Daniel Bovet, "Sapienza" University of Rome, 00185 Rome, Italy

* Correspondence: adamaria.tata@uniroma1.it;

Abstract: Multiple sclerosis (MS) is an autoimmune and demyelinating disease of the central nervous system. Although the etiology of MS is still unknown, both genetic and environmental factors contribute to the pathogenesis of the disease. Acetylcholine participates in the modulation of central and peripheral inflammation. The cells of the immune system, as well as microglia, astrocytes and oligodendrocytes express cholinergic markers and receptors of muscarinic and nicotinic type. The role played by acetylcholine in MS has been recently investigated. In the present review, we summarize the evidence indicating the cholinergic dysfunction in serum and cerebrospinal fluid of relapsing–remitting (RR)-MS patients and in the brains of the MS animal model experimental autoimmune encephalomyelitis (EAE). The correlation between the increased activity of the cholinergic hydrolyzing enzymes acetylcholinesterase and butyrylcholinesterase, the reduced levels of acetylcholine and the increase of pro-inflammatory cytokines production were recently described in immune cells of MS patients. Moreover, the genetic polymorphisms for both hydrolyzing enzymes and the possible correlation with the altered levels of their enzymatic activity have been also reported. Finally, the changes in cholinergic markers expression in the central nervous system of EAE mice in peak and chronic phases suggest the involvement of the acetylcholine also in neuro-inflammatory processes.

Keywords: cholinergic system; acetylcholine; multiple sclerosis; inflammation; cytokines; EAE

---

1. Acetylcholine and Immune System

Acetylcholine (ACh) is known as one of the main neurotransmitters in the central (CNS) and the peripheral nervous system (PNS) [1]. It plays relevant roles in several organisms: in multicellular organisms and in particular in mammalian species, it mediates the communication between the nervous system and several peripheral organs such as muscle cells, heart, glands, gut, etc.....[2,3]. Interestingly, ACh can be produced also by non-neuronal cells, such as keratinocytes and endothelial cells, contributing to local regulation of the cell physiology [4–6].

Evidence has been accumulated over the past 20 years on the ability of immune cells to respond to cholinergic stimuli, focusing on the cholinergic modulation of the immune response and inflammatory processes both in the immune system and in the brain [7,8].

The first evidence suggested that the vagus nerve was responsible of the control of immune cells responses by inflammatory reflex mediated by the cholinergic stimulation [9]. Albeit the vagus nerve stimulation can modulate the peripheral inflammation, it has been proposed that it may control ACh production directly by the immune cells in the spleen or in other lymphoid organs through adrenergic stimulation [10,11]. This hypothesis appears more realistic considering that the ACh has an extremely short half-life in vivo as a consequence of the ubiquitous distribution of its hydrolytic enzymes acetylcholinesterase (AChE) and butirylcholinesterase (BChE) [12], which rapidly degrade it. Therefore, the cholinergic source of ACh must be very close to the site of action (paracrine function). It has been shown that several immune cells are able to produce ACh and to respond to cholinergic stimuli. T and B cells, macrophages and dendritic cells (DCs) express most of the components of the cholinergic system [13,14]. The presence of choline acetyltransferase (ChAT) and AChE in immune cells has been demonstrated by different techniques [8,15,16]. Immunological activation of T cells up-regulates cholinergic activity, as well as the toll-like receptor activation by selective agonists, induces ChAT expression in DCs and macrophages [7]. These data support a clear cholinergic involvement in the regulation of the immune functions.

The acetylcholine signaling in the immune system is mediated by two types of cholinergic receptors: the muscarinic and nicotinic receptors.

The muscarinic receptors (mAChRs) are metabotropic receptors able to activate different signal transduction pathways [17]. The immune cells express muscarinic receptors whose selective activation modulates the synthesis and production of pro-inflammatory cytokines contributing to modulating the inflammatory processes and, albeit they are not involved in the regulation of the antibodies' synthesis, they favor the antibody class switching from IgM to IgG1 [18,19].

Nicotinic receptors (nAChRs) are classical ionotropic receptors. The immune cells express different nicotinic receptor subunits ($\alpha 2$, $\alpha 4$, α 5, $\alpha 9$, $\alpha 7$ and $\beta 1$, $\beta 2$) whose combination contributes to the hetero- or homopentameric receptor subtype formation. The expression of these receptors is differently distributed in the immune cells and in some cases correlates with their differentiation state [20]. The homopentameric $\alpha 7$ nAChR is the best characterized nicotinic receptor subtype in the immune system. This receptor appears mainly involved in the inhibition of inflammatory processes modulating the production of the anti-inflammatory cytokine, suppressing dendritic cells and macrophage activity and leading to the suppression of T cell differentiation [21,22].

Considering the relevant role of the ACh and its receptors in immune cells functions and in the modulation of the inflammatory processes, it is not difficult to hypothesize that a better understanding of the roles played by ACh and its receptors in inflammatory-related diseases such as neurodegenerative diseases, is of great clinical relevance.

In the present review, we summarize the data indicating the possible involvement of ACh also in demyelinating disease such as multiple sclerosis (MS), reporting recent data demonstrating how the alteration of the cholinergic system activity is present in MS patients and in experimental autoimmune encephalomyelitis (EAE) mice, may be correlated with the immune system dysfunction and alterations of the neuro-inflammatory processes characterizing the MS pathology.

2. Cholinergic Dysfunction in Multiple Sclerosis

MS is an autoimmune disease characterized by demyelination and chronic inflammation. The progressive phases of the disease are associated with myelin sheets alteration and degradation and decreased oligodendrocyte differentiation. The involvement of the cholinergic system in MS is poorly known. However, several studies on EAE mice have suggested how the treatment with cholinesterase inhibitors may improve motor and cognitive impairment and reduce the neuro-inflammation [23]. These effects were significantly abolished by $\alpha 7$ nAChR antagonists [24]. Moreover, as reviewed by Nizri and Brenner [25], the $\alpha 7$ nAChRs also play a relevant role in the immune system where they control the number of dendritic cells and the proliferation of the autoreactive T cells [26].

According to this evidence, the ACh production and cholinergic marker expression and activity in serum and cerebrospinal fluid (CSF) of MS patients were reported [27]. The first data have demonstrated that ACh levels were significantly lower in MS patients with a relapsing–remitting course of the disease

(RR-MS) compared with healthy subjects (HS), both in sera and CSF [27,28]. However, no relationship was found between ACh levels and patient gender or demographic and clinical aspects [27].

Interestingly the enzymatic activity of the ACh hydrolyzing enzymes AChE and BChE resulted significantly increased in sera of MS patients [29]. The studies of the expression of AChE and BChE transcripts in peripheral blood mononuclear cells (PBMC) of MS patients have demonstrated an increase in the transcript levels of both hydrolyzing enzymes, in particular for BChE [28,29]. Moreover, the levels of ACh biosynthetic enzyme ChAT were higher in MS patients compared with HS. Finally, the expression of transcript for OCTN-1 and mediatophore, the two proteins typically expressed in immune cells and responsible for the non-vesicular ACh release were also upregulated in MS patients [29].

These results suggest that the decreased levels of ACh observed in MS patients, may mainly be dependent on the increased expression and activity of cholinergic hydrolyzing enzyme BChE and AChE (Figure 1).

The dysregulated homeostasis of ACh has already been described in other neurological and neurodegenerative diseases (i.e., schizophrenia, Alzheimer's, Parkinson diseases) [30]. For these pathologies, as well as for MS, it is difficult to understand whether the cholinergic dysregulation is the cause or the effect of the pathology.

Interestingly, also some autoimmune diseases present alterations of cholinergic receptors expression or activity (i.e., Sjogren's disease, sepsis, myasthenia gravis) [31–33], confirming a relevant role of cholinergic receptors also in immune system activity. Thus, the MS may be a new pathology possibly correlated with cholinergic dysfunction.

3. The Interface between Cholinergic System and Inflammatory Cytokines in MS

Cytokines orchestrate all phases of immune responses, act in highly complex and dynamic networks in a paracrine and/or autocrine manner and often perform overlapping and partly redundant functions through multicomponent molecules that can be shared by different cell types. For the homeostatic balance, a dynamic equilibrium between pro and anti-inflammatory cytokines is required. Cytokines play a key role in the pathogenesis of MS through the activation of the immune system in the periphery and in the central nervous system. Aberrant immune responses occur in MS and it is likely that the spectrum of the cytokines produced decisively influences the outcome of the disease, as evidenced by the cytokine profiles altered in the central nervous system [34] and in the biological fluid of MS patients. As reported above, the serum levels of ACh were found to be lower in MS patients with respect to levels detected in HS. Considering that ACh plays a central role in the crosstalk between the immune and nervous system and that may act as a suppressor of inflammatory responses, the relationship between the ACh synthesizing and degrading enzymes and pro-inflammatory cytokines was evaluated. Interestingly, AChE and BChE are present at high levels in MS patients, contributing to alter the steady-state equilibrium of the ACh [29]. The balance between the levels of pro- and anti-inflammatory cytokines and their sequential release can be decisive for the severity of inflammatory responses. Alteration of this balance can convert a beneficial effect into a pathological inflammatory reaction. The well-known contribution of the inflammatory component to the progression of multiple sclerosis has led to new attempts to discover ways to attenuate inflammation. The cholinergic system has been suggested as a mediator of the crosstalk between the immune and nervous systems playing an important role as a modulator of immune responses. The effect of dysregulated balance between ACh, AChE and BChE on cytokines levels was studied in order to understand the role of the cholinergic system on inflammatory environment present in MS patients. In the CSF and sera of RR-MS patients and control subjects, the levels of IL-10 and IL-4 were evaluated and no statistical differences were detected [27]. Conversely in both CSF and serum from RR-MS patients, the levels of IL-1β were significantly higher than those detected in CSF and serum of control subjects. Interesting, in both MS and control groups, also the mean level of IL-17 was higher in the CSF than in serum, and serum levels of IL-1β were about four times higher than in CSF of MS subjects. These data confirmed the active pro-inflammatory state characterizing the MS patients [27,28,35]. Moreover, significant differences in TNFα, IL-12/IL-23p40 and IL-18 levels were observed between MS patients and controls. However, a not significant association between ACh hydrolyzing enzymes and the levels of these cytokines was found [27,29].

However, in the serum of MS patients undergoing IFN-β treatment substantially lower levels of IL-1β, IL-12/23p40, IL-18, TNF-α, and HMGB-1 and higher levels of IL-18BP and ACh were detected. These results, other than reinforce the previous observation that a reduction in ACh levels is involved in RR-MS and that ACh and circulating cytokines are mutually influenced [29], have suggested the ability of IFN-β to modulate inflammatory cytokines also by restoring of the ACh levels [36].

ACh was present in inflammatory sites, probably synthesized from immune cells, and cytokines produced to represent an inflammatory input signal to activate afferent vagus nerve fibers that transmit information to the brain. Therefore, the cytokines produced by blood peripheral cells might affect the function of the CNS by crossing the blood–brain barrier (BBB) for direct interaction with CNS tissue. On the other hand, the cells of the immune systems may respond to neurotransmitters released by autonomic nerves and communicate through neurotransmitters [11].

The higher gene expression level of several cytokines, such as IL-1β, IL-12/IL-23p40, IL-17, IL-18 and TNFα was detected in RR-MS compared to HS, according to with the levels measured in the serum; this confirms the relationship between expression and production of pro-inflammatory cytokines in MS patients [35].

These results led to evaluating which components of the cholinergic system could be relevant in terms of the therapeutic tool in controlling the inflammatory state in MS patients. It is known that α7 nicotinic receptors stimulate the cholinergic anti-inflammatory pathway [37]. The expression of α7 and α4 nicotinic receptor subunits, in RR-MS patients and HS, was documented [35]. The expression of the α7 receptor protein by western blot analysis, confirmed the gene expression data, showing higher protein levels in MS patients. The stimulation with phytohaemagglutinin (PHA) was also able to differently modulate the α7 nicotinic receptor expression in RR-MS patients and HS. In fact, PHA stimulation significantly decreased mRNA levels for the α7 receptor subunit only in RR-MS patients. Instead, the increased α7 nAChR expression after nicotine stimulation in PBMC of RR-MS patients correlated with a reduction of the pro-inflammatory cytokines [35]. In fact, the ability of nicotine to modulate the inflammatory cytokines in RR-MS patients was also evaluated. The effects of nicotine on the production of IL-1β and IL-17 from PHA-stimulated PBMC of RR-MS and HS were described. In both groups, nicotine decreased the levels of IL-1β and IL-17 released, but a more significant decrease was observed in RR-MS patients. The expression of the cytokine transcript levels after nicotine treatment was also evaluated [35]. In particular, the treatment of PBMC with PHA plus nicotine significantly reduced the expression of IL-1β, especially in MS patients. Interestingly the co-treatment of PBMC with PHA and 10 μM nicotine did not modify the expression of α7 subunit mRNA in HS, while inducing a significant increase of α7 transcript levels in RR-MS patients [35]. Globally, these data suggest that the locally expressed and released components of the non-neuronal cholinergic system may play paracrine or autocrine effects and contribute to modulate inflammatory cytokines (Figure 1). This may suggest strategies involving the use of selective agonists of α7 nAChRs in the modulation of the inflammatory responses also in demyelinating disease.

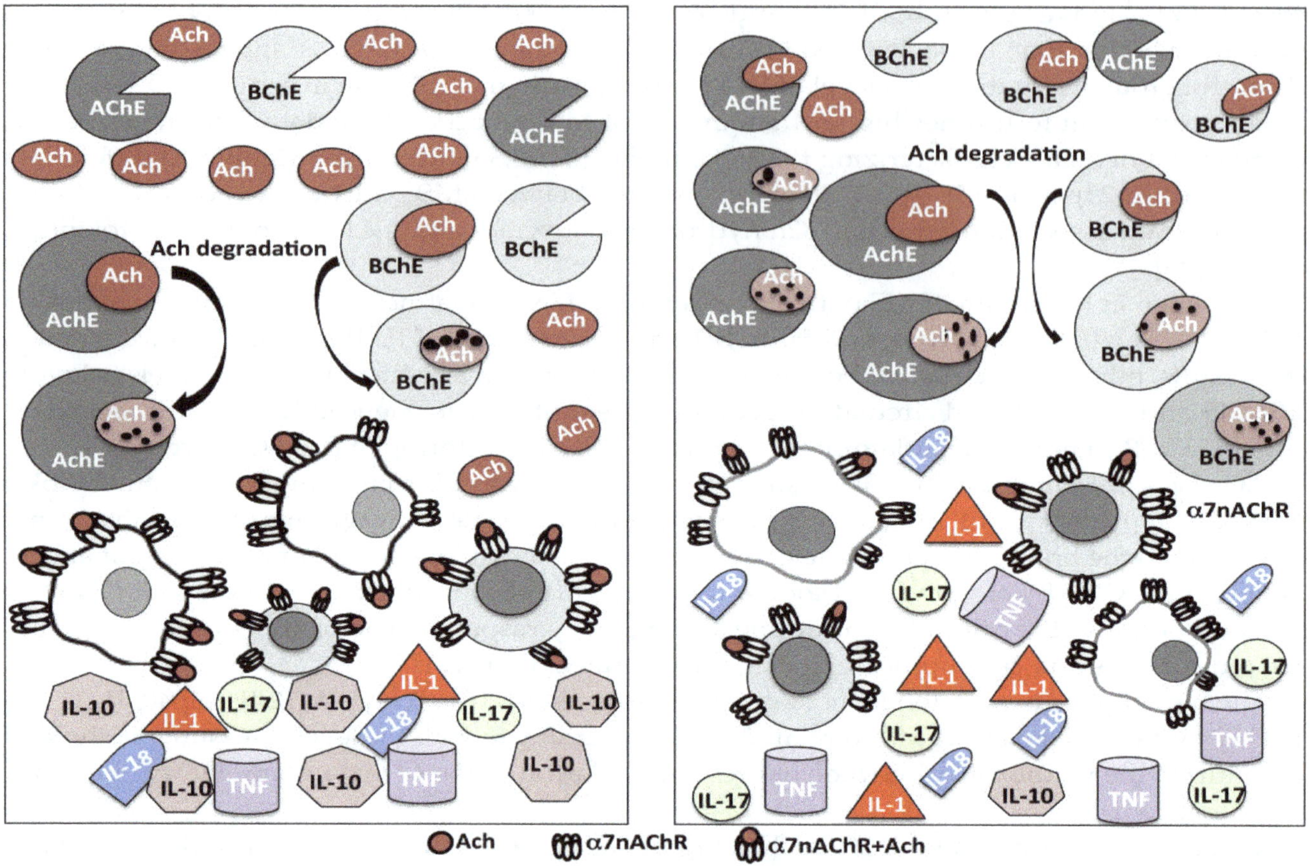

Figure 1. Schematic representation of the mechanism associated with Acetylcholine (Ach) degradation by acetylcholinesterase (AChE) and butirylcholinesterase (BChE) (see arrows), in healthy (left) and multiple sclerosis patients' immune cells (right). The decreased ACh levels may contribute to a reduced α-7 nicotinic receptor activation and a consequent increase of pro-inflammatory cytokines.

4. Genetic Polymorphisms for BChE and AChE and MS

The etiology of MS can be considered multifactorial, based on the interaction between genetic and several environmental factors (Figure 2). A hereditary basis of MS is suggested by epidemiological studies. This can be supported by the recurrence risk of MS in twins, siblings, conjugal MS individuals, and lower recurrence risk in adoptees [38–40]. In the general population, the risk of developing MS is about 0.00125%, including the variability for geographic areas. Overall, about 15% of the patients with MS have an affected relative. Studies in twins reveal a concordance of 25% in monozygotic twins and only 2.4% in dizygotic twins [41]. Recently, the following meta-analysis estimate was reported: 0.50 (95% CI: 0.39–0.61) for heritability, 0.21 (95% CI: 0.11–0.30) for shared environmental component and 0.29 (95% CI: 0.26–0.33) for unique environmental component [42]. The authors conclude that these results support the efforts to fill the gap of 'missing heritability' by genome-wide association studies (GWAS) on large populations as well as massive sequencing analysis by next-generation sequencing (NGS). The risk of developing the disease is 15-fold higher when MS is present in a first-degree relative. Siblings of patients with MS have a risk of ~2.6%, parents have a risk of 1.8% and sons have a risk of ~1.5%. Accordingly, considering the distinction between monogenic and complex traits, no single gene or environmental factor causes MS and it does not follow the Mendelian model.

MS is believed to be dependent on multiple independent or interacting polymorphism genes with small or moderate effects, as well as their interaction with behavioral and environmental factors (Figure 2) [43]. Several studies also aim to disclose the genetic basis of MS. For decades, only several variants of the *HLA* antigen were known to have the strongest effect on the risk of MS [44,45]. Carrying *HLA-DRB1*1501* is associated with about three-fold greater odds of developing MS, while carrying

*HLA-A*02* is associated with meaningfully reduced odds. So far, genome-wide association studies, carried out in populations worldwide, provided strong evidence for the association of approximately >230 genetic variants. All these variants only account for 20% to 30% of MS heritability, suggesting that its remaining part is likely related to epigenetic factors and gene-gene or gene-environment interactions. Considerable attention has been focused on studies evaluating disease-modifying effects in MS that identified genes such as the *APOE, CXCR5, IL2RA, IL7R, IL7, IL12RB1, IL22RA2, IL12A, IL12B, IRF8, TNFRSF1A, TNFRSF14, TNFSF14, CBLB, GPR65, MALT1, RGS1, RIC3, STAT3, TAGAP, TYK2, CYP27B1* and *CYP24A1* [44,45].

Recently, it was reported in genome-wide association studies, that the implication of RIC3, a chaperone of nAChRs, in multiple sclerosis (MS) and neuroinflammatory disease. RIC3 promotes the functional expression of α7 nAChR, and it was shown a dynamic regulation of RIC3 in macrophages and in lymphocytes, following an immune activation in human and murine cells.

Moreover, increased average expression of *RIC3* and *CHRNA7* in lymphocytes from MS patients but not in healthy donors was observed. These data are consistent with a role for RIC3 and in its regulated expression in inflammatory processes and in neuroinflammatory diseases [45].

The variation in some genes of the cholinergic system, such as those encoding BChE (gene *BChE*, chrom. 3q26.1–q26.2) and AChE (gene *AChE*, chrom. 7q22.1) [http://www.genatlas.org] has also been studied in MS patients in relation to altered levels of their enzymatic activity.

Variants in these genes have been largely investigated in relation to the onset of Alzheimer's disease [46,47], since the levels of these enzymes were found increased in the brains of patients, as well as a number of low-grade systemic inflammation pathologies [48,49].

In particular, two specific polymorphisms within these genes have been studied, namely rs1803274 for *BChE* and rs2571598 for *AChE*. It is reported that rs1803274 for *BChE* is able to reduce the enzymes' activity by about 30%–50% [50]. The *BChE* rs1803274 is characterized by a G/A substitution inducing the Ala/Tr change at the codon 539 and it produces the so-called K-allele. This variation causes the reduction of 30%–60% of ACh's hydrolyzing activity and 30% of the capacity to hydrolyze butyryl-thiocholine. *BChE* K-carriers, showing lowered hydrolytic activity of *BChE* K-allele, could potentially improve cholinergic activity.

There are 19 single nucleotide polymorphisms (SNPs) for *AChE* [51]. The only rs1799806 on exon 6, a functional intronic C/T substitution, was associated with activity changes. The AChE activity of homozygote Pro/Pro genotype was significantly lower than Arg/Arg genotypes. The presence of these variants is controversially considered a risk factor for Alzheimer's disease, as well as other conditions such as stroke, Parkinson's disease and related dementia [52,53]. Even if cholinergic neurotransmission regulates the immune response and inhibits cytokine release after stroke, only the variant alleles of *BChE* have been identified as risk factors for ischemic stroke [54] and associated with reduced BChE activity in patients with post-stroke dementia (PSD) [49], while *AChE* rs1799806 do not influence the AChE activity.

As above-described the ACh levels in serum of RR-MS patients were inversely correlated with the increased activity of the hydrolyzing enzymes AChE and BChE [29]. The observed lower circulating ACh levels in sera of MS patients are probably dependent on the higher activity of cholinergic hydrolyzing enzymes [29].

In this context, it was recently investigated whether lower ACh concentration observed in RR-MS compared to HS may be related to the ability to regulate the extracellular ACh levels, when needed, or to the variation of AChE or BChE activity related to the association with rs1803274 for *BChE* and rs2571598 for *AChE* genetic variations [55]. An association between the *BChE* K-allele and *AChE* rs2571598 in 102 relapsing remitting-MS patients compared to 117 healthy controls was reported. These data underlined that in RR-MS patients carrying the K-allele, higher BChE activity was observed [55]. Although this is in contrast with the reported role of this SNP in *BChE* gene, this excess of circulating BChE removes ACh, negatively influencing the levels of all investigated pro-inflammatory cytokines (Figure 1). Conceivably, other pathways, such as increased transduction of BChE, microRNAs or other gene modulators acting in combination with BChE-K, could be involved in the balance of the BChE as well as a higher BChE enzymatic activity induced by the presence of the polymorphic allele may reduce the amounts of circulating ACh.

These evidences may suggest that specific genetic endo-phenotypes are able to modulate the pro-inflammatory immune responses in MS patients, altering the activity of AChE through ACh hydrolysis. These data highlight the potential role of the non-neuronal cholinergic system in immune cell function, even if studies on larger populations are needed in order to better discover MS etiology and progression and to develop new disease-modifying therapies for MS with AChE and ACh as targets.

The reported literature about genetic biomarkers in MS is not always consistent in the worldwide population. The detection of a single nucleotide polymorphism related to MS pathogenesis is very hard given that several genetic polymorphisms are implicated, each with a small contribution to the susceptibility or resistance to MS. Although numerous causal genes have been detected by genome-wide association studies (GWAS), these susceptibility genes are linked to relatively low disease risk, indicating the important role of environmental factors in the pathogenesis of the disease. Next-generation sequencing (NGS) technology, with high-throughput capacity and accuracy, could be a powerful tool to discover the genetic basis of MS. NGS can be applied to sequence analysis in any part of the genome and the resulting transcriptome, including the whole genome, exons, and other interesting regions, and accordingly can be roughly classified as whole-genome sequencing (WGS), whole-exome sequencing (WES), RNA sequencing (RNA-seq), and DNA methylation sequencing. So far, only rare variants of modest effect on MS risk affecting a subset of patients have been detected by NGS including *CYP27B1* and *TYK2* genes [56,57]. Epigenetic mechanisms that have been detected for MS pathogenesis are DNA methylation, histone modification and some microRNAs' alternations. Several cellular processes including apoptosis, differentiation and evolution can be modulated along with epigenetic changes [58]. All these data support the idea of a complex basis of MS with clear gene–environment interactions and epigenetic alterations triggered by environmental exposures in individuals with a particular genetic profile (Figure 2) [59].

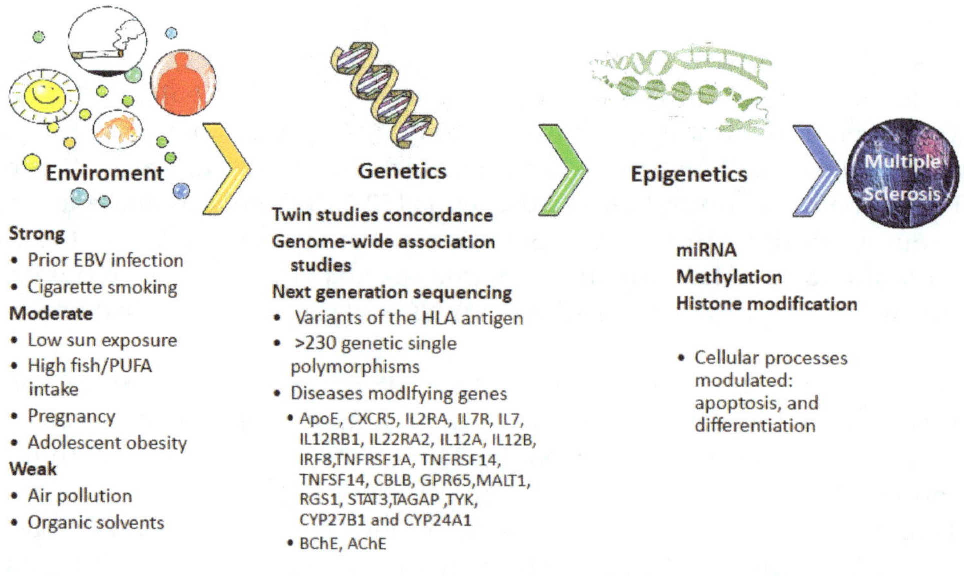

Figure 2. Risk factors for multiple sclerosis (MS). A hereditary basis of MS is suggested by epidemiological studies and recurrence risk of MS in twins, siblings, conjugal MS individuals. MS is believed to result from multiple independent or interacting polymorphism genes as well as their interaction with behavioral and environmental factors with strong, moderate, or weak effects. Epigenetic mechanisms that have been detected for MS pathogenesis are DNA methylation, histone modification and some microRNAs alternations.

5. Cholinergic Markers Alteration in the Brain of EAE Mice

One of the animal models of MS, EAE can be obtained after active immunization with myelin oligodendrocyte glycoprotein (MOG) 35–55 peptide as antigen in C57BL6 mice, and reproduces many pathological features observed in MS [60]. Several days after immunization, it is possible to observe immune cells infiltrating the CNS and activation of microglia. These events take place predominantly in the spinal cord but also in other brain structures such as the cerebellum and the optic tract [61], which lead to axonal damage and demyelination [62]. The $MOG_{35\text{-}55}$-induced model of EAE is characterized by the peak inflammatory phase, followed by a chronic phase of neurological deficit.

ACh may play a role in the development or in the remission of MS. Recent analyses of cholinergic markers in the brain and spinal cord of EAE mice revealed specific alterations in their expression in different brain areas and cellular populations associated to the different phases of the disease [63]. The mRNA coding for ChAT, the enzyme responsible for the synthesis of ACh from choline and acetyl-CoA that serves as a marker of cholinergic cells, presents alterations in the expression levels in different brain regions and spinal cord and in different disease phases of EAE mice [63]. Several cholinergic nuclei of EAE mice in the chronic phase present an increment in ChAT expression levels and an increase of the AChE activity and mRNA expression at peak of disease, suggesting that the balance of ACh levels may contribute to the chronicity of the disease.

The BChE activity, a non-selective cholinesterase enzyme that catalyzes the ACh hydrolysis, is altered in the habenula and solitary nucleus in both disease phases of EAE mice and in higher proportion in astroglia and microglia/macrophage cells in the chronic group [63]. BChE activity is detected in both glial cell populations and presents a significant increment in EAE animals in the chronic phase compared to the peak phase or control brains. The high ratio of BChE to AChE found in astrocytes of EAE mice in peak phase [63] may suggest this ratio as a potential marker for brain areas selectively vulnerable to this neuropathology as it was described for Alzheimer's disease brains [64]. However, the treatment of EAE mice with a BChE/AChE inhibitor (rivastigmine) resulted in an amelioration of the clinical symptoms associated also with a reduction in the demyelination [24], supporting the role of BChE in neuroinflammation and demyelination (Figure 3).

As reported above, several studies show that $\alpha7$ nAChR is the key subtype involved in nAChR-mediated immune regulation [20,26,65]. $\alpha7$ nAChR mRNA expression in the EAE chronic group is increased in habenula and decreased in the dorsal tegmental nucleus. Conversely, the mRNA levels of this receptor are increased in the dorsal tegmental nucleus of animals in the peak phase [63]. The altered expression of this receptor subunit in EAE mice during the chronic phase compared to the peak phase of the disease may sustain its role in the neuro-inflammation regulation also in the brain (Figure 3).

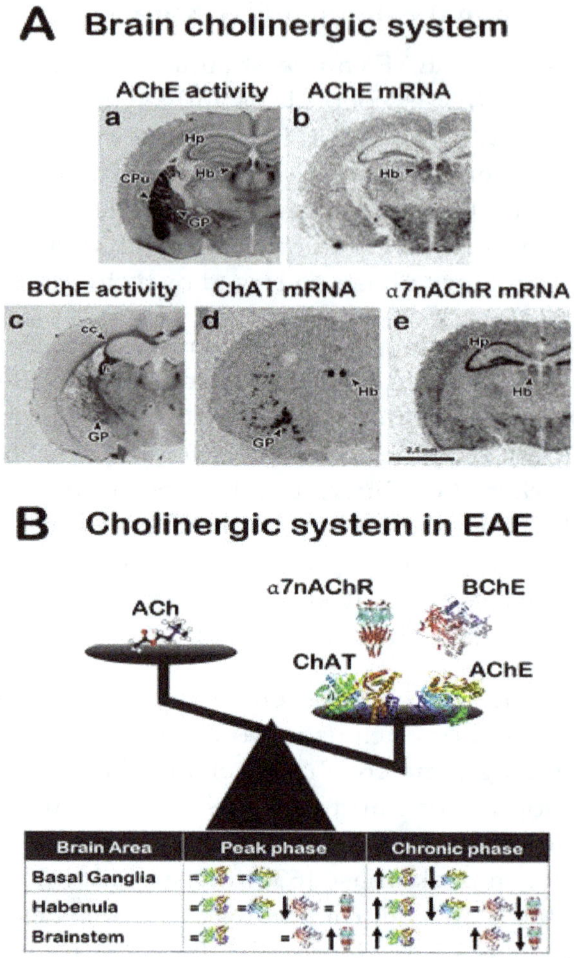

Figure 3. Cholinergic system changes in some brain areas (basal ganglia, habenula, and nuclei of the brainstem) of experimental autoimmune encephalomyelitis (EAE) mice at peak and chronic phases of the disease. (**A**) Photomicrographs showing AChE (**a**) and BChE (**c**) enzymatic activities stained histological brain sections and photomicrographs from autoradiograms of control mouse brain tissue sections visualizing brain areas expressing mRNAs coding for *AChE* (**b**), *ChAT* (**d**) and *α7nAChR* (**e**). (**B**) Representation of the homeostatic balance of cholinergic markers expression in brain areas of EAE mice. The table summarizes the quantification of enzymatic activities and mRNAs expression of cholinergic markers at peak and chronic phases of the disease. Abbreviations and symbols: CPu, caudate-putamen; CC, cerebral cortex; fi, fimbria; GP, globus pallidus; Hb, habenula; Hp, hippocampus; 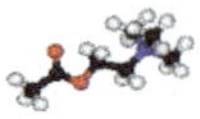, ACh; 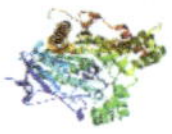, AChE; 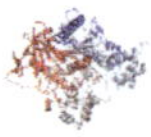, BChE, 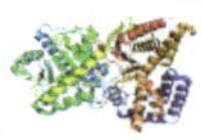 ChAT; 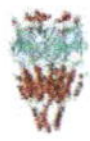, α7nAChR.

6. Cholinergic Receptors in the Glial Cells

New ideas have emerged during the past several years on how the neurotransmitters, including Ach, can actively participate in neuron–glia cross talk. This interaction is relevant both during nervous system development to improve and address neuron and glial cell survival, proliferation and differentiation, and in adulthood, to maintain axonal function and myelin integrity [66]. It is now known that glial cells express receptors for different neurotransmitters, suggesting that these molecules, most probably when released in extra-synaptic regions [67–69], may modulate glial cell survival, proliferation, and myelination [67,70].

The expression of ACh receptors has been reported in several glial cells indicating these cells as potential targets for ACh action [70,71]. Oligodendrocyte (OLs), the main target in MS, express muscarinic receptors whose activation triggers different signal transduction pathways [67,70,72–74]. The presence of nicotinic receptor subunits (*α*3, *a*4, *a*5, *a*7, *β*2, and β4) was also revealed by RT-PCR and immunocytochemistry in oligodendrocytes precursor cells (OPC), but not in mature cells [75]. Oligodendrocytes express also acetylcholine muscarinic receptors. M1, M3, and M4 ACh receptors were the muscarinic subtypes expressed in OPCs, whereas all five muscarinic receptor subtypes were found to be expressed at low levels in mature OLs; thus muscarinic receptors favor the maintenance of immature proliferating progenitor cells and counteract progression toward a mature state [75]. Accordingly, with this evidence, more recent research demonstrated that antagonists of muscarinic receptors promote oligodendrocyte differentiation and rescue of the lesions in white matter in EAE mice [76]. In fact benztropine, a typical muscarinic antagonist used as a drug for Parkinson's disease treatment has been proposed for MS treatment considering that MS symptoms in the EAE mouse model were reverted [76,77]. Moreover, the benztropine appears to favor oligodendrocyte differentiation and myelination by a specific antagonism of M1 and M3 receptors on oligodendrocyte precursor cells (OPCs) [76]. Another important aspect to consider is that muscarinic receptors are able to modulate pro-inflammatory cytokine production [18,28], so it may be possible to hypothesize that the antagonism of muscarinic receptors can support not only oligodendrocyte differentiation but also the neuro-inflammation decrease.

The presence of muscarinic receptors was demonstrated in cultured astrocytes [78] as well as the expression of functional nAChRs subunits ($\alpha4$, $\alpha7$, $\beta2$, $\beta3$) has been reported in rat astrocytes [39,79]. In particular, the expression of $\alpha7$ nAChR in astrocytes plays a relevant role in neuroprotection in several neurodegenerative diseases (i.e., Alzheimer and Parkinson) [80,81].

Finally, microglia also express both muscarinic and nicotinic receptors. Zhang and collaborators [82] described for the first time the expression of functional muscarinic receptors in human microglia. Interestingly the upregulated expression of M3 receptor subtype in these cells causes an increase of MHC-I and MHC-II expression, suggesting the pro-inflammatory microglia phenotype [83]. Microglia also display nicotinic receptors, with a prevalence of $\alpha7$ subunit [84–87]. For these reasons, this nicotinic receptor subtype may be considered an interesting therapeutic target for several neurological disorders considering its ability to modulate the cholinergic anti-inflammatory pathway and the synaptic plasticity.

Taking all these into account, it cannot be excluded that cholinergic stimulation in the brain may influence a complex network controlling both neuronal and glial functions and play a relevant role in the control of the neuro-inflammation.

7. Conclusions

Understanding the mechanisms leading to aberrant immune response and the severe neuro-inflammation in MS plays a relevant role in the development of new treatments directed to decrease pro-inflammatory cytokine production and to ameliorate the clinical symptoms, slowing the disease outcome and delaying or arresting the onset of the disabilities. In this review we have presented recent data in EAE mice and in MS patients, supporting the role of ACh in MS. The dysregulated ACh homeostasis in MS, suggest how its altered functions might represent an additional pathogenetic mechanism negatively influencing the cytokines production with consequent disease outcome.

Interestingly, using the EAE mice model, it has also been described as the alteration of ACh synthesis or degradation may impact on neuron function, contributing to the motor and cognitive disabilities characteristics of MS patients, also influencing the glia network, the differentiation and survival of the oligodendrocytes, and triggering the neuro-inflammation.

The relevant role played by ACh in this context, is supported by the evidence that modulating the cholinergic system activity or cholinergic receptor functions, the clinical disabilities, at least in mice, are significantly reduced. In fact, the altered balance of ACh also in cholinergic area of the brain or spinal cord of EAE mice (i.e., basal ganglia or spinal motoneuros), suggested that the decreased ACh levels may influence the MS motor disabilities both reducing the levels of the neurotransmitter in the cholinergic neurons and increasing the neuro-inflammation with consequent impact on myelin disruption and axonal conduction [63,76,77].

This aspect appears supported by additional studies performed with conventional drugs used in the treatment of MS, as INFβ or dimethyl fumarate [36,88], that demonstrate a significant amelioration of the cholinergic activity with a possible consequent reduction of the clinical symptoms-MS associated. Therefore, further studies will be necessary to evaluate the impact of different immune modulators on the cholinergic system activity both in the immune system and in the brain.

In conclusion, the data described in this review highlight as ACh and its receptors may be implicated in MS pathogenesis. However, further investigation on the genetic aspects and epigenetic modulation of cholinergic markers gene expression could significantly improve the knowledge about MS onset and progression as well as to contribute to identifying new possible therapeutic strategies.

Author Contributions: Conceptualization A.M.T., Original draft preparation, writing—review and editing V.G., G.M., M.R., A.M.T. All authors have read and agreed to the published version of the manuscript.

References

1. Mesulam, M.M. Central cholinergic pathways: Neuroanatomy and some behavioral implications. In *Neurotransmitters and Cortical Function*; Avoli, M., Reader, T.A., Dikes, R.W., Gloor, P., Eds.; Plenum Publishing: New York, NY, USA, 1988; pp. 237–260.
2. Wessler, I.; Kilbinger, H.; Bittinger, F.; Unger, R.; Kirkpatrick, C.J. The biological role of non-neuronal acetylcholine in plants and humans. *Jpn. J. Pharmacol.* **2001**, *85*, 2–10. [CrossRef] [PubMed]
3. Picciotto, M.R.; Higley, M.J.; Mineur, Y.S. Acetylcholine as a neuromodulator: Cholinergic signaling shapes nervous system function and behavior. *Neuron* **2012**, *76*, 116–129. [CrossRef] [PubMed]
4. Kawashima, K.; Fujii, T. Basic and clinical aspects of non-neuronal acetylcholine: Overview of non-neuronal cholinergic systems and their biological significance. *J. Pharmacol. Sci.* **2008**, *106*, 167–173. [CrossRef] [PubMed]
5. Furchgott, R.F.; Carvalho, M.H.; Khan, M.T.; Matsunaga, K. Evidence for endothelium-dependent vasodilation of resistance vessels by acetylcholine. *Blood Vessel.* **1987**, *24*, 145–149. [CrossRef]
6. Grando, S.A.; Pittelkow, M.R.; Schellreunter, K.U. Adrenergic and cholinergic control in the biology of epidermis: Physiological and clinical Significance. *J. Invest. Dermatol.* **2006**, *126*, 1948–1965. [CrossRef]
7. Cox, M.A.; Bassi, C.; Saunders, M.E.; Nechanitzky, R.; Morgado-Palacin, I.; Zheng1, C.; Mak, T.W. Beyond neurotransmission: Acetylcholine in immunity and inflammation. *J. Int. Med.* **2020**, *287*, 120–133. [CrossRef]
8. Fujii, T.; Mashimo, M.; Moriwaki, Y.; Misawa, H.; Ono, S.; Horiguchi, K.; Kawashima, K. Physiological functions of the cholinergic system in immune cells. *J. Pharmacol. Sci.* **2017**, *134*, 1–21. [CrossRef]
9. Borovikova, L.V.; Ivanova, S.; Zhang, M.; Yang, H.; Botchkina, G.I.; Watkins, L.R.; Wang, H.; Abumrad, N.; Eaton, J.W.; Tracey, K.J. Vagus nerve stimulation attenuates the systemic inflammatory response to endotoxin. *Nature* **2000**, *405*, 458–462. [CrossRef]
10. Carnevale, D.; Perrotta, M.; Pallante, F.; Fardella, V.; Iacobucci, R.; Fardella, S.; Carnevale, L.; Carnevale, R.; de Lucia, M.; Cifelli, G.; et al. A cholinergic sympathetic pathway primes immunity in hypertension and mediates brain-to-spleen communication. *Nat. Commun.* **2016**, *7*, 13035. [CrossRef]
11. Rosas-Ballina, M.; Olofsson, P.S.; Ochani, M.; Valdés-Ferrer, S.I.; Levine, Y.A.; Reardon, C.; Tusche, M.W.; Pavlov, V.A.; Andersson, U.; Chavan, S.; et al. Acetylcholine-synthesizing T cells relay neural signals in a vagus nerve circuit. *Science* **2011**, *334*, 98–101. [CrossRef]
12. Soreq, H.; Seidman, S. Acetylcholinesterase–new roles for an old actor. *Nat. Rev. Neurosci.* **2001**, *2*, 294–302. [CrossRef] [PubMed]
13. Kawashima, K.; Fujii, T. The lymphocytic cholinergic system and its contribution to the regulation of immune activity. *Life Sci.* **2003**, *74*, 675–696. [CrossRef] [PubMed]
14. Fujii, T.; Mashimo, M.; Moriwaki, Y.; Misawa, H.; Ono, S.; Horiguchi, K.; Kawashima, K. Expression and Function of the Cholinergic System in Immune Cells. *Front. Immunol.* **2017**, *8*, 1085. [CrossRef] [PubMed]
15. Ogawa, H.; Fujii, T.; Watanabe, Y.; Kawashima, K. Expression of multiple mRNA species for choline acetyltransferase in human T-lymphocytes. *Life Sci.* **2003**, *72*, 2127–2130. [CrossRef]

16. Kawashima, K.; Fujii, T. Extraneuronal cholinergic system in lymphocytes. *Pharmacol. Ther.* **2000**, *86*, 29–48. [CrossRef]
17. Tata, A.M. Muscarinic acetylcholine receptors: New potential therapeutic targets in antinociception and in cancer therapy. *Rec Pat. CNS Drug Discov.* **2008**, *3*, 94–103. [CrossRef]
18. Kawashima, K.; Fujii, T.; Watanabe, Y.; Misawa, H. Acetylcholine synthesis and muscarinic receptor subtype mRNA expression in T-lymphocytes. *Life Sci.* **1998**, *62*, 1701–1705. [CrossRef]
19. Fujii, T.; Watanabe, Y.; Inoue, T.; Kawashima, K. Upregulation of mRNA encoding the M5 muscarinic acetylcholine receptor in human T- and B-lymphocytes during immunological responses. *Neurochem. Res.* **2003**, *28*, 423–429. [CrossRef]
20. Wang, H.; Yu, M.; Ochani, M.; Amella, C.A.; Tanovic, M.; Susarla, S.; Li, J.H.; Wang, H.; Yang, H.; Ulloa, L.; et al. Nicotinic acetylcholine receptor [alpha] 7 subunit is an essential regulator of inflammation. *Nature* **2003**, *421*, 384–388. [CrossRef]
21. Skok, M.V.; Grathe, K.; Agenes, F.; Changeux, P.J. The role of nicotinic receptorsi in B-lymphocites development and activation. *Life Sci.* **2007**, *80*, 2324–2336. [CrossRef]
22. Kawashima, K.; Fuji, T.; Moriwaki, Y.; Misawa, H.; Horiguchi, K. Non-neuronal cholinergic system in regulation of immune function with a focus on α7 nAChRs. *Int. Immunopharmacol.* **2015**, *29*, 127–134. [CrossRef] [PubMed]
23. Nizri, E.; Hamra-Amitay, Y.; Sicsic, C.; Lavon, I.; Brenner, T. Anti-inflammatory properties of cholinergic up-regulation: A new role for acetylcholinesterase inhibitors. *Neuropharmacology* **2006**, *50*, 540–547. [CrossRef] [PubMed]
24. Nirzi, E.; Jromy-Tir-Sinai, M.; Faranesh, N.; Layon, I.; Lavi, E.; Weinstock, M.; Brenner, T. Supprssion of neuroinflammationby the acetylcholinesterase inhibitor rivastigamine. *J. Neuroimmunol.* **2008**, *203*, 12–22.
25. Nirzi, E.; Brenner, T. Modulation of inflammatory pathways by the immune-cholinergic system. *Amino Acids* **2013**, *45*, 75–85.
26. Nizri, E.; Irony-Tur-Sinai, M.; Lory, O.; Orr-Urtreger, A.; Lavi, E.; Brenner, T. Activation of the cholinergic anti-inflammatory system by nicotine attenuates neuroinflammation via suppression of Th1 and Th17 responses. *J. Immunol.* **2010**, *183*, 6681–6688. [CrossRef] [PubMed]
27. Reale, M.; De Angelis, F.; Di Nicola, M.; Capello, E.; Di Ioia, M.; De Luca, G.; Lugaresi, A.; Tata, A.M. Relation Between Pro-Inflammatory Cytokines and Acetylcholine Levels in Relapsing-Remitting Multiple Sclerosis Patients. *Int. J. Mol. Sci.* **2012**, *13*, 12656–12664. [CrossRef]
28. Di Bari, M.; Di Pinto, G.; Reale, M.; Mengod, G.; Tata, A.M. Cholinergic system and neuroinflammation: Implication in multiple sclerosis. *CNS Agents Med. Chem.* **2017**, *17*, 109–115. [CrossRef]
29. Di Bari, M.; Reale, M.; Di Nicola, M.; Orlando, V.; Galizia, S.; Porfilio, I.; Costantini, E.; D'Angelo, C.; Ruggieri, S.; Biagioni, S.; et al. Dysregulated homeostasis of acetylcholine levels in immune cells of RR-multiple sclerosis patients. *Int. J. Mol. Sci.* **2016**, *17*, E2009. [CrossRef]
30. Tata, A.M.; Velluto, L.; D'Angelo, C.; Reale, M. Cholinergic system dysfunctions and neurodegenerative diseases: Cause or effect? *CNS Neurol. Disord. Drug Targets* **2014**, *13*, 1294–1303. [CrossRef]
31. Yilmaz, V.; Oflazer, P.; Aysal, F.; Durmus, H.; Poulas, K.; Yentur, S.P.; Gulsen-Parman, Y.; Tzartos, S.; Marx, A.; Tuzun, E.; et al. Differential Cytokine Changes in Patients with Myasthenia Gravis with Antibodies against AChR and MuSK. *PLoS ONE* **2015**, *10*, e0123546. [CrossRef]
32. Baggi, F.; Antozzi, C.; Toscani, C.; Cordiglieri, C. Acetylcholine receptor-induced experimental myasthenia gravis: What have we learned from animal models after three decades? *Arch. Immunol. Ther. Exp.* **2012**, *60*, 19–30. [CrossRef] [PubMed]
33. Peña, G.; Cai, B.; Ramos, L.; Vida, G.; Deitch, E.A.; Ulloa, L. Cholinergic regulatory lymphocytes re-establish neuromodulation of innate immune responses in sepsis. *J. Immunol.* **2011**, *187*, 718–725. [CrossRef] [PubMed]
34. Wang, K.; Song, F. The Properties of Cytokines in Multiple Sclerosis: Pros and Cons. *Am. J. Med. Sci.* **2018**, *356*, 552–560. [CrossRef] [PubMed]
35. Reale, M.; Di Bari, M.; Di Nicola, M.; D'Angelo, C.; De Angelis, F.; Velluto, L.; Tata, A.M. Nicotinic receptor activation negatively modulates pro-inflammatory cytokine production in multiple sclerosis patients. *Int. Immunopharmacol.* **2015**, *29*, 152–157. [CrossRef] [PubMed]
36. D'Angelo, C.; Reale, M. IFN-β-Treatment and Canonical and Non-Traditional Cytokine Levels. *Front. Immunol.* **2018**, *9*, 1240. [CrossRef] [PubMed]

37. Báez-Pagán, C.A.; Delgado-Vélez, M. Activation of the Macrophage α7 Nicotinic Acetylcholine Receptor and Control of Inflammation. *J. Neuroimmune Pharmacol.* **2015**, *10*, 468–476. [CrossRef]
38. Marrosu, M.G.; Lai, M.; Cocco, E.; Loi, V.; Spinicci, G.; Pischedda, M.P.; Massole, S.; Marrosu, G.; Contu, P. Genetic factors and the founder effect explain familial MS in Sardinia. *Neurology* **2002**, *58*, 283–288. [CrossRef]
39. Kahana, E. Epidemiologic studies of multiple sclerosis: A review. *Biomed. Pharmacother.* **2000**, *54*, 100–112. [CrossRef]
40. Carton, H.; Vlietinck, R.; Debruyne, J.; De, K.J.; D'Hooghe, M.B.; Loos, R.; Medaer, R.; Truyen, L.; Yee, I.M.; Sadovnick, A.D. Risks of multiple sclerosis in relatives of patients in Flanders, Belgium. *J. Neurol. Neuros. Psych.* **1997**, *62*, 329–333. [CrossRef]
41. Miller, J.R. Esclerose múltipla. In *Tratado de Neurologia*, 10th ed.; Sociedad de Neurología: Santiago, Chile, 2002; pp. 670–686.
42. Buscarinu, M.C.; Fornasiero, A.; Ferraldeschi, M.; Romano, S.; Reniè, R.; Morena, E.; Romano, C.; Pellicciari, G.; Landi, A.C.; Fagnani, C.; et al. Disentangling the molecular mechanisms of multiple sclerosis: The contribution of twin studies. *Neurosci. Biobehav. Rev.* **2020**, *111*, 194–198. [CrossRef]
43. Hollenbach, J.A.; Oksenberg, J.R. The immunogenetics of multiple sclerosis: A comprehensive review. *J. Autoimmun.* **2015**, *64*, 13–25. [CrossRef] [PubMed]
44. Kallaur, A.P.; Kaimen-Maciel, D.R.; Morimoto, H.K.; Watanabe, M.A.; Georgeto, S.M.; Reiche, E.M. Genetic polymorphisms associated with the development and clinical course of multiple sclerosis. *Int. J. Mol. Med.* **2011**, *28*, 467–479. [PubMed]
45. Ben-David, Y.; Kagan, S.; Cohen Ben-Ami, H.; Rostami, J.; Mizrahi, T.; Kulkarni, A.R.; Thakur, G.A.; Vaknin-Dembinsky, A.; Healy, L.M.; Brenner, T.; et al. RIC3, the cholinergic anti-inflammatory pathway, and neuroinflammation. *Int. Immunopharmacol.* **2020**, *83*, 106381. [CrossRef] [PubMed]
46. Jasiecki, J.; Wasąg, B. Butyrylcholinesterase Protein Ends in the Pathogenesis of Alzheimer's Disease-Could BCHE Genotyping Be Helpful in Alzheimer's Therapy. *Biomolecules* **2019**, *9*, 592. [CrossRef]
47. Jasiecki, J.; Limon-Sztencel, A.; Żuk, M.; Chmara, M.; Cysewski, D.; Limon, J.; Wasąg, B. Synergy between the alteration in the N-terminal region of butyrylcholinesterase K variant and apolipoprotein E4 in late-onset Alzheimer's disease. *Sci. Rep.* **2019**, *9*, 5223. [CrossRef]
48. Scacchi, R.; Ruggeri, M.; Corbo, R.M. Variation of the butyrylcholinesterase (BChE) and acetylcholinesterase (AChE) genes in coronary artery disease. *Clin. Chim. Acta* **2011**, *412*, 1341–1344. [CrossRef]
49. Chen, Y.C.; Chou, W.H.; Fang, C.P.; Liu, T.H.; Tsou, H.H.; Wang, Y.; Liu, Y.L. Serum Level and Activity of Butylcholinesterase: A Biomarker for Post-Stroke Dementia. *J. Clin. Med.* **2019**, *8*, 1778. [CrossRef]
50. Lockridge, O.; Norgren, R.B., Jr.; Johnson, R.C.; Blake, T.A. Naturally Occurring Genetic Variants of Human Acetylcholinesterase and Butyrylcholinesterase and Their Potential Impact on the Risk of Toxicity from Cholinesterase Inhibitors. *Chem. Res. Toxicol.* **2016**, *29*, 1381–1392. [CrossRef]
51. Valle, A.M.; Radic, Z.; Rana, B.K.; Mahboubi, V.; Wessel, J.; Shih, P.A.; Rao, F.; O'Connor, D.T.; Taylor, P. Naturally occurring variations in the human cholinesterase genes: Heritability and association with cardiovascular and metabolic traits. *J. Pharmacol. Exp. Ther.* **2011**, *338*, 125–133. [CrossRef]
52. Santarpia, L.; Grandone, I.; Contaldo, F.; Pasanisi, F. Butyrylcholinesterase as a prognostic marker: A review of the literature. *J. Cachexia Sarcopenia Muscle* **2013**, *4*, 31–39. [CrossRef]
53. Dong, M.X.; Xu, X.M.; Hu, L.; Liu, Y.; Huang, Y.J.; Wei, Y.D. Serum Butyrylcholinesterase Activity: A Biomarker for Parkinson's Disease and Related Dementia. *BioMed. Res. Int.* **2017**, *2017*, 1524107. [CrossRef] [PubMed]
54. Oguri, M.; Kato, K.; Yokoi, K.; Yoshida, T.; Watanabe, S.; Metoki, N.; Yoshida, H.; Satoh, K.; Aoyagi, Y.; Tanaka, M.; et al. Association of a polymorphism of BCHE with ischemic stroke in Japanese individuals with chronic kidney disease. *Mol. Med. Rep.* **2009**, *2*, 779–785. [PubMed]
55. Reale, M.; Costantini, E.; Di Nicola, M.; D'Angelo, C.; Franchi, S.; D'Aurora, M.; Di Bari, M.; Orlando, V.; Galizia, S.; Ruggieri, S.; et al. Butyrylcholinesterase and Acetylcholinesterase polymorphisms in Multiple Sclerosis patients: Implication in peripheral inflammation. *Sci. Rep.* **2018**, *8*, 1319. [CrossRef] [PubMed]
56. Dyment, D.A.; Cader, M.Z.; Chao, M.J.; Lincoln, M.R.; Morrison, K.M.; Disanto, G.; Morahan, J.M.; De Luca, G.C.; Sadovnick, A.D.; Lepage, P.; et al. Exome sequencing identifies a novel multiple sclerosis susceptibility variant in the TYK2 gene. *Neurology* **2012**, *79*, 406–411. [CrossRef]

57. Ramagopalan, S.V.; Dyment, D.A.; Cader, M.Z.; Morrison, K.M.; Disanto, G.; Morahan, J.M.; Berlanga-Taylor, A.J.; Handel, A.; de Luca, G.C.; Sadovnick, D.P.A.D.; et al. Rare variants in the CYP27B1 gene are associated with multiple sclerosis. *Ann. Neurol.* **2011**, *70*, 881–886. [CrossRef]
58. Jamebozorgi, K.; Rostami, D.; Pormasoumi, H.; Taghizadeh, E.; Barreto, G.E.; Sahebkar, A. Epigenetic aspects of multiple sclerosis and future therapeutic options. *Int. J. Neurosci.* **2020**, 1–15. [CrossRef]
59. Waubant, E.; Lucas, R.; Mowry, E.; Graves, J.; Olsson, T.; Alfredsson, L.; Langer-Gould, A. Environmental and genetic risk factors for MS: An integrated review. *Ann. Clin. Transl. Neurol.* **2019**, *9*, 1905–1922. [CrossRef]
60. Swanborg, R.H. Experimental autoimmune encephalomyelitis in rodents as a model for human demyelinating disease. *Clin. Immunol. Immunopathol.* **1995**, *77*, 4–13. [CrossRef]
61. Brown, D.A.; Sawchenko, P.E. Time course and distribution of inflammatory and neurodegenerative events suggest structural bases for the pathogenesis of experimental autoimmune encephalomyelitis. *J. Comp. Neurol.* **2007**, *502*, 236–260. [CrossRef]
62. Soulika, A.M.; Lee, E.; McCauley, E.; Miers, L.; Bannerman, P.; Pleasure, D. Initiation and progression of axonopathy in experimental autoimmune encephalomyelitis. *J. Neurosci.* **2009**, *29*, 14965–14979. [CrossRef]
63. Di Pinto, G.; Di Bari, M.; Martin-Alvarez, R.; Sperduti, S.; Serrano-Acedo, S.; Gatta, V.; Tata, A.M.; Mengod, G. Comparative study of the expression of cholinergic system components in the CNS of experimental autoimmune encephalomyelitis mice: Acute vs. remitting phase. *Eur. J. Neurosci.* **2018**, *48*, 2165–2181. [CrossRef] [PubMed]
64. Wright, C.I.; Geula, C.; Mesulam, M.M. Neuroglial cholinesterases in the normal brain and in Alzheimer's disease: Relationship to plaques, tangles, and patterns of selective vulnerability. *Ann. Neurol.* **1993**, *34*, 373–384. [CrossRef] [PubMed]
65. Jiang, W.; St Pierre, S.; Roy, P.; Morley, B.J.; Hao, J.; Simard, A.R. Infiltration of CCR2+Ly6Chigh Proinflammatory Monocytes and Neutrophils into the Central Nervous System Is Modulated by Nicotinic Acetylcholine Receptors in a Model of Multiple Sclerosis. *J. Immunol.* **2016**, *196*, 2095–2108. [CrossRef] [PubMed]
66. Taveggia, C.; Feltri, M.L.; Wrabetz, L. Signals to promote myelin formation and repair. *Nat. Rev. Neurol.* **2010**, *6*, 276–287. [CrossRef] [PubMed]
67. Karadottir, R.; Attwell, D. Neurotrasmitter receptors in the life and death of oligodendrocytes. *Neuroscience* **2007**, *145*, 1426–1438. [CrossRef] [PubMed]
68. Corsetti, V.; Mozzetta, C.; Biagioni, S.; Augusti Tocco, G.; Tata, A.M. Acetylcholine release: The mechanisms and the site of release during chick dorsal root ganglia ontogenesis. *Life Sci.* **2012**, *91*, 783–788. [CrossRef]
69. Bernardini, N.; Srubek Tomassy, G.; Tata, A.M.; Augusti Tocco, G.; Biagioni, S. Detection of basal and potassium-evoked acetylcholine release from embryonic DRG explants. *J. Neurochem.* **2004**, *88*, 1533–1539. [CrossRef]
70. Jamebozorgi, K.; Rostami, D.; Pormasoumi, H.; Taghizadeh, E.; Barreto, G.E.; Sahebkar, A. Cholinergic signaling in myelination. *Glia* **2017**, *65*, 687–698.
71. Magnaghi, V.; Procacci, P.; Tata, A.M. Novel pharmacological approaches to Schwann cells as neuroprotective agents for peripheral nerve regeneration. *Int. Rev. Neurobiol.* **2009**, *87*, 295–315.
72. Larocca, J.N.; Almazan, G. Acetylcholine Agonists Stimulate Mitogen-Activated Protein Kinase in Oligodendrocyte Progenitors by Muscarinic Receptors. *J. Neurosci. Res.* **1997**, *50*, 743–754. [CrossRef]
73. Ragheb, F.; Molina-Holgado, E.; Cui, Q.L.; Khorchid, A.; Liu, H.N.; Larocca, J.N.; Almazan, G. Pharmacological and functional characterization of muscarinic receptor subtypes in developing oligodendrocytes. *J. Neurochem.* **2001**, *77*, 1396–1406. [CrossRef] [PubMed]
74. Molina-Holgado, E.; Khorchid, A.; Liu, H.; Almazan, G. Regulation of muscarinic receptor function in developing oligodendrocytes by agonist exposure. *Br. J. Pharmacol.* **2003**, *138*, 47–56. [CrossRef] [PubMed]
75. De Angelis, F.; Bernardo, A.; Magnaghi, V.; Minghetti, L.; Tata, A.M. Muscarinic receptor subtypes as potential targets to modulate oligodendrocyte progenitor survival, proliferation and differentiation. *Dev. Neurobiol.* **2012**, *72*, 713–728. [CrossRef] [PubMed]
76. Deshmukh, V.A.; Tardif, V.; Lyssiotis, C.A.; Green, C.C.; Kerman, B.; Kim, H.J.; Padmanabhan, K.; Swoboda, J.G.; Ahmad, I.; Kondo, T.; et al. The regenerative approaches for the treatment of multiple sclerosis. *Nature* **2013**, *502*, 327–332. [CrossRef] [PubMed]

77. Thompson, K.K.; Nissen, J.C.; Pretory, A.; Tsirka, S.E. Tuftis combines with remyelinating therapy and improves outcomes in models of CNS demyelinating disease. *Front. Immunol.* **2018**, *9*, 2784. [CrossRef] [PubMed]
78. Hertz, L.; Schousboe, I.; Hertz, L.; Schousboe, A. Receptor expression in primary cultures of neurons or astrocytes. *Prog Neuropsychopharmacol. Biol. Psych.* **1984**, *8*, 521–527. [CrossRef]
79. Lykhmus, O.; Voytenko, L.P.; Lips, K.S.; Bergen, I.; Krasteva-Christ, G.; Vetter, D.E.; Kummer, W.; Skok, M. Nicotinic acetylcholine receptor $\alpha 9$ and $\alpha 10$ subunits are express in the brain of mice. *Front. Cell Neurosci.* **2017**, *11*, 282. [CrossRef]
80. Zhang, X.; Lao, K.; Qiu, Z.; Rahman, M.S.; Zhang, Y.; Gou, X. Potential Astrocytic receptors and transporters in the pathogenesis of Alzheimer's disease. *J. Alzheimers Dis.* **2019**, *67*, 1109–1122. [CrossRef]
81. Kume, T.; Takada-Takatori, Y. Nicotinic acetylcholine receptor signaling: Roles in neuroprotection. In *Nicotinic Acetylcholine Receptor Signaling in Neuroprotection*; Akaike, A., Shimohama, S., Misu, Y., Eds.; Springer: Singapore, 2018.
82. Zhang, L.; McLarnon, J.G.; Goghari, V.; Lee, Y.B.; Kim, S.U.; Krieger, C. Cholinergic agonists increase intracellular Ca2+ in cultured human microglia. *Neurosci. Lett.* **1998**, *255*, 33–36. [CrossRef]
83. Pannell, M.; Meier, M.A.; Szulzewsky, F.; Matyash, V.; Endres, M.; Kronenberg, G.; Prinz, V.; Waiczies, S.; Wolf, S.A.; Kettenmann, H. The subpopulation of microglia expressing functional muscarinic acetylcholine receptors expands in stroke and Alzheimer's disease. *Brain Struct. Funct.* **2016**, *221*, 1157–1172. [CrossRef]
84. Shytle, R.D.; Mori, T.; Townsend, K.; Vendrame, M.; Sun, N.; Zeng, J.; Ehrhart, J.; Silver, A.A.; Sanberg, P.R.; Tan, J. Cholinergic modulation of microglial activation by a7 nicotinic receptors. *J. Neurochem.* **2004**, *89*, 337–343. [CrossRef] [PubMed]
85. Ke, P.; Shao, B.Z.; Xu, Z.Q.; Chen, X.W.; Wei, W.; Liu, C. Activation of $\alpha 7$ nicotinic acetylcholine receptor inhibits NLRP3 inflammasome through reulation of β-arrestin. *Neurosci. Ther.* **2017**, *23*, 875–884. [CrossRef] [PubMed]
86. De Simone, R.; Ajimone-Cat, M.A.; Carnevale, D.; Minghetti, L. Activation of $\alpha 7$ nicotinic acetylcholine receptor by nicotine selectively upregulates ciclooxigenase 2 and prostaglandin E2 in rat microglial cultures. *J. Neuroinflamm.* **2005**, *2*, 1–10. [CrossRef] [PubMed]
87. Egea, J.; Buendia, I.; Parada, E.; Navarro, E.; Leon, R.; Lopea, M.G. Anty inflammatory role of microglia $\alpha 7$ nAChRs and its role in neuroprotection. *Biochem. Pharmacol.* **2015**, *97*, 463–472. [CrossRef]
88. Nicoletti, C.G.; Landi, D.; Monteleone, F.; Mataluni, G.; Albanese, M.; Lauretti, B.; Rocchi, C.; Simonelli, I.; Boffa, L.; Buttari, F.; et al. Treatment with Dimethyl Fumarate Enhances Cholinergic Transmission in Multiple Sclerosis. *CNS Drugs* **2019**, *33*, 1133–1139. [CrossRef]

14

Daclizumab: Mechanisms of Action, Therapeutic Efficacy, Adverse Events and its Uncovering the Potential Role of Innate Immune System Recruitment as a Treatment Strategy for Relapsing Multiple Sclerosis

Stanley L. Cohan [1,*], Elisabeth B. Lucassen [1], Meghan C. Romba [1] and Stefanie N. Linch [2]

1 Providence Multiple Sclerosis Center, Providence Brain and Spine Institute, Portland, OR 97225, USA; elisabeth.lucassen@providence.org (E.B.L.); meghan.romba@providence.org (M.C.R.)
2 Providence Health and Services, Regional Research Department, Portland, OR 97213, USA; stefanie.linch@providence.org
* Correspondence: Stanley.Cohan@Providence.org;

Abstract: Daclizumab (DAC) is a humanized, monoclonal antibody that blocks CD25, a critical element of the high-affinity interleukin-2 receptor (IL-2R). DAC HYP blockade of CD25 inhibits effector T cell activation, regulatory T cell expansion and survival, and activation-induced T-cell apoptosis. Because CD25 blockade reduces IL-2 consumption by effector T cells, it increases IL-2 bioavailability allowing for greater interaction with the intermediate-affinity IL-2R, and therefore drives the expansion of CD56^{bright} natural killer (NK) cells. Furthermore, there appears to be a direct correlation between CD56^{bright} NK cell expansion and DAC HYP efficacy in reducing relapses and MRI evidence of disease activity in patients with RMS in phase II and phase III double-blind, placebo- and active comparator-controlled trials. Therapeutic efficacy was maintained during open-label extension studies. However, treatment was associated with an increased risk of rare adverse events, including cutaneous inflammation, autoimmune hepatitis, central nervous system Drug Reaction with Eosinophilia Systemic Symptoms (DRESS) syndrome, and autoimmune Glial Fibrillary Acidic Protein (GFAP) alpha immunoglobulin-associated encephalitis. As a result, DAC HYP was removed from clinical use in 2018. The lingering importance of DAC is that its use led to a deeper understanding of the underappreciated role of innate immunity in the potential treatment of autoimmune disease.

Keywords: daclizumab; relapsing multiple sclerosis; CD25; innate immune system; interleukin-2; drug reaction with eosinophilia systemic symptoms; DRESS; autoimmunity

1. Introduction

Daclizumab (DAC) is a humanized monoclonal antibody that blocks CD25, the α-subunit of the high-affinity interleukin-2 receptor (IL-2R-HA). DAC was initially developed as an intravenous therapy (Zenapax, Hoffman-LaRoche, Nutley, New Jersey) to prevent transplant organ rejection and to treat T cell leukemia and severe uveitis [1–4]. Subcutaneous DAC, often referred to as DAC High Yield Process (DAC HYP; Zinbryta, Biogen, Cambridge MA and AbbVie, Chicago Il), demonstrated efficacy in reducing both clinical and MRI measures of disease activity in patients with relapsing forms of multiple sclerosis (RMS) and was approved to treat RMS in 2016 [5–8]. Unfortunately, secondary autoimmune disease directed primarily against the central nervous system (CNS), liver, and skin resulted in serious adverse events (SAE) leading to its withdrawal in 2018. However, investigations of its mechanisms of therapeutic action and immunomodulatory activity have revealed insights into heretofore underappreciated relationships between innate and adaptive immunity in autoimmune diseases, particularly RMS. Future exploitation of these relationships may provide further therapeutic opportunities. This review will discuss known and proposed, direct and indirect effects of DAC HYP upon the immune system and how these effects are potentially related to its therapeutic impact in RMS. To better appreciate the multiple mechanisms by which DAC may impact autoimmunity, a brief description of the major immune system components that it is believed to affect, and the downstream impact of those actions, will be reviewed.

2. Immunologic Background for DAC Efficacy

2.1. IL-2 and IL-2R Signaling

IL-2 is a trophic cytokine expressed predominantly by activated T cells, which occurs upon cognate antigen recognition by the T cell receptor. While IL-2 promotes proliferation and survival of both activated effector and naïve T cells, it also promotes the expansion of regulatory T cells (T_{reg} cells), and some authors have reported that IL-2 activation may also promote apoptosis of antigen-activated T cells, thereby contributing to the maintenance of immune homeostasis [9–15]. Although most IL-2 is produced by activated T cells, it is also produced by myeloid dendritic cells (mDC) and macrophages [16,17].

IL-2 activity is primarily mediated through binding to the IL-2 high-affinity receptor (IL-2R-HA), which, in addition to IL-2, is comprised of three subunits: the α-subunit (CD25), the β-subunit (CD122), and the common γ-chain subunit (CD132), as shown in Figure 1. CD122 and CD132 can also combine to form an intermediate-affinity IL-2R (IL-2R-IA). CD132 is expressed on all lymphoid cells, whereas CD122 is constitutively expressed on natural killer (NK) and CD8 memory T cells, and can be induced on naïve T cells following antigen recognition. CD25 expression is much more tightly restricted; it is absent on naïve and memory cells, but is induced following antigen activation [17,18]. Furthermore, CD25 is constitutively expressed at very high levels on T_{reg} cells and is vital for the development and peripheral maintenance of the T_{reg} cell population [19]. It is also expressed on mDC, which may assist in T cell activation by using CD25 to "trans-present" IL-2 to a CD25-deficient IL-2R expressed on recently activated T cells, thus converting it to the IL-2R-HA [20].

Although both CD122 and CD132 are constitutively expressed on lymphocytes, IL-2 must be bound to CD25 to recruit these subunits to form the IL-2R-HA complex [21,22]. While IL-2 can also bind and signal through the IL-2R-IA, receptor affinity increases 1000-fold following its association with CD25 [18]. Furthermore, in the absence of CD25, the IL-2R-IA requires up to 50 times the IL-2 available at basal physiological states [23]. IL-2 bound to the IL-2R-HA results in rapid internalization and degradation of the high-affinity receptor complex. This latter step, terminating IL-2-induced T cell activation via the intracellular domain of CD122, may be initiated by activation of the intracellular domain of the CD132 portion of the IL-2R, thereby regulating IL-2 effects [24–26]. Subsequently, CD25 can be recycled back to the surface of the cell for future engagement with CD122, CD132, and IL-2 [27,28].

2.2. Innate Lymphoid Cells (ILC)

Innate lymphoid cells (ILC) arise from a hematopoietic $CD34^{+}$ cell line, which is considered the common progenitor for all ILC [29]. Multiple subsets of ILC have been identified, of which several are relevant to the potential immunoregulatory actions of DAC: group 1, which includes ILC1 and $CD56^{bright}$ NK cells; group 2, comprised of ILC2, to which we will return later; and group 3, which includes ILC3 and pro-inflammatory lymphoid tissue inducer (LTi) cells [30–33]. NK cells constitutively express CD122 and CD132. Notably, $CD56^{bright}$ NK cells have 10-fold greater expression of CD122 relative to the pro-inflammatory $CD56^{dim}$ NK cells [34]. IL-2 stimulation of the IL-2R-IA has been reported to drive ILC toward anti-inflammatory $CD56^{bright}$ NK cell production, possibly at the expense of the pro-inflammatory LTi cell pathway [11,35,36].

There is considerable evidence to support a role for CD56^{bright} NK cells in auto-regulation and tolerance. CD56^{bright} NK cells can destroy activated immune cells through direct contact, including autologous antigen-activated CD4^{+} and CD8^{+} T cells, which play a critical role in autoimmune responses [34,37,38]. In support of this concept, reduced CD56^{bright} NK cell cytotoxicity was observed in patients with MS as early as the 1980s [39–42]. Subsequently, investigators demonstrated that CD56^{bright} NK cells are directly cytotoxic to auto-antigen-specific T cells [34,38]. Of note and expanded upon below, there is a strong correlation between DAC-induced up-regulation of CD56^{bright} NK cells and the therapeutic efficacy of DAC HYP in RMS [34,43,44].

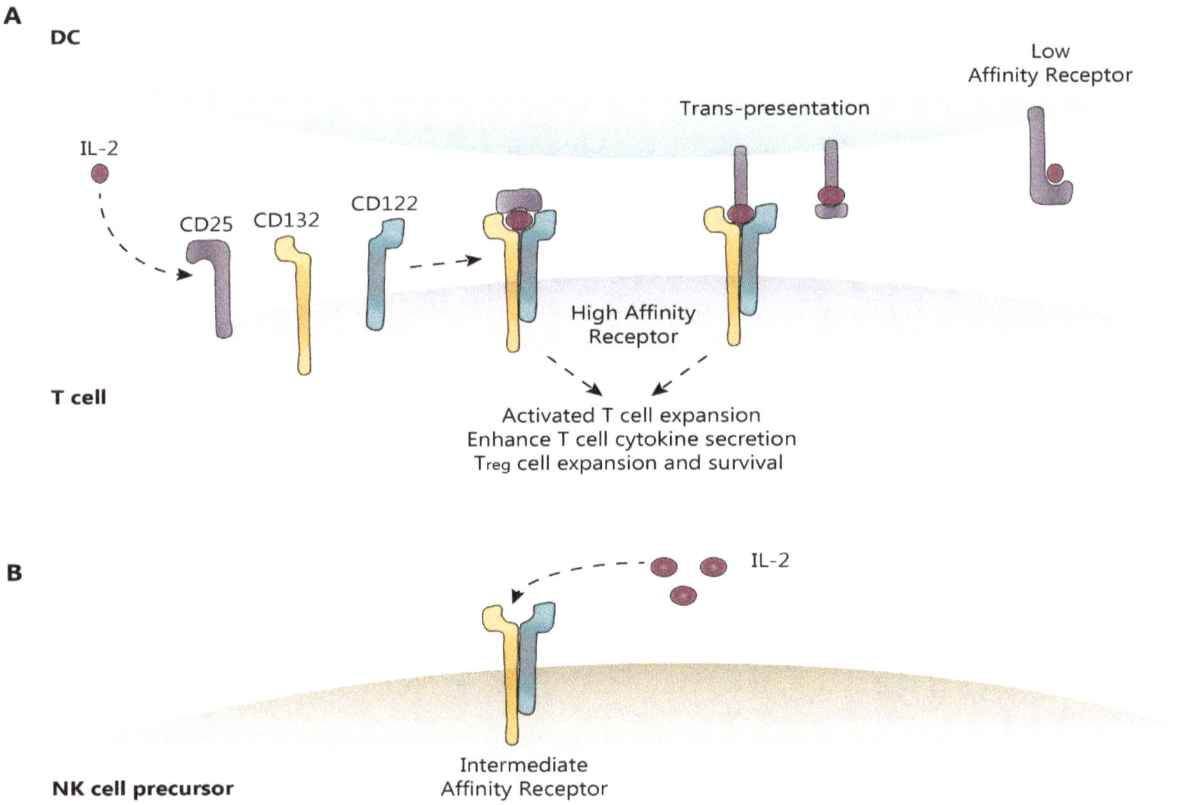

Figure 1. IL-2 receptor (IL-2R) subunits. (**A**) CD25 (α-subunit) is the low-affinity IL-2R and is expressed on activated T cells, T_{reg} cells, and mDC. Once IL-2 is bound to CD25 on the cell surface, CD132 (γ) and CD122 (β) are recruited to form the high-affinity IL-2R. CD132 and CD122 are the only subunits capable of intracellular signaling. (**B**) Other cell types such as NK cells express the intermediate-affinity IL-2R, comprised of CD132 and CD122 only. This receptor requires elevated levels of IL-2 for signaling, such as those found in a local draining lymph node, due to reduced binding affinity for IL-2. DC-dendritic cell; IL-2-interleukin-2; NK-natural killer. Dotted lines show the sequence of events following IL-2 binding to its receptor.

3. DAC Mechanisms of Action: Known and Proposed

DAC reversibly binds to CD25, preventing the interaction of IL-2 with the IL-2R-HA, leaving more IL-2 available to induce IL-2R-IA signaling. As noted above, the IL-2R requires CD25 to render it high-affinity. By blocking the formation of IL-2R-HA, DAC blocks IL-2 consumption by activated effector T cells, causing a moderate decrease in the frequency of CD4^{+} and CD8^{+} T cells in the periphery and increasing the availability of IL-2 to interact with the IL-2R-IA [34,37,43,45]. As might be expected with a reduction in IL-2 consumption, IL-2 concentrations in the serum were elevated following DAC treatment by approximately 50% [46]. Because expansion of T_{reg} cells is dependent upon IL-2 interaction with the IL-2R-HA, as predicted, DAC treatment also resulted in a 50–60% decrease in peripheral T_{reg} cells [37,46–48], as shown in Figure 2. By blocking the IL-2R-HA, DAC may also potentially prevent activation-induced T cell apoptosis, paradoxically inhibiting auto-regulation by allowing the survival of activated effector T cells recognizing "self" antigens [10,11]. DAC HYP administration has also been reported to normalize previously elevated intrathecal $CD4^+$, $CD8^+$ and HLA-DR-expressing $CD4^+$ T cells and B cells in patients with RMS [35]. In some patients, the effect of DAC on effector T and T_{reg} cells may not be adequately compensated for by $CD56^{bright}$ NK cell expansion, as is observed in patients with spontaneously occurring autoimmunity due to genetic variants that delete CD25 [49,50]. These resultant autoimmunity-promoting circumstances may also explain, in part, the paradoxical increase risk of autoimmune adverse events (AE) observed in some DAC HYP-treated RMS patients (see below).

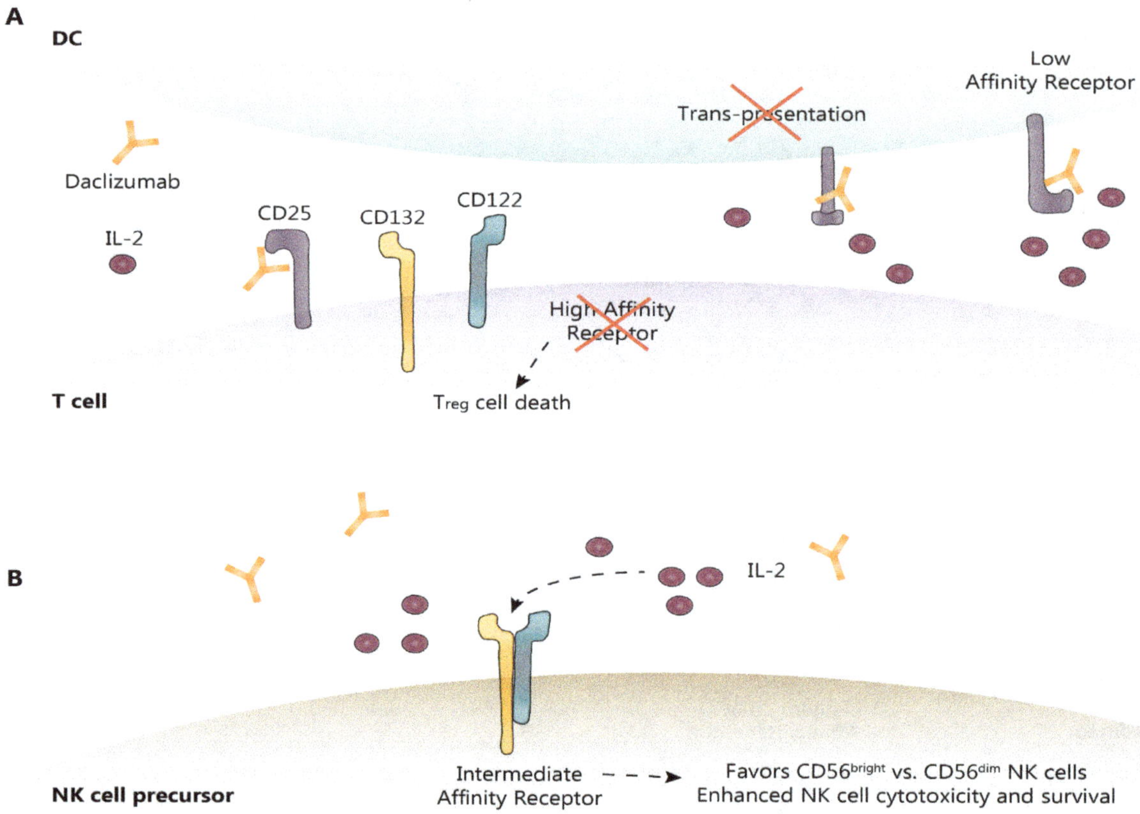

Figure 2. Known and proposed DAC mechanisms of action. (**A**) DAC binds to CD25 blocking its association with CD132 and CD122. This prevents trans-presentation of CD25 from mDC to T cells and ultimately results in effector T cell and T_{reg} cell death; (**B**) As a result of CD25 blockade, serum IL-2 levels are elevated allowing for NK cell activation through the intermediate-affinity receptor, CD132 and CD122, and promoting $CD56^{bright}$ NK cell cytotoxicity and survival. DC-dendritic cell; IL-2-interleukin-2; NK-natural killer. Dotted lines show the sequence of events following IL-2 binding to its receptor.

Although part of the anti-inflammatory activity of DAC is through selective inhibition of IL-2-driven effector T cell activation and expansion, it is evident that this does not entirely account for its therapeutic efficacy [37]. Innate immune components also play an essential role in auto-tolerance and autoimmunity. As mentioned above, $CD56^{bright}$ NK cells from multiple sclerosis patients exhibit reduced cytotoxicity. This is important because $CD56^{bright}$ NK cells are believed to be directly cytotoxic to auto-antigen activated T cells [34,38]. $CD56^{bright}$ NK cells also express high levels of cell surface IL-2R-IA, and IL-2 activation of the IL-2R-IA through DAC resulted in $CD56^{bright}$ NK cell expansion, which was abolished by IL-2 inhibition [37]. IL-2 may also enhance CD56^{bright} NK cell maturation and reduce NK cell death, and further increase NK cell cytotoxicity, through enhanced killing efficiency [37,51] as shown in Figure 2. In prospective clinical studies, DAC HYP treatment resulted in an expansion of CD56^{bright} NK cells in up to 90% of DAC HYP-treated patients, with a 5-fold elevation of CD56^{bright} NK cell counts seen by 52 weeks of treatment that was sustained thereafter [44]. By blocking consumption of IL-2 by the IL-2R-HA, IL-2 levels increase systemically, thereby increasing the bioavailability of IL-2 to interact with the IL-2R-IA and preferentially promoting the expansion of anti-inflammatory CD56^{bright} NK cells via CD122 intracellular signaling [52].

It has also been reported that DAC reduces the expansion of pro-inflammatory LTi, as shown in Figure 3 [34]. By orienting the innate CD34^{+} progenitor cell line away from the pro-inflammatory LTi cell line, DAC may indirectly reduce the formation or activity of meningeal lymphoid follicle-like structures, which have been observed overlying cortical areas of demyelination [53–55]. Consistent with this concept, DAC HYP administration reportedly normalized previously elevated LTi cell numbers in the spinal fluid of patients with RMS [35]. One study found that the total number of ILC was reduced in DAC HYP-treated patients; however, this remains controversial and has not been replicated by subsequent research [31,35,36,56,57].

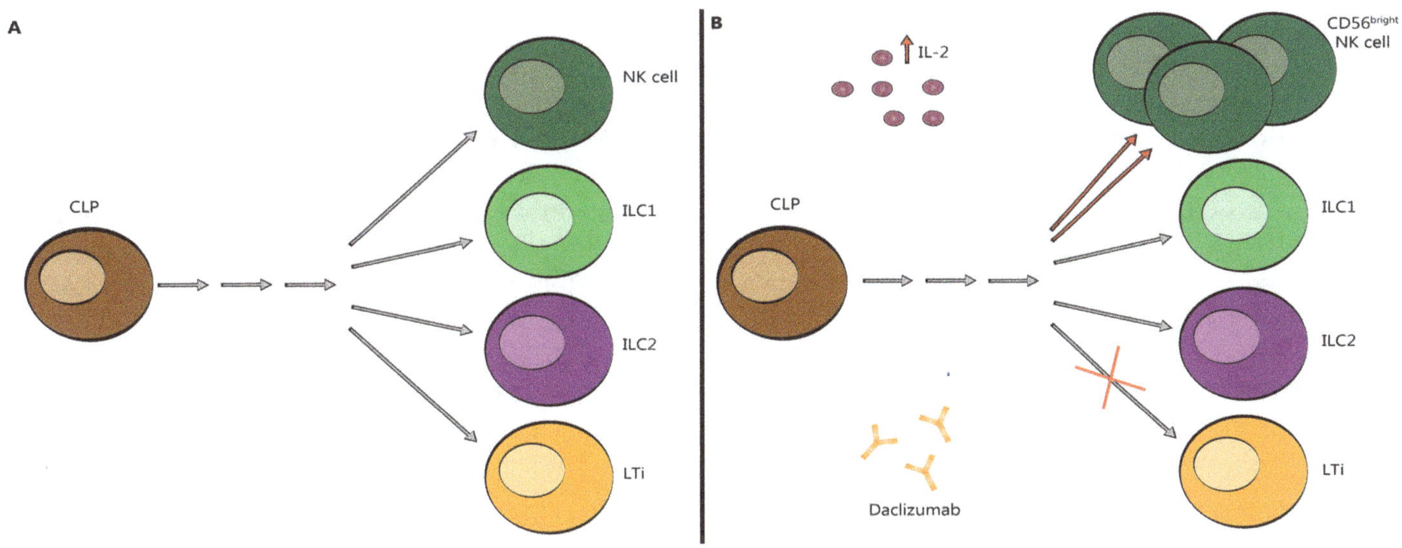

Figure 3. Innate Lymphoid Cells skewed toward CD56^{bright} NK cells following DAC treatment. (**A**) DAC binds to CD25 blocking association with CD132 and CD122. This prevents trans-presentation of CD25 from mDC to T cells and results in effector T cell and T_{reg} cell death. (**B**) As a result of CD25 blockade, serum IL-2 levels are elevated allowing for NK cell activation through the intermediate-affinity receptor, CD132 and CD122, and promoting CD56^{bright} NK cell cytotoxicity and survival (red arrows). It may also redirect the commitment of LTi cells (red ×). CLP-common lymphoid progenitor; NK-natural killer; ILC-innate lymphoid cell; LTi-lymphoid tissue-inducer cell; IL-2-interleukin-2. Grey arrows indicate a series of differentiation steps not depicted in this figure.

Because CD25 is also expressed on mDC, which may use CD25 to "trans-present" IL-2 to CD25-deficient T cells, it is possible that may block mDC potentiation of IL-2R-HA signaling on effector T cells, as shown in Figure 2a [20]. There is also some preclinical evidence to suggest that the modulation of cytokine production by mDC may also be a target of DAC therapy [58]. Further research is needed to confirm these reported effects of DAC on mDC.

In summary, activated effector T cell expansion is dependent upon IL-2 interaction with IL-2R-HA expressed on the cell surface. To perform as a high-affinity receptor, the IL-2R requires CD25, which is blocked by DAC, reducing IL-2 utilization by T cells. This drives IL-2 towards IL-2R-IA and CD56^{bright} NK cell expansion, which destroy activated effector T cells by direct contact. As will become evident from the paragraphs that follow, there is a direct correlation between the DAC-induced decrease in activated effector T cells and $CD56^{bright}$ NK cell expansion with both clinical and MRI efficacy of DAC. However, there is also a reduction in T_{reg} cells, and possibly a decrease in activated T cell apoptosis, both of which may paradoxically promote the up-regulation of heightened autoimmunity, leading to SAE which will be discussed further below.

4. Pharmacokinetics and Pharmacodynamics of DAC HYP

Initial studies of DAC HYP in healthy adult subjects (ages 18–65) showed that the maximum serum concentration (C_{max}) was 7 days while the $t^{1/2}$ of elimination was 24 days [59]. In a subsequent study in adults with RMS, C_{max} was achieved in 5–7 days, and the $t^{1/2}$ of elimination was approximately 21 days after the last injection [60]. Maximum CD25 saturation by DAC HYP was reached by 7 h and was sustained as long as DAC HYP serum concentration was 5.0 mcg/mL or higher. Baseline CD25 saturation was achieved in approximately 24 weeks following DAC HYP discontinuation, in parallel with a serum DAC HYP concentration of 1.0 mcg/mL or less. During treatment with DAC HYP (150 mg every 4 weeks), maximum $CD56^{bright}$ NK cell level is reached by approximately 36 weeks, achieving a maximum 5-fold increase over baseline [47]. For patients treated with 300 mg DAC HYP, the changes in NK cell and T_{reg} frequency were nearly identical; no other results were reported separately for this group [47].

Several other studies examined various immune parameters in pooled DAC HYP-treated patients (150 mg and 300 mg) from the SELECT, SELECTION, and DECIDE trials. Following DAC HYP cessation, in both 150 mg DAC HYP alone and pooled (150 mg and 300 mg) DAC HYP groups $CD56^{bright}$ NK cells return to pre-treatment levels by 24 weeks after the last injection. In parallel with increased $CD56^{bright}$ NK cells, serum IL-2 levels increased by roughly 50% within 4 weeks of DAC HYP treatment and T_{reg} cell counts fell by 50–60% within 4 days of a 150 mg DAC HYP injection and returned to pre-treatment levels approximately 20 weeks after the last DAC HYP injection [34,44,46,47]. $CD4^{+}$ and $CD8^{+}$ T lymphocyte counts were decreased by 7–10% after 52 weeks and by 15–18% after 96 weeks of DAC HYP treatment [7]. Importantly, there was also a roughly 25% decrease in HLA-DR2-expressing activated effector $CD4^{+}$ T cells, in DAC HYP treatment in patients with RMS in both the 150 mg and 300 mg groups similarly [61]. This coincides with the timing of maximum inflammatory lesion reductions observed in the CHOICE study and provides further evidence of the down-regulation of the pro-inflammatory activity of DAC HYP [5].

5. DAC Efficacy: Controlled Clinical Trial Data

As noted in the section on mechanisms of action, DAC administration expands immunoregulatory $CD56^{bright}$ natural killer cells, reduces whole blood and intrathecal pro-inflammatory T cells and T_{reg} cells. Based on its immunologic effects, subcutaneous use of DAC HYP was approved by the United States Food and Drug Administration for RMS in May 2016 and the European Medicines Agency (EMA) in July 2016 [62].

Several small open-label studies evaluating intravenous DAC in RMS demonstrated improvement in several outcome measures [43,63,64]. Due to cell-mediated toxicities reported with intravenous DAC preparations, it was subsequently reformulated to DAC HYP, facilitating subcutaneous administration [59]. CHOICE was a randomized phase II double-blind, placebo-controlled trial in which DAC HYP was an add-on therapy to interferon beta (IFNβ) versus placebo plus IFNβ. CHOICE demonstrated that DAC HYP administered at 2 mg/kg with IFNβ resulted in a 72% decrease in the number of contrast-enhancing lesions relative to IFNβ with placebo ($p = 0.004$) [5], as shown in Table 1.

Table 1. Selected Clinical and MRI Outcomes of DAC HYP Treatment in RMS Controlled Trials.

	Clinical Trials									
	CHOICE		SELECT			SELECTION			DECIDE	
	DAC [1]	pl	150 mg	300 mg	pl	Continuous [2]	Switch [3]	Washout [4]	DAC	IFNβ
Parameters										
ARR	0.27	0.41	0.21	0.23	0.46	0.165	0.179 ****	0.302	0.22	0.39
Risk Reduction, %	34		54 ****	50 ***					45 ***	
PPRF, %	52	55	81 ****	80 ***	64	86.4	82.4 ****	75.9	67	51
CDP, %										
12 weeks	NR	NR	6*	8	13	7	8 ****	10	16	20
24 weeks	NR	NR	NR	NR	NR	NR	NR	NR	13 *	18
New Gd+	1.32 **	4.75	0.3 ****	0.2 ****	1.4	0.2	0.2 ****	0.2	0.4 ***	1.0
Reduction, %	72		79	86		NR	NR	NR	60	
T2 Lesions										
New/enlarging	1.1 **	3.4	2.4 ****	1.7 ****	8.1	1.2	2.1 ****	3.3	4.3	9.4
Reduction, %	68		70	79					54 ***	
Volume change, %	ND		−11.1 ****	−12.5 ****	−27.3	−6.9	−8.1 ****	−3.1	0.2 ***	8.6
Brain Volume, % change	NR	NR	−0.79	−0.70	−0.74	−0.536	−0.830	−0.551	−0.559 ***	−0.585 ***
NEDA%	NR	NR	NR	NR	NR	NR	NR	NR	13 ***	22

DAC—daclizumab; HYP—high-yield process; pl—placebo; RMS—relapsing forms of multiple sclerosis; ARR—annualized relapse rate; CDP—confirmed disability progression; PPRF—proportion of patients relapse-free; Gd^+—gadolinium-enhancing lesions; IFNβ—interferon beta-1a; NR—not reported; ND—no difference. [1] Data reported are for patients receiving high-dose DAC (2 mg/kg); both DAC and placebo received IFNβ; [2] Continuous-patients receiving DAC HYP 150 or 300 mg every 4 weeks during SELECT continued their same dose of DAC HYP through additional 52 weeks of SELECTION; [3] Switch-patients receiving placebo during SELECT were placed on either 150 or 300 mg DAC HYP for the 52 weeks of SELECTION; [4] Washout-patients receiving either 150 or 300 mg of DAC HYP during SELECT were placed on placebo for 20 weeks followed by resumption of their previous dose of DAC HYP administered during SELECT; **** $p < 0.0001$; *** $p < 0.001$; ** $p < 0.01$; * $p < 0.05$.

DAC HYP was subsequently studied in two large, pivotal phase III clinical trials in patients with RMS; a 52-week placebo-controlled trial (SELECT) and an active comparator trial (DECIDE) of DAC HYP versus IFNβ. The primary endpoint of the SELECT and DECIDE trials was the annualized relapse rate (ARR). Secondary and tertiary outcomes measured include: impact on 3 month confirmed disability progression, T2 lesion burden and gadolinium-enhancing (Gd^+) lesions, safety, measurement of markers of immune activity; and in DECIDE, changes in cognitive status and patient-reported outcomes [6,7,65].

5.1. SELECT

In SELECT, patients with RMS were randomized 1:1:1 to subcutaneous DAC HYP 150 mg, DAC HYP 300 mg, or placebo every four weeks for 52 weeks. The primary endpoint was met with a 54% relative reduction in ARR (95% CI 33–68%; $p < 0.0001$) in the group treated with DAC HYP 150 mg (ARR 0.21) and 50% reduction (95% CI 28–65%; $p < 0.0001$) in those treated with DAC HYP 300 mg (ARR 0.23) in comparison to placebo (ARR 0.46). At 52 weeks, the three-month sustained disability progression decreased by 57% in the DAC HYP 150 mg group and 43% in the DAC HYP 300 mg group compared to placebo [7], as shown in Table 1.

Subcutaneous DAC HYP also demonstrated effects on brain MRI measures in SELECT. There was a statistically significant relative decrease in the number of Gd^+ lesions ($p < 0.0001$) at week 52, with a 69% reduction in the DAC HYP 150 mg group versus 78% reduction in the DAC HYP 300 mg group compared to placebo. The number of new/newly enlarging T2 hyperintense lesions were also significantly reduced at week 52 ($p < 0.0001$) in the 150 mg group by 70% versus 79% in the 300 mg group compared to placebo [7], as shown in Table 1. The mean percentage of brain volume loss was not significantly different between the treatment arms in SELECT. Exploratory studies performed in SELECT demonstrated a strong correlation between early increases in $CD56^{bright}$NK cells and decrease in new and enlarging T2 lesions at 24 and 52 weeks of DAC HYP treatment, and DAC HYP patients in the highest CD56bright NK cell quartile had 62% fewer new and enlarging T2 lesions than those in the lowest quartile [44].

5.2. SELECTION

SELECTION was a double-blind extension of SELECT, designed to further assess the risks of AE associated with prolonged DAC HYP therapy (52 weeks), the impact of discontinuing DAC HYP, and to determine if early efficacy was sustained. Placebo-treated patients in SELECT were randomized 1:1 to initiate either 150 mg or 300 mg DAC HYP subcutaneously every four weeks ("Switch" in Table 1). The patients who received DAC HYP during SELECT either continued the same medication dose through SELECTION for a total of 104 weeks of continuous therapy, or underwent a blinded, placebo-treated washout that lasted for a total of 20 weeks, followed by resumption of their prior DAC HYP dose for the remaining 32 weeks of their participation in SELECTION [8]. Therapeutic efficacy achieved by DAC HYP therapy in SELECT was measured by: ARR, proportion of patients experiencing a relapse (PPRF), 12-week confirmed disability worsening, number of new Gd^+ lesions, number of new and enlarging T2 lesions, volume of T2 lesions, mean and total T1 lesion volume was sustained by week 52 of SELECTION (104 weeks of total DAC HYP therapy).

For patients treated with placebo in SELECT, treatment with DAC HYP during SELECTION resulted in a statistically significant decrease in ARR, the proportion of patients having relapses, the number of Gd^+ enhancing lesions, new and enlarging T2, and the volume of T2 lesions. No significant differences were observed in T1 lesion measurements or whole brain volume, as shown in Table 1. For DAC HYP-treated patients in SELECT who underwent the 20-week washout period in SELECTION, clinical and MRI end-points were similar after 52 weeks in SELECTION to those patients who received DAC HYP for the entire 52 weeks in SELECTION, as shown in Table 1. By the end of the washout period, CD56^{bright} NK counts had returned to baseline values, but at the conclusion of SELECTION (32 weeks of DAC HYP treatment), CD56^{bright} NK numbers were similar to those found in patients who had been continuously treated with DAC HYP through the 104 weeks of SELECT and SELECTION.

5.3. DECIDE

DECIDE was a double-blind and double-dummy, active-comparator, phase III study, and compared efficacy in patients with RMS, randomized 1:1 to either subcutaneous DAC HYP 150 mg every four weeks plus weekly intramuscular placebo, or to IFNβ (30 μg, intramuscularly) once weekly, and placebo subcutaneously every four weeks, for up to 144 weeks [6]. The primary end point was met with a 45% reduction in annualized relapse rate (ARR 0.22) in the DAC HYP treated group compared to the IFNβ group (ARR 0.32) $p < 0.001$. The DAC HYP group also demonstrated a significant reduction in the annualized rate of severe relapses (38% reduction, $p = 0.002$). The number of patients who remained relapse-free at week 144 was 67% in the DAC HYP group and 51% in the IFNβ group. Three-month confirmed disability progression measured at week 144 revealed a 16% relative risk reduction in the DAC HYP cohort compared to IFNβ, which did not reach statistical significance. However, the risk of 24-week confirmed disability worsening demonstrated DAC HYP significantly reduced disability worsening by 27% compared to IFNβ ($p = 0.03$)

There was a 75% relative decrease ($p < 0.001$) in new Gd$^+$ lesions and a 54% relative reduction ($p < 0.001$) in the number of new or newly enlarged T2 hyperintense brain MRI lesions over a 96-week period in patients treated with DAC HYP compared to IFNβ ($p < 0.001$). There was also a statistically significant decrease in brain volume loss in DAC HYP versus IFNβ treated patients after two years of treatment ($p < 0.01$). No evidence of disease activity (NEDA) over 96 weeks, as measured by no relapses, no disability progression, no new/enlarged T2 or Gd$^+$ lesions, was seen in 22% of DAC HYP and 13% of IFNβ-treated patients ($p < 0.001$).

Investigators also observed a 7–10% drop in total CD4$^+$ and CD8$^+$ T lymphocyte counts over 52 weeks in the DAC HYP treated group in SELECT versus 15–18% over 96 weeks among the DAC HYP treated group in the DECIDE trial. The ratio of CD4$^+$ to CD8$^+$ T cells remained stable in the DAC HYP group in both SELECT and DECIDE. No correlation was found between the reduced CD4$^+$ and CD8$^+$ T cells and the infection rate in the DECIDE trial [6].

A tertiary outcome in DECIDE was the assessment of cognitive outcomes, as measured by changes in the orally administered Symbol Digit Modalities Test (SDMT). At 96 weeks, there was a significantly greater ($p = 0.0274$) improvement from baseline SDMT in DAC HYP-treated patients compared to IFNβ treated patients [65]. Furthermore, a significantly greater number of DAC HYP-treated patients experienced clinically meaningful improvement ($p = 0.0366$) and a significantly smaller number of patients experienced a clinically-meaningful decline ($p = 0.0103$) in their SDMT scores.

5.4. SELECTED

SELECTED was a single-armed open-label extension trial of DAC HYP 150 mg, for which any patient completing SELECT and SELECTION qualified [66]. Although the primary outcomes dealt with AE (see below), adjusted ARR was calculated every six months from the time the patient received their first dose of DAC HYP dose in either SELECT or SELECTION up to 144 weeks; changes in the number of new/enlarging T2 lesions and brain volume (percentage) compared to baseline, were obtained on yearly MRI scans. ARR varied from 0.21 in patients having received DAC HYP for 0–24 weeks and gradually declined to 0.15 in patients receiving DAC HYP for 121–144 weeks. The adjusted mean number of new/enlarging T2 lesions was 1.96 after year 1, 1.62 at year 2 and 1.26 at year 3. The annualized median decrease in brain volume from the first dose of DAC HYP was 0.77 at year 1, 0.57 at year 2, and 0.32 at year 3. As in all single arm open-label studies, efficacy outcomes may have been affected by selection bias arising from dropout of poor responders, and subjects with AE.

5.5. Patient-Reported Outcomes

The DAC HYP treatment groups in both SELECT and DECIDE demonstrated significant benefits in patient-reported outcomes, when utilizing the 29-item Multiple Sclerosis Impact Scale (MSIS-29), which evaluates the impact of MS on physical (PHYS) and psychological health (psychological impact scale), as well as EuroQol 5-Dimensions (EQ-5D), which is used to examine overall health status using five domains. In SELECT, there was a significant improvement in MSIS-29 PHYS score at week 52 in the subcutaneous DAC HYP 150 mg compared with placebo ($p = 0.00082$), but not with the DAC HYP 300 mg group. There was also a statistically significant benefit for subcutaneous DAC HYP 150 mg for EQ-5D index ($p = 0.0091$) compared to placebo in SELECT.

In DECIDE, DAC HYP 150mg treated patients showed a greater improvement compared to IFNβ at 96 weeks in regards to MSIS-29 PHYS ($p < 0.001$), MSIS-29 psychological impact scale ($p = 0.04$), and EQ-5D index ($p = 0.005$). Clinically meaningful worsening was defined as an increase in ≥7.5 points in the patient-reported outcomes at 96 weeks. As measured by MSIS-29 physical subscale, worsening was 19% in the DAC HYP group versus 23% in the interferon IFNβ group (NS). DECIDE also demonstrated a greater improvement in Multiple Sclerosis Functional Composite (MSFC) at 96 weeks in patients treated with DAC HYP compared to IFNβ in DECIDE ($p < 0.001$) [6].

6. Adverse Events with DAC: Prospective Clinical Trial Data

6.1. SELECT

In the randomized, double-blind, placebo-controlled SELECT trial, SAE excluding relapse was similar between groups, as shown in Table 2. Nine (2%) patients treated with DAC HYP developed serious infections, one of whom discontinued treatment, while six resumed treatment after the resolution of infection. No placebo-treated patients had serious infections. The frequency of oral herpes and herpes zoster infections was similar in all groups.

Table 2. Adverse Event Incidence for DAC treated patients in Controlled Trials of DAC HYP.

	Clinical Trials						
	SELECT		SELECTION			DECIDE	SELECTED
			Continuous [1]	Switch [2]	Washout [3]		
DAC Dose	**150 mg**	**300 mg**	**150 mg, 300 mg**	**150 mg, 300 mg**	**150 mg, 300 mg**	**150 mg**	**150 mg**
AE							
Infection (%)	104 (50)	112 (54)	36 (42),36 (41)	34 (40), 31 (37)	34 (40), 38 (43)	595 (65)	205 (50)
Serious Infection (%)	6 (3)	3 (1)	2 (2), 2 (2)	3 (3), 1 (1)	3 (3), 2 (2)	40 (4)	13 (3)
Hepatic TA (%)	NR	NR	NR	NR	NR	144 (16)	61 (15)
AST/ALT:							
1–3× ULN (%)	54 (26)	62 (30)	30 (35), 30 (34)	23 (27), 22 (26)	21 (24), 26 (30)	NR	NR
3–5× ULN (%)	7 (3)	6 (3)	1 (1), 5 (6)	0, 2 (2)	2 (2), 0	96 (10)	37 (9)
>5× ULN (%)	9 (4)	8 (4)	0, 3 (3)	1 (1), 1 (1)	2 (2), 4 (5)	59 (6)	18 (4)
Hepatic SAE (%)	NR	NR	0, 0	0, 0	0, 1 (<1)	6 (1)	5 (1)
Malignancy (%)	1 (<1)	2 (<1)	0, 0	0, 1 (1)	0, 0	7 (1)	4 (1)
Death (%)	1 (<1)	0	0, 0	0, 0	0, 1 (<1)	1 (<1)	0

DAC—daclizumab; HYP—high-yield process; TA—transaminases; AST—aspartate aminotransferase; ALT—alanine aminotransferase; AE—adverse events; ULN—upper limit of normal; NR—not reported. [1] Continuous-patients receiving DAC HYP 150 or 300 mg every 4 weeks during SELECT continued their same dose of DAC HYP through additional 52 weeks of SELECTION; [2] Switch-patients receiving placebo during SELECT were placed on either 150 or 300 mg DAC HYP for the 52 weeks of SELECTION; [3] Washout-patients receiving either 150 or 300 mg of DAC HYP during SELECT were placed on placebo for 20 weeks followed by resumption of their previous dose of DAC HYP administered during SELECT.

Four malignancies were reported during the trial, including two cervical carcinomas (one in the placebo, one in DAC HYP 150 mg) and two melanomas in the DAC HYP 300 mg group. Two patients in the DAC HYP 150 mg group and three in the DAC HYP 300 mg group, had serious cutaneous events, including rash, atopic and allergic dermatitis, ex-foliative dermatitis, and erythema nodosum, as shown in Table 3. While recovering from a serious rash, one DAC HYP (150 mg) patient died due to a psoas abscess. No serious cutaneous events were seen in the placebo group. More patients in the DAC HYP groups had liver transaminase increases of greater than five times the upper limit of normal (>5× ULN). These increases had a median onset at 308 (±SD) treatment days. Continued DAC HYP dosing did not increase recovery time of transaminase abnormalities, and 7/17 patients with elevated alanine aminotransferase levels >5× ULN continued or resumed DAC HYP after enzyme recovery, and did not experience a recurrence of liver function test abnormalities in the five months that followed [7].

Table 3. Cutaneous AE Incidence for DAC treated patients in Controlled Trials of DAC HYP.

	SELECT		Clinical Trials SELECTION Continuous [1]	Switch [2]	Washout [3]	DECIDE	SELECTED	Post Approval [4]
DAC Dose	**150 mg**	**300 mg**	**150 mg, 300 mg**	**150 mg, 300 mg**	**150 mg, 300 mg**	**150 mg**	**150 mg**	
Cutaneous Events								
AE (%)	38 (18)	45 (22)	15 (17), 21 (24)	17 (20), 11 (13)	19 (22), 16 (18)	344 (37)	114 (28)	23 (77)
SAE (%)	2 (<1)	3 (<1)	0, 3 (3)	2 (2), 0	1 (1), 0	14 (2)	8 (2)	6 (19)

DAC-daclizumab; HYP-high-yield process; AE-adverse event; SAE-serious adverse event. [1] Continuous-patients receiving DAC HYP 150 or 300 mg every 4 weeks during SELECT continued their same dose of DAC HYP through additional 52 weeks of SELECTION; [2] Switch-patients receiving placebo during SELECT were placed on either 150 or 300 mg DAC HYP for the 52 weeks of SELECTION; [3] Washout-patients receiving either 150 or 300 mg of DAC HYP during SELECT were placed on placebo for 20 weeks followed by resumption of their previous dose of DAC HYP administered during SELECT; [4] Cortese et al., open-label study.

6.2. SELECTION

In the multicenter, randomized, double-blind SELECT extension trial (SELECTION), frequencies of AEs and SAEs were similar between the patients switched from placebo to DAC HYP treatment and the continuous DAC HYP treatment groups, as shown in Table 2. Infections were reported in 42% of patients; 3% were considered serious infections. The only serious infection occurring in more than one patient was bronchitis. All infections were resolved with standard-of-care.

Breast cancer was reported in one (<1%) patient, which investigators did not believe was treatment-related. Cutaneous events occurred in up to 24% of patients as shown in Table 3. Serious cutaneous events were reported in six (1%) patients. These events included drug eruption, eczema, pityriasis rubra pilaris, exfoliative dermatitis, and urticaria. Alanine or aspartate aminotransferase levels of >5× ULN were observed in 11 patients (2%) and resolved in a median of 84.5 days. Of these patients, 10 resumed DAC HYP without recurrence; one did not resume treatment. One patient died due to autoimmune hepatitis following re-initiation of 300 mg DAC HYP; this was confirmed by liver histology upon autopsy. The contribution of DAC HYP could not be ruled out [8].

6.3. DECIDE

In the double-blind, active-controlled, randomized phase III DECIDE trial comparing DAC HYP 150 mg with IFNβ weekly injections, the overall incidence of AEs was similar among all groups, leading to discontinuation in 14% of DAC HYP-treated patients and 9% in the IFNβ treated group, as shown in Table 2. SAEs (excluding relapse) occurred in 15% of the patients treated with DAC HYP and in 10% of those treated with IFNβ. One patient in the DAC HYP group and four in the IFNβ died, but none of these deaths was considered to be related to study treatment according to investigators.

Infections occurred in 65% of DAC HYP patients and 57% of IFNβ patients. Five DAC HYP patients (1%) and three (<1%) IFNβ patients discontinued treatment due to infection. Common infections included nasopharyngitis (25% in DAC HYP group; 21% in IFNβ group), upper respiratory infection (16% and 13%, respectively), and urinary tract infection (UTI; 10% and 11%, respectively). The incidence of herpes virus infections, including herpes zoster, was similar in both treatment groups. Serious infections were reported in 4% of patients in the DAC HYP group and in 2% of the IFNβ group, including UTI, cellulitis, appendicitis, pneumonia, and viral infection. There were no reported cases of progressive multifocal leukoencephalopathy or infectious encephalitis.

Malignancies were found in seven DAC HYP patients and eight IFNβ patients, and no deaths related to treatment [6]. Cutaneous events occurred in 37% of DAC HYP patients and 19% of IFNβ patients, leading to treatment discontinuation in 5% and 1% of patients, respectively, as shown in Table 3. The most frequent cutaneous events were rash (7% in DAC HYP and 3% in IFNβ) and eczema (4% and 1%, respectively). Serious cutaneous events were observed in 2% of DAC HYP patients and <1% of IFNβ patients, and included dermatitis and angioedema. Hepatic events occurred in 16% of DAC HYP- and 14% of IFNβ-treated patients (serious events in 1% and <1%, respectively). Transaminase elevations >5× ULN occurred in 6% of DAC HYP and 3% of IFNβ patients. Elevations of transaminase levels were more common during the first year of IFNβ treatment, but were distributed evenly throughout DAC HYP treatment.

6.4. SELECTED

In SELECTED, the open-label DAC HYP extension study, SAEs (not including MS relapse) occurred in 16%. Discontinuation of treatment due to AEs including MS relapse occurred in 12% of patients, as shown in Table 2. The most common AEs (not including MS relapse) included nasopharyngitis and upper respiratory infection (both 12%). The most common SAEs (not including MS relapse) included elevated hepatic enzymes, ulcerative colitis, pneumonia, and UTI (<1% for each). Infections were observed in 50% of patients; 3% were considered serious. The infection incidence did not increase over time, and less than 1% of discontinuations were as a result of infection. Serious infections included UTI, pneumonia, and bronchitis. There were two reports of opportunistic infection—vulvovaginal candidiasis and pulmonary tuberculosis.

Malignancies were reported in four (1%) patients and included breast cancer, basal cell carcinoma, anal cancer, and a pulmonary carcinoid tumor. Investigators believed the anal cancer and pulmonary carcinoma cases were related to DAC HYP treatment, though there was no observed pattern in malignancies [66]. Cutaneous events occurred in 28% of patients, with the most frequent cutaneous AEs being rash (7%), allergic dermatitis (5%), and eczema (3%). Cutaneous events in 3% of patients led to treatment discontinuation as shown in Table 3. Serious cutaneous events occurred in 2% of patients: urticaria was reported in two patients; and Stevens–Johnson Syndrome (SJS) in one case, which was not validated by a dermatologist and did not meet standard SJS diagnostic criteria. Drug-related hepatic disorders were found in 15% of patients, only 1% of which were serious.

Gastrointestinal AEs were observed in 16% of patients, six (1%) of which were serious inflammatory gastrointestinal events, including ulcerative colitis (three patients), and colitis, Crohn's disease, and hemorrhagic enterocolitis (one patient each). Overall the safety profile in the SELECTED open-label extension was felt to be comparable to that observed in the SELECT trial, and the risks associated with DAC HYP did not appear to increase with longer durations of therapy [66].

7. Adverse Events: DAC HYP Post-Marketing

7.1. Cutaneous Events

A prospective open-label study evaluated the risk of development of cutaneous AEs over a 42-month period, as shown in Table 3 [67]. Twenty-three participants (77%) developed new or recurring cutaneous AEs. The majority of cutaneous eruptions presented with localized eczematous and in some cases progressive patches. All moderate to severe rashes (6/23) had psoriaform features, which persisted in later stages. Six patients developed mucosal lesions, the most common of which were recurring aphthous ulcers. Non-eczematous facial rashes included eyelid edema with erythema or diffuse facial erythema. Scalp involvement resembling seborrheic dermatitis was observed in six patients. Eight patients presented cyclic exacerbations of skin symptoms. Skin manifestations developed in most patients within the first 12 months of treatment, and commonly recurred two weeks after DAC HYP injection. There was no correlation between duration of DAC HYP treatment and rash development, and was not associated with MS disease course or with efficacy of DAC HYP therapy in suppressing CNS inflammation. However, a predisposing factor was a prior history of eczema or seborrheic dermatitis.

Biopsies from eight patients showed features of eczematous dermatitis, including scattered $CD25^+$ and T_{reg} $FOXP3^+$ cells. A consistent finding, most notable in moderate and severe rashes, was a robust population of $CD56^+$ cells, but the degree of $CD56^+$ infiltration did not correlate with the degree of expansion of this cell population in peripheral blood.

The cyclic pattern of eruptions and/or their temporal relationship to DAC HYP dosing in 8/31 patients (25.8%), including three patients with severe cutaneous AEs, led the authors to conclude that these events may be drug-related, and that by altering normal immune networks, DAC HYP could induce adverse cutaneous reactions resulting in the expansion of $CD56^+$ cells, the hallmark of DAC HYP-related skin inflammation. As previously noted, $CD56^{bright}$ NK cells are part of the ILC lineage, and ILC are strategically placed at pathogen entry locations such as skin and mucous membranes. Since DAC typically skews differentiation of common ILC precursors toward $CD56^{bright}$ NK cells, DAC-driven changes in ILC differentiation, while beneficial for CNS inflammatory disease, might in some patients lead paradoxically to enhanced skin reactivity. Because DAC prevents the expansion of T_{reg} cells, this may further contribute to heightened skin reactivity in affected patients [67]. Contrary to most of the literature on drug-induced cutaneous and systemic reactions, which has been attributed to the adaptive immune system, SAE to DAC HYP might suggest a larger role for $CD56^{bright}$ NK cells and the innate immune system in this process [68–70]. Further study in this area is warranted.

7.2. Drug Reaction with Eosinophilia and Systemic Symptoms (DRESS Syndrome)

The EMA reported on March 6, 2018 that four DAC HYP-treated patients developed exanthema/skin reactions with the involvement of other organs and eosinophilia, and five additional patients developed multi-organ failure that were possibly immune-mediated and later recognized as DRESS syndrome. DRESS is a life-threatening syndrome manifesting with cutaneous lesions and internal organ involvement; it has a 10% mortality rate. The time of onset of DRESS varies, typically from 2 and 12 weeks following drug exposure, though diagnosis may be missed or unnoticed due to its rare and varied presentation [71]. Typical features include eosinophilia, fever, extensive cutaneous lesions, atypical lymphocytosis, lymphadenopathy, hepatic injury, and renal failure. Lung, cardiac, and CNS involvement with meningitis and/or encephalitis may also occur, including brain edema, rhombencephalitis, and high cerebrospinal fluid (CSF) cell count [71,72]. Brain biopsy in one case contained demyelinating lesions showing conspicuous inflammation, and an abundance of T cells, plasma cells, eosinophils and eosinophilic/lymphocytic/plasma cellular meningitis, leading to a diagnosis of DAC-induced DRESS syndrome of the CNS. In marked contrast to typical DRESS syndrome, DAC-induced DRESS appears to occur principally within the CNS. Though CNS DRESS is exceptionally rare and usually presents with a pattern resembling vasculitis, it is likely that five of the patients with CNS complications in the EMA report had CNS DRESS syndrome [72]. Reduced IL-2 consumption due to DAC HYP blockade of IL-2R-HA may increase the opportunity for IL-2 to interact with ILC2 lineage cells, promoting IL-5 secretion and expansion of eosinophils, offering a potential pathway to CNS DRESS in rare cases [73].

7.3. Glial Fibrillary Acidic Protein (GFAP)-α Immunoglobulin (IgG)-Associated Encephalitis and Other Severe Encephalopathy Syndromes

Of the 12 patients with severe encephalopathy syndromes cited in the EMA report, one patient had CNS vasculitis, and several cases were reported as anti-N-methyl-D-aspartate (NMDA) receptor encephalitis. One patient was described who developed GFAP-α IgG-associated encephalitis [74]. This patient presented with behavioral and cognitive changes eight months after starting DAC HYP treatment. CSF contained oligoclonal bands and intrathecal immunoglobulin A (IgA) synthesis. Immunostaining showed GFAP-IgG antibodies in CSF. Although anti-GFAP-IgG may occur in isolation, it has also been in the setting of anti-NMDA receptor encephalitis or CNS vasculitis. Although one-third of cases with GFAP-IgG are paraneoplastic, malignancy was not found with this DAC HYP-treated patient.

As a consequence of these 12 cases of severe encephalopathy, four of which had a fatal outcome, DAC HYP was withdrawn from the market in February 2018. Although the precise mechanisms of these disorders are yet to be illuminated, it is reasonable to postulate that inhibition of T_{reg} cell expansion without an adequate concomitant expansion of immunoregulatory $CD56^{bright}$ NK cells or general immune suppression by depletion of activated effector $CD25^{+}$ T cells may have played a role. These latter cases suggest that redirecting IL-2 away from its high-affinity receptor may reduce activation and expansion of pro-inflammatory effector T cells, but in some cases does so at the expense of T_{reg} cells to such an extent that it may result in severe, paradoxical secondary autoimmune attack on multiple organs, including the CNS [74].

7.4. DAC: Is There a Future?

Although efficacious in controlled trials, the SAE leading to DAC withdrawal may preclude it from ever returning to clinical use. Even in a head-to-head trial against IFN-β, its therapeutic benefit was modest compared to more recently approved medications for the treatment of RMS [75–78]. At perhaps the simplest level, given the immunogenicity of the subcutaneous space, would intravenous administration of DAC have been preferable? Would this have reduced the likelihood of SAE?

The frequency of autoimmune cutaneous AE, and rarer but very serious autoimmune hepatitis and CNS events, including CNS DRESS and anti-NMDA encephalitis, reduce the likelihood of DAC returning as a therapeutic agent. Although SAE are also observed with other RMS medications, these can be prevented through the adoption of risk stratification strategies, such as detection and monitoring for John Cunningham virus infection in patients treated with natalizumab, exclusionary co-morbidities in patients receiving fingolimod or ocrelizumab, or frequent monitoring and early detection of side effects with use of alemtuzumab [79–82]. However, no risk stratification emerged for patients treated with DAC, with the possible exception of a prior history of hepatic disease, psoriasis, or eczema.

The time and expense of additional research to determine biomarkers for risk and efficacy are considerable barriers to pursuing the continued use of DAC. Despite these obstacles, the ability to modify disease activity in RMS, and possibly other autoimmune diseases, via innate immune system expansion should be recognized as a topic of potential scientific and therapeutic importance and thus justify further investigation into the development of biomarkers of risk or modified treatment protocols. If changes in immune cell parameters—the reduction in T_{reg} cell numbers, combined with the modest percentage decrease in $CD4^{+}$ and $CD8^{+}$ T cells and the expansion in $CD56^{bright}$ NK cells—resulting from DAC treatment contribute to autoimmune AE, this data could theoretically be used to develop an index table which might predict risk for developing secondary autoimmune AE. Data obtained from patients in already executed clinical trials and knowledge of their clinical outcomes could be used to develop such an index. However, the calculation of the risk index value in an individual patient would probably require treating them with DAC long enough to obtain steady state T_{reg}, $CD4^{+}/CD8^{+}$ T cell and $CD56^{bright}$ NK cell levels, which in of itself might place the patient at significant risk of an autoimmune AE. At a more complex and expensive level, transcriptomic and microRNA analyses of still stored serum samples from patients treated with DAC in past clinical trials could reveal valid predictive biomarkers for both efficacy and risk susceptibility.

The current standard of care for multiple sclerosis, at least as it pertains to disease process modifying drugs, relies upon adaptive immune system manipulation. This ranges from immune pathway alterations, immune cell expansion and maturation, reducing oxidative stress, immune cell sequestration and/or migration into the CNS, to outright antibody-directed lymphocyte and monocyte destruction. Unfortunately, the opportunity to expand therapeutic immune modulation into the potentially promising innate system arena has, at least for the present, been stymied by the SAE profile that accompanied DAC use in RMS. Targeting innate immune system expansion, without suppressing IL-2-dependent T_{reg} expansion through activation of IL-2R-IA directly via a CD122 agonist, might be employed as a strategy to expand the $CD56^{bright}$NK cell population. Nevertheless, at least for the present, we do not anticipate that the lessons learned from DAC will positively impact the process of future agent development, and instead may discourage attempts at further development of agents targeting innate immune modulation for RMS. Despite these challenges, developing additional strategies to promote innate immune system expansion should be employed in preclinical models of RMS, with the hope of developing novel therapeutic agents targeting innate immune pathways.

8. Conclusions

DAC HYP was efficacious for the treatment of RMS, demonstrating a reduction in relapse rate and disability progression, a reduction in MRI markers of disease activity, and an improvement in patient-reported outcome measures. DAC HYP may reduce autoimmune reactivity by obstructing IL-2 interaction with its high-affinity receptor on lymphoid cells, thus reducing activation and expansion of effector T cell-driven inflammation. However, most of the evidence to date would suggest that the impact of DAC on the innate immune system is largely responsible for its therapeutic efficacy. Unique to RMS therapeutic agents, DAC drives the innate immune system through the expansion of $CD56^{bright}$ NK cells, further reducing T cell-driven auto-reactivity in RMS. Both these actions appear to underlie DAC HYP efficacy in RMS. However, DAC significantly impairs T_{reg} cell expansion, and, possibly, activation-induced T cell apoptosis, both of which depend on IL-2 interacting with its high-affinity receptor on lymphoid lineage cells, and may largely explain the susceptibility of DAC HYP-treated patients to develop the severe secondary autoimmune disorders that resulted in its removal from clinical use in patients with RMS. Hopefully, this will not dissuade future research into the potential utility of innate immune system modulation in the treatment of autoimmune disorders.

Author Contributions: Writing—original draft preparation, S.L.C., E.B.L., M.C.R.; writing—review and editing, S.L.C., E.B.L., M.C.R., and S.N.L.; visualization, S.L.C., E.B.L., S.N.L.

References

1. Nussenblatt, R.B.; Fortin, E.; Schiffman, R.; Rizzo, L.; Smith, J.; Van Veldhuisen, P.; Sran, P.; Yaffe, A.; Goldman, C.K.; Waldmann, T.A.; et al. Treatment of noninfectious intermediate and posterior uveitis with the humanized anti-Tac mAb: A phase I/II clinical trial. *Proc. Natl. Acad. Sci. USA* **1999**, *96*, 7462–7466. [CrossRef] [PubMed]
2. Waldmann, T.A.; Goldman, C.K.; Bongiovanni, K.F.; Sharrow, S.O.; Davey, M.P.; Cease, K.B.; Greenberg, S.J.; Longo, D.L. Therapy of patients with human T-cell lymphotrophic virus I-induced adult T-cell leukemia with anti-Tac, a monoclonal antibody to the receptor for interleukin-2. *Blood* **1988**, *72*, 1805–1816. [PubMed]
3. Vincenti, F.; Kirkman, R.; Light, S.; Bumgardner, G.; Pescovitz, M.; Halloran, P.; Neylan, J.; Wilkinson, A.; Ekberg, H.; Gaston, R.; et al. Interleukin-2-receptor blockade with daclizumab to prevent acute rejection in renal transplantation. Daclizumab Triple Therapy Study Group. *N. Engl. J. Med.* **1998**, *338*, 161–165. [CrossRef] [PubMed]
4. Bumgardner, G.L.; Hardie, I.; Johnson, R.W.; Lin, A.; Nashan, B.; Pescovitz, M.D.; Ramos, E.; Vincenti, F. Phase III Daclizumab Study Group. Results of 3-year phase III clinical trials with daclizumab prophylaxis for prevention of acute rejection after renal transplantation. *Transplantation* **2001**, *72*, 839–845. [CrossRef] [PubMed]
5. Wynn, D.; Kaufman, M.; Montalban, X.; Vollmer, T.; Simon, J.; Elkins, J.; O'Neill, G.; Neyer, L.; Sheridan, J.; Wang, C.; et al. Daclizumab in active relapsing multiple sclerosis (CHOICE study): A phase 2, randomised, double-blind, placebo-controlled, add-on trial with interferon beta. *Lancet Neurol.* **2010**, *9*, 381–390. [CrossRef]
6. Kappos, L.; Wiendl, H.; Selmaj, K.; Arnold, D.L.; Havrdova, E.; Boyko, A.; Kaufman, M.; Rose, J.; Greenberg, S.; Sweetser, M.; et al. Daclizumab HYP versus Interferon Beta-1a in Relapsing Multiple Sclerosis. *N. Engl. J. Med.* **2015**, *373*, 1418–1428. [CrossRef] [PubMed]
7. Gold, R.; Giovannoni, G.; Selmaj, K.; Havrdova, E.; Montalban, X.; Radue, E.W.; Stefoski, D.; Robinson, R.; Riester, K.; Rana, J.; et al. Daclizumab high-yield process in relapsing-remitting multiple sclerosis (SELECT): A randomised, double-blind, placebo-controlled trial. *Lancet* **2013**, *381*, 2167–2175. [CrossRef]
8. Giovannoni, G.; Gold, R.; Selmaj, K.; Havrdova, E.; Montalban, X.; Radue, E.W.; Stefoski, D.; McNeill, M.; Amaravadi, L.; Sweetser, M.; et al. Daclizumab high-yield process in relapsing-remitting multiple sclerosis (SELECTION): A multicentre, randomised, double-blind extension trial. *Lancet Neurol.* **2014**, *13*, 472–481. [CrossRef]

9. Lenardo, M.J. Interleukin-2 programs mouse alpha beta T lymphocytes for apoptosis. *Nature* **1991**, *353*, 858–861. [CrossRef] [PubMed]
10. Baan, C.C.; Balk, A.H.; van Riemsdijk, I.C.; Vantrimpont, P.J.; Maat, A.P.; Niesters, H.G.; Zondervan, P.E.; van Gelder, T.; Weimar, W. Anti-CD25 monoclonal antibody therapy affects the death signals of graft-infiltrating cells after clinical heart transplantation. *Transplantation* **2003**, *75*, 1704–1710. [CrossRef] [PubMed]
11. Bielekova, B. Daclizumab therapy for multiple sclerosis. *Neurotherapeutics* **2013**, *10*, 55–67. [CrossRef] [PubMed]
12. Richter, G.H.; Mollweide, A.; Hanewinkel, K.; Zobywalski, C.; Burdach, S. CD25 blockade protects T cells from activation-induced cell death (AICD) via maintenance of TOSO expression. *Scand. J. Immunol.* **2009**, *70*, 206–215. [CrossRef] [PubMed]
13. Ku, C.C.; Murakami, M.; Sakamoto, A.; Kappler, J.; Marrack, P. Control of homeostasis of CD8+ memory T cells by opposing cytokines. *Science* **2000**, *288*, 675–678. [CrossRef] [PubMed]
14. Lenardo, M.; Chan, K.M.; Hornung, F.; McFarland, H.; Siegel, R.; Wang, J.; Zheng, L. Mature T lymphocyte apoptosis–immune regulation in a dynamic and unpredictable antigenic environment. *Annu. Rev. Immunol.* **1999**, *17*, 221–253. [CrossRef] [PubMed]
15. Li, X.C.; Demirci, G.; Ferrari-Lacraz, S.; Groves, C.; Coyle, A.; Malek, T.R.; Strom, T.B. IL-15 and IL-2: A matter of life and death for T cells in vivo. *Nat. Med.* **2001**, *7*, 114–118. [CrossRef] [PubMed]
16. Granucci, F.; Feau, S.; Angeli, V.; Trottein, F.; Ricciardi-Castagnoli, P. Early IL-2 production by mouse dendritic cells is the result of microbial-induced priming. *J. Immunol.* **2003**, *170*, 5075–5081. [CrossRef] [PubMed]
17. Malek, T.R. The biology of interleukin-2. *Annu. Rev. Immunol.* **2008**, *26*, 453–479. [CrossRef] [PubMed]
18. Waldmann, T.A. The multi-subunit interleukin-2 receptor. *Annu. Rev. Biochem.* **1989**, *58*, 875–911. [CrossRef] [PubMed]
19. Setoguchi, R.; Hori, S.; Takahashi, T.; Sakaguchi, S. Homeostatic maintenance of natural Foxp3(+) CD25(+) CD4(+) regulatory T cells by interleukin (IL)-2 and induction of autoimmune disease by IL-2 neutralization. *J. Exp. Med.* **2005**, *201*, 723–735. [CrossRef] [PubMed]
20. Wuest, S.C.; Edwan, J.H.; Martin, J.F.; Han, S.; Perry, J.S.; Cartagena, C.M.; Matsuura, E.; Maric, D.; Waldmann, T.A.; Bielekova, B. A role for interleukin-2 trans-presentation in dendritic cell-mediated T cell activation in humans, as revealed by daclizumab therapy. *Nat. Med.* **2011**, *17*, 604–609. [CrossRef] [PubMed]
21. Roessler, E.; Grant, A.; Ju, G.; Tsudo, M.; Sugamura, K.; Waldmann, T.A. Cooperative interactions between the interleukin 2 receptor alpha and beta chains alter the interleukin 2-binding affinity of the receptor subunits. *Proc. Natl. Acad. Sci. USA* **1994**, *91*, 3344–3347. [CrossRef] [PubMed]
22. Takeshita, T.; Asao, H.; Ohtani, K.; Ishii, N.; Kumaki, S.; Tanaka, N.; Munakata, H.; Nakamura, M.; Sugamura, K. Cloning of the gamma chain of the human IL-2 receptor. *Science* **1992**, *257*, 379–382. [CrossRef] [PubMed]
23. Gaffen, S.L. Signaling domains of the interleukin 2 receptor. *Cytokine* **2001**, *14*, 63–77. [CrossRef] [PubMed]
24. Duprez, V.; Cornet, V.; Dautry-Varsat, A. Down-regulation of high affinity interleukin 2 receptors in a human tumor T cell line. Interleukin 2 increases the rate of surface receptor decay. *J. Biol. Chem.* **1988**, *263*, 12860–12865. [PubMed]
25. Fujii, M.; Sugamura, K.; Nakai, S.; Tanaka, Y.; Tozawa, H.; Hinuma, Y. High- and low-affinity interleukin 2 receptors: Distinctive effects of monoclonal antibodies. *J. Immunol.* **1986**, *137*, 1552–1556. [PubMed]
26. Morelon, E.; Dautry-Varsat, A. Endocytosis of the common cytokine receptor gammac chain. Identification of sequences involved in internalization and degradation. *J. Biol. Chem.* **1998**, *273*, 22044–22051. [CrossRef] [PubMed]
27. Hemar, A.; Subtil, A.; Lieb, M.; Morelon, E.; Hellio, R.; Dautry-Varsat, A. Endocytosis of interleukin 2 receptors in human T lymphocytes: Distinct intracellular localization and fate of the receptor alpha, beta, and gamma chains. *J. Cell Biol.* **1995**, *129*, 55–64. [CrossRef] [PubMed]
28. Malek, T.R.; Yu, A.; Scibelli, P.; Lichtenheld, M.G.; Codias, E.K. Broad programming by IL-2 receptor signaling for extended growth to multiple cytokines and functional maturation of antigen-activated T cells. *J. Immunol.* **2001**, *166*, 1675–1683. [CrossRef] [PubMed]
29. Freud, A.G.; Becknell, B.; Roychowdhury, S.; Mao, H.C.; Ferketich, A.K.; Nuovo, G.J.; Hughes, T.L.; Marburger, T.B.; Sung, J.; Baiocchi, R.A.; et al. A human CD34(+) subset resides in lymph nodes and differentiates into CD56bright natural killer cells. *Immunity* **2005**, *22*, 295–304. [CrossRef] [PubMed]

30. Spits, H.; Cupedo, T. Innate lymphoid cells: Emerging insights in development, lineage relationships, and function. *Annu. Rev. Immunol.* **2012**, *30*, 647–675. [CrossRef] [PubMed]
31. Spits, H.; Di Santo, J.P. The expanding family of innate lymphoid cells: Regulators and effectors of immunity and tissue remodeling. *Nat. Immunol.* **2011**, *12*, 21–27. [CrossRef] [PubMed]
32. Artis, D.; Spits, H. The biology of innate lymphoid cells. *Nature* **2015**, *517*, 293–301. [CrossRef] [PubMed]
33. Huang, Q.; Seillet, C.; Belz, G.T. Shaping Innate Lymphoid Cell Diversity. *Front. Immunol.* **2017**, *8*, 1569. [CrossRef] [PubMed]
34. Bielekova, B.; Catalfamo, M.; Reichert-Scrivner, S.; Packer, A.; Cerna, M.; Waldmann, T.A.; McFarland, H.; Henkart, P.A.; Martin, R. Regulatory CD56(bright) natural killer cells mediate immunomodulatory effects of IL-2Ralpha-targeted therapy (daclizumab) in multiple sclerosis. *Proc. Natl. Acad. Sci. USA* **2006**, *103*, 5941–5946. [CrossRef] [PubMed]
35. Lin, Y.C.; Winokur, P.; Blake, A.; Wu, T.; Romm, E.; Bielekova, B. Daclizumab reverses intrathecal immune cell abnormalities in multiple sclerosis. *Ann. Clin. Transl. Neurol.* **2015**, *2*, 445–455. [CrossRef] [PubMed]
36. Perry, J.S.; Han, S.; Xu, Q.; Herman, M.L.; Kennedy, L.B.; Csako, G.; Bielekova, B. Inhibition of LTi cell development by CD25 blockade is associated with decreased intrathecal inflammation in multiple sclerosis. *Sci. Transl. Med.* **2012**, *4*, 145ra106. [CrossRef] [PubMed]
37. Martin, J.F.; Perry, J.S.; Jakhete, N.R.; Wang, X.; Bielekova, B. An IL-2 paradox: Blocking CD25 on T cells induces IL-2-driven activation of CD56(bright) NK cells. *J. Immunol.* **2010**, *185*, 1311–1320. [CrossRef] [PubMed]
38. Xu, W.; Fazekas, G.; Hara, H.; Tabira, T. Mechanism of natural killer (NK) cell regulatory role in experimental autoimmune encephalomyelitis. *J. Neuroimmunol.* **2005**, *163*, 24–30. [CrossRef] [PubMed]
39. Benczur, M.; Petranyl, G.G.; Palffy, G.; Varga, M.; Talas, M.; Kotsy, B.; Foldes, I.; Hollan, S.R. Dysfunction of natural killer cells in multiple sclerosis: A possible pathogenetic factor. *Clin. Exp. Immunol.* **1980**, *39*, 657–662. [PubMed]
40. Merrill, J.; Jondal, M.; Seeley, J.; Ullberg, M.; Siden, A. Decreased NK killing in patients with multiple sclerosis: An analysis on the level of the single effector cell in peripheral blood and cerebrospinal fluid in relation to the activity in the disease. *Clin. Exp. Immunol.* **1982**, *47*, 419–430. [PubMed]
41. Neighbour, P.A.; Grayzel, A.I.; Miller, A.E. Endogenous and interferon-augmented natural killer cell activity of human peripheral blood mononuclear cells in vitro. Studies of patients with multiple sclerosis, systemic lupus erythematosus or rheumatoid arthritis. *Clin. Exp. Immunol.* **1982**, *49*, 11–21. [PubMed]
42. Oger, J.; Kastrukoff, L.F.; Li, D.K.; Paty, D.W. Multiple sclerosis: In relapsing patients, immune functions vary with disease activity as assessed by MRI. *Neurology* **1988**, *38*, 1739–1744. [CrossRef] [PubMed]
43. Bielekova, B.; Howard, T.; Packer, A.N.; Richert, N.; Blevins, G.; Ohayon, J.; Waldmann, T.A.; McFarland, H.F.; Martin, R. Effect of anti-CD25 antibody daclizumab in the inhibition of inflammation and stabilization of disease progression in multiple sclerosis. *Arch. Neurol.* **2009**, *66*, 483–489. [CrossRef] [PubMed]
44. Elkins, J.; Sheridan, J.; Amaravadi, L.; Riester, K.; Selmaj, K.; Bielekova, B.; Parr, E.; Giovannoni, G. CD56(bright) natural killer cells and response to daclizumab HYP in relapsing-remitting MS. *Neurol. NeuroImmunol. Neuroinflamm.* **2015**, *2*, e65. [CrossRef] [PubMed]
45. Oh, U.; Blevins, G.; Griffith, C.; Richert, N.; Maric, D.; Lee, C.R.; McFarland, H.; Jacobson, S. Regulatory T cells are reduced during anti-CD25 antibody treatment of multiple sclerosis. *Arch. Neurol.* **2009**, *66*, 471–479. [CrossRef] [PubMed]
46. Huss, D.J.; Mehta, D.S.; Sharma, A.; You, X.; Riester, K.A.; Sheridan, J.P.; Amaravadi, L.S.; Elkins, J.S.; Fontenot, J.D. In vivo maintenance of human regulatory T cells during CD25 blockade. *J. Immunol.* **2015**, *194*, 84–92. [CrossRef] [PubMed]
47. Diao, L.; Hang, Y.; Othman, A.A.; Mehta, D.; Amaravadi, L.; Nestorov, I.; Tran, J.Q. Population PK-PD analyses of CD25 occupancy, CD56(bright) NK cell expansion, and regulatory T cell reduction by daclizumab HYP in subjects with multiple sclerosis. *Br. J. Clin. Pharmacol.* **2016**, *82*, 1333–1342. [CrossRef] [PubMed]
48. Rech, A.J.; Mick, R.; Martin, S.; Recio, A.; Aqui, N.A.; Powell, D.J., Jr.; Colligon, T.A.; Trosko, J.A.; Leinbach, L.I.; Pletcher, C.H.; et al. CD25 blockade depletes and selectively reprograms regulatory T cells in concert with immunotherapy in cancer patients. *Sci. Transl. Med.* **2012**, *4*, 134ra162. [CrossRef] [PubMed]
49. Roifman, C.M. Human IL-2 receptor alpha chain deficiency. *Pediatr. Res.* **2000**, *48*, 6–11. [CrossRef] [PubMed]

50. Sharfe, N.; Dadi, H.K.; Shahar, M.; Roifman, C.M. Human immune disorder arising from mutation of the alpha chain of the interleukin-2 receptor. *Proc. Natl. Acad. Sci. USA* **1997**, *94*, 3168–3171. [CrossRef] [PubMed]
51. Fehniger, T.A.; Bluman, E.M.; Porter, M.M.; Mrozek, E.; Cooper, M.A.; VanDeusen, J.B.; Frankel, S.R.; Stock, W.; Caligiuri, M.A. Potential mechanisms of human natural killer cell expansion in vivo during low-dose IL-2 therapy. *J. Clin. Investig.* **2000**, *106*, 117–124. [CrossRef] [PubMed]
52. Sheridan, J.P.; Zhang, Y.; Riester, K.; Tang, M.T.; Efros, L.; Shi, J.; Harris, J.; Vexler, V.; Elkins, J.S. Intermediate-affinity interleukin-2 receptor expression predicts CD56(bright) natural killer cell expansion after daclizumab treatment in the CHOICE study of patients with multiple sclerosis. *Mult. Scler.* **2011**, *17*, 1441–1448. [CrossRef] [PubMed]
53. Howell, O.W.; Reeves, C.A.; Nicholas, R.; Carassiti, D.; Radotra, B.; Gentleman, S.M.; Serafini, B.; Aloisi, F.; Roncaroli, F.; Magliozzi, R.; et al. Meningeal inflammation is widespread and linked to cortical pathology in multiple sclerosis. *Brain* **2011**, *134*, 2755–2771. [CrossRef] [PubMed]
54. Magliozzi, R.; Howell, O.; Vora, A.; Serafini, B.; Nicholas, R.; Puopolo, M.; Reynolds, R.; Aloisi, F. Meningeal B-cell follicles in secondary progressive multiple sclerosis associate with early onset of disease and severe cortical pathology. *Brain* **2007**, *130*, 1089–1104. [CrossRef] [PubMed]
55. Serafini, B.; Rosicarelli, B.; Magliozzi, R.; Stigliano, E.; Aloisi, F. Detection of ectopic B-cell follicles with germinal centers in the meninges of patients with secondary progressive multiple sclerosis. *Brain Pathol.* **2004**, *14*, 164–174. [CrossRef] [PubMed]
56. Gillard, G.O.; Saenz, S.A.; Huss, D.J.; Fontenot, J.D. Circulating innate lymphoid cells are unchanged in response to DAC HYP therapy. *J. NeuroImmunol.* **2016**, *294*, 41–45. [CrossRef] [PubMed]
57. Sawa, S.; Cherrier, M.; Lochner, M.; Satoh-Takayama, N.; Fehling, H.J.; Langa, F.; Di Santo, J.P.; Eberl, G. Lineage relationship analysis of RORgammat+ innate lymphoid cells. *Science* **2010**, *330*, 665–669. [CrossRef] [PubMed]
58. Mnasria, K.; Lagaraine, C.; Velge-Roussel, F.; Oueslati, R.; Lebranchu, Y.; Baron, C. Anti-CD25 antibodies affect cytokine synthesis pattern of human dendritic cells and decrease their ability to prime allogeneic CD4+ T cells. *J. Leukoc. Biol.* **2008**, *84*, 460–467. [CrossRef] [PubMed]
59. Othman, A.A.; Tran, J.Q.; Tang, M.T.; Dutta, S. Population pharmacokinetics of daclizumab high-yield process in healthy volunteers: Integrated analysis of intravenous and subcutaneous, single- and multiple-dose administration. *Clin. Pharm.* **2014**, *53*, 907–918. [CrossRef] [PubMed]
60. Tran, J.Q.; Othman, A.A.; Mikulskis, A.; Wolstencroft, P.; Elkins, J. Pharmacokinetics of daclizumab high-yield process with repeated administration of the clinical subcutaneous regimen in patients with relapsing-remitting multiple sclerosis. *Clin. Pharmacol.* **2016**, *8*, 9–13. [CrossRef] [PubMed]
61. Zhang, Y.; McClellan, M.; Efros, L.; Shi, D.; Bielekova, B.; Tang, M.T.; Vexler, V.; Sheridan, J.P. Daclizumab reduces CD25 levels on T cells through monocyte-mediated trogocytosis. *Mult. Scler.* **2014**, *20*, 156–164. [CrossRef] [PubMed]
62. Soelberg Sorensen, P. Safety concerns and risk management of multiple sclerosis therapies. *Acta Neurol. Scand.* **2017**, *136*, 168–186. [CrossRef] [PubMed]
63. Bielekova, B.; Richert, N.; Howard, T.; Blevins, G.; Markovic-Plese, S.; McCartin, J.; Frank, J.A.; Wurfel, J.; Ohayon, J.; Waldmann, T.A.; et al. Humanized anti-CD25 (daclizumab) inhibits disease activity in multiple sclerosis patients failing to respond to interferon beta. *Proc. Natl. Acad. Sci. USA* **2004**, *101*, 8705–8708. [CrossRef] [PubMed]
64. Rose, J.W.; Burns, J.B.; Bjorklund, J.; Klein, J.; Watt, H.E.; Carlson, N.G. Daclizumab phase II trial in relapsing and remitting multiple sclerosis: MRI and clinical results. *Neurology* **2007**, *69*, 785–789. [CrossRef] [PubMed]
65. Benedict, R.H.; Cohan, S.; Lynch, S.G.; Riester, K.; Wang, P.; Castro-Borrero, W.; Elkins, J.; Sabatella, G. Improved cognitive outcomes in patients with relapsing-remitting multiple sclerosis treated with daclizumab beta: Results from the DECIDE study. *Mult. Scler.* **2018**, *24*, 795–804. [CrossRef] [PubMed]
66. Gold, R.; Radue, E.W.; Giovannoni, G.; Selmaj, K.; Havrdova, E.; Stefoski, D.; Sprenger, T.; Montalban, X.; Cohan, S.; Umans, K.; et al. Safety and efficacy of daclizumab in relapsing-remitting multiple sclerosis: 3-year results from the SELECTED open-label extension study. *BMC Neurol.* **2016**, *16*, 117. [CrossRef] [PubMed]
67. Cortese, I.; Ohayon, J.; Fenton, K.; Lee, C.C.; Raffeld, M.; Cowen, E.W.; DiGiovanna, J.J.; Bielekova, B. Cutaneous adverse events in multiple sclerosis patients treated with daclizumab. *Neurology* **2016**, *86*, 847–855. [CrossRef] [PubMed]

68. Zawodniak, A.; Lochmatter, P.; Yerly, D.; Kawabata, T.; Lerch, M.; Yawalkar, N.; Pichler, W.J. In vitro detection of cytotoxic T and NK cells in peripheral blood of patients with various drug-induced skin diseases. *Allergy* **2010**, *65*, 376–384. [CrossRef] [PubMed]
69. Porebski, G. In Vitro Assays in Severe Cutaneous Adverse Drug Reactions: Are They Still Research Tools or Diagnostic Tests Already? *Int. J. Mol. Sci.* **2017**, *18*, 1737. [CrossRef] [PubMed]
70. Peter, J.G.; Lehloenya, R.; Dlamini, S.; Risma, K.; White, K.D.; Konvinse, K.C.; Phillips, E.J. Severe Delayed Cutaneous and Systemic Reactions to Drugs: A Global Perspective on the Science and Art of Current Practice. *J. Allergy Clin. Immunol. Pract.* **2017**, *5*, 547–563. [CrossRef]
71. Scheibe, F.; Metz, I.; Radbruch, H.; Siebert, E.; Wolf, S.; Kohnlein, M.; Harms, L.; Meisel, A. Drug reaction with eosinophilia and systemic symptoms after daclizumab therapy in MS. *Neurol. NeuroImmunol. Neuroinflamm.* **2018**, *5*, e479. [CrossRef] [PubMed]
72. Avasarala, J. DRESS Syndrome and Daclizumab Failure-Were Potentially Dangerous Signs Missed in Clinical Trials? *Drug Target. Insights* **2018**, *12*, 1177392818785136. [CrossRef] [PubMed]
73. Van Gool, F.; Molofsky, A.B.; Morar, M.M.; Rosenzwajg, M.; Liang, H.E.; Klatzmann, D.; Locksley, R.M.; Bluestone, J.A. Interleukin-5-producing group 2 innate lymphoid cells control eosinophilia induced by interleukin-2 therapy. *Blood* **2014**, *124*, 3572–3576. [CrossRef] [PubMed]
74. Luessi, F.; Engel, S.; Spreer, A.; Bittner, S.; Zipp, F. GFAPalpha IgG-associated encephalitis upon daclizumab treatment of MS. *Neurol. NeuroImmunol. Neuroinflamm.* **2018**, *5*, e481. [CrossRef] [PubMed]
75. Polman, C.H.; O'Connor, P.W.; Havrdova, E.; Hutchinson, M.; Kappos, L.; Miller, D.H.; Phillips, J.T.; Lublin, F.D.; Giovannoni, G.; Wajgt, A.; et al. A Randomized, Placebo-Controlled Trial of Natalizumab for Relapsing Multiple Sclerosis. *N. Engl. J. Med.* **2006**, *354*, 899–910. [CrossRef] [PubMed]
76. Kappos, L.; Li, D.; Calabresi, P.A.; O'Connor, P.; Bar-Or, A.; Barkhof, F.; Yin, M.; Leppert, D.; Glanzman, R.; Tinbergen, J.; et al. Ocrelizumab in relapsing-remitting multiple sclerosis: A phase 2, randomised, placebo-controlled, multicentre trial. *Lancet* **2011**, *378*, 1779–1787. [CrossRef]
77. Alemtuzumab vs. Interferon Beta-1a in Early Multiple Sclerosis. *N. Engl. J. Med.* **2008**, *359*, 1786–1801. [CrossRef]
78. Kappos, L.; Radue, E.-W.; O'Connor, P.; Polman, C.; Hohlfeld, R.; Calabresi, P.; Selmaj, K.; Agoropoulou, C.; Leyk, M.; Zhang-Auberson, L.; et al. A Placebo-Controlled Trial of Oral Fingolimod in Relapsing Multiple Sclerosis. *N. Engl. J. Med.* **2010**, *362*, 387–401. [CrossRef] [PubMed]
79. Kappos, L.; Bates, D.; Hartung, H.P.; Havrdova, E.; Miller, D.; Polman, C.H.; Ravnborg, M.; Hauser, S.L.; Rudick, R.A.; Weiner, H.L.; et al. Natalizumab treatment for multiple sclerosis: Recommendations for patient selection and monitoring. *Lancet Neurol.* **2007**, *6*, 431–441. [CrossRef]
80. Ayzenberg, I.; Hoepner, R.; Kleiter, I. Fingolimod for multiple sclerosis and emerging indications: Appropriate patient selection, safety precautions, and special considerations. *Ther. Clin. Risk Manag.* **2016**, *12*, 261–272. [CrossRef] [PubMed]
81. Cossburn, M.; Pace, A.A.; Jones, J.; Ali, R.; Ingram, G.; Baker, K.; Hirst, C.; Zajicek, J.; Scolding, N.; Boggild, M.; et al. Autoimmune disease after alemtuzumab treatment for multiple sclerosis in a multicenter cohort. *Neurology* **2011**, *77*, 573–579. [CrossRef]
82. Montalban, X.; Hauser, S.L.; Kappos, L.; Arnold, D.L.; Bar-Or, A.; Comi, G.; de Seze, J.; Giovannoni, G.; Hartung, H.P.; Hemmer, B.; et al. Ocrelizumab versus Placebo in Primary Progressive Multiple Sclerosis. *N. Engl. J. Med.* **2017**, *376*, 209–220. [CrossRef] [PubMed]

15

Therapeutic Plasma Exchange in Multiple Sclerosis and Autoimmune Encephalitis: A Comparative Study of Indication, Efficacy, and Safety

Tobias Moser [1], Gayane Harutyunyan [1], Anush Karamyan [1], Ferdinand Otto [1], Carola Bacher [1], Vaclav Chroust [1], Markus Leitinger [1], Helmut F. Novak [1], Eugen Trinka [1] and Johann Sellner [1,2,3,*]

1 Department of Neurology, Christian Doppler Medical Center, Paracelsus Medical University, 5020 Salzburg, Austria; t.moser@salk.at (T.M.); gayane.harutyunyan@stud.pmu.ac.at (G.H.); anush.karamyan@stud.pmu.ac.at (A.K.); f.otto@salk.at (F.O.); ca.bacher@salk.at (C.B.); info@neurologie-chroust.at (V.C.); ma.leitinger@salk.at (M.L.); h.novak@salk.at (H.F.N.); e.trinka@salk.at (E.T.)

2 Department of Neurology, Klinikum rechts der Isar, Technische Universität München, 81675 München, Germany

3 Department of Neurology, Landesklinikum Mistelbach-Gänserndorf, 2130 Mistelbach, Austria

* Correspondence: j.sellner@salk.at;

Abstract: Therapeutic plasma exchange (TPE) is a well-established method of treatment for steroid-refractory relapses in multiple sclerosis (MS) and neuromyelitis optica spectrum disorders (NMOSD). Little is known about indications and clinical responses to TPE in autoimmune encephalitis and other immune-mediated disorders of the central nervous system (CNS). We performed a retrospective chart review of patients with immune-mediated disorders of the CNS undergoing TPE at our tertiary care center between 2003 and 2015. The response to TPE within a 3- to 6-month follow-up was scored with an established rating system. We identified 40 patients including 21 patients with multiple sclerosis (MS, 52.5%), 12 with autoimmune encephalitis (AE, 30%), and 7 with other immune-mediated CNS disorders (17.5%). Among patients with AE, eight patients had definite AE (Immunolobulin G for N-methyl-D-aspartate receptor $n = 4$, Leucine-rich, glioma inactivated 1 $n = 2$, Ma 2 $n = 1$, and Alpha-amino-3-hydroxy-5-methyl-4-isoxazolepropionic Acid $n = 1$). Intravenous immunoglobulins had been given prior to TPE in all but one patient with AE, and indications were dominated by acute psychosis and epileptic seizures. While TPE has a distinct place in the treatment sequence of different immune-mediated CNS disorders, we found consistent efficacy and safety. Further research should be directed toward alternative management strategies in non-responders.

Keywords: multiple sclerosis; autoimmune encephalitis; plasma exchange; autoimmunity; immunotherapeutics; clinical outcomes

---

1. Introduction

Apheresis therapies separate patients' plasma from the whole blood by using centrifugation devices or highly permeable filters. In this regard, therapeutic plasma exchange (TPE) aims to eliminate pathogenic antibodies and other proinflammatory mediators from the patient's circulation. This procedure is an established treatment for steroid-refractory relapses in multiple sclerosis (MS) [1]. Several studies corroborated its efficacy in about 66%–86% of patients undergoing TPE, after conventional high-dose glucocorticoid (GC) treatment had failed [2–4]. The rationale for treatment of acute and recurrent attacks in neuromyelitis optica spectrum disorders (NMOSD) is based upon evidence that humoral autoimmunity plays a key role in the pathogenesis. Of note, the interest to achieve rapid remission in NMOSD is driven by the high attack-related disability and -mortality [5]. Therefore, a more aggressive treatment concept based on immunosuppression, pulsed immunotherapy, or targeted disruption of the immunological cascade leading to neuroaxonal injury is maintained in NMOSD in order to preserve long-term neurological function [6].

The spectrum of immune-mediated disorders of the CNS widened over the recent decade. There is emerging evidence that GCs are less effective in B-cell-mediated diseases, including autoimmune encephalitis, and TPE is likely to be effective from a pathophysiological viewpoint in the treatment of antibody-mediated immune processes [7,8]. Autoimmune encephalitis (AE) is a clinical challenge, since presentation is unspecific, and therefore diagnostic consideration is often delayed. Moreover, some patients require treatment at the intensive care unit (ICU), and outcomes can be devastating [9]. Notably, due to the relatively recent discovery of anti-neuronal antibodies and the rarity of AE, treatment recommendations are based on retrospective reports and expert opinion. In a study of 30 patients with AE, 67% improved with TPE by at least 1 point in the modified ranking scale (mRS) [10]. There are, however, two other components of treatment of AE [11]. These include intravenous immunoglobulins (IVIG) and tumor removal. Of note, the ideal sequence for GC, IVIG, and TPE has not been established yet. In addition, there is emerging evidence for the efficacy of rituximab, a CD20 depleting antibody, for achieving long-term remission [12]. Moreover, TPE is not without risks and should only be carried out in conditions where there is good evidence of its effectiveness. Side-effects include disturbances of coagulation, vasovagal episodes, fluid overload or under-replacement, and allergic or anaphylactic reactions due to plasma infusion [13]. Immunoadsorption (IA) is a selective technique for the removal of autoantibodies and immune complexes with less adverse effects in contrast to TPE, which is a non-selective extracorporeal blood purification process with elimination of plasma and subsequent substitution. Recent studies have shown that IA is not only effective in GC-unresponsive MS relapses but also in exacerbations related to NMOSD [14,15].

Here, we hypothesized that TPE is effective in autoimmune encephalitis and therefore studied indication, efficacy, and safety in comparison with MS and other immune-mediated disorders of the CNS.

2. Materials and Methods

2.1. Study Design

We performed a retrospective chart review of all patients with immune-mediated disorders of the CNS who underwent TPE at the 9-bed neurological intensive care unit (NICU) of a tertiary university hospital (Christian Doppler Medical Center, Paracelsus Medical University, Salzburg, Austria). The study protocol was reviewed and approved by the local Ethics Committee (Ethikkommission für das Bundesland Salzburg; 415-EP/73/534-2015).

2.2. Study Population and Data Collection

We reviewed the electronic records for demographic data, neurological diagnosis, symptoms, complications, number of TPE cycles, and outcome and included patients according to the following inclusion criteria:

- acute immune-mediated disorder of the CNS
- TPE during the period of January 2003 to December 2015
- sufficient clinical documentation on underlying disease, indication, procedures, and complications

Multiple sclerosis was diagnosed according to the McDonald's criteria revised in 2010 [16]. For AE, we followed the diagnostic criteria set up by Graus and coworkers [4]. Briefly, diagnosis can be made when all three of the following criteria have been met:

- subacute onset (rapid progression of less than three months) of working memory deficits (short-term memory loss), altered mental status, or psychiatric symptoms

- at least one of the following: new focal CNS findings, seizures not explained by a previously known seizure disorder, CSF pleocytosis (white blood cell count of more than five cells per μL), MRI features suggestive of encephalitis

The cohort of patients with "other immune-mediated CNS disorders" comprised acute disseminated encephalomyelitis (ADEM), CNS lupus, optic neuritis not related to MS, and NMOSD. MS patients with progressive multifocal leukoencephalopathy (PML, $n = 3$) who received TPE for elimination of natalizumab were excluded. Three patients with AE were excluded for lack of sufficient follow-up (Figure 1).

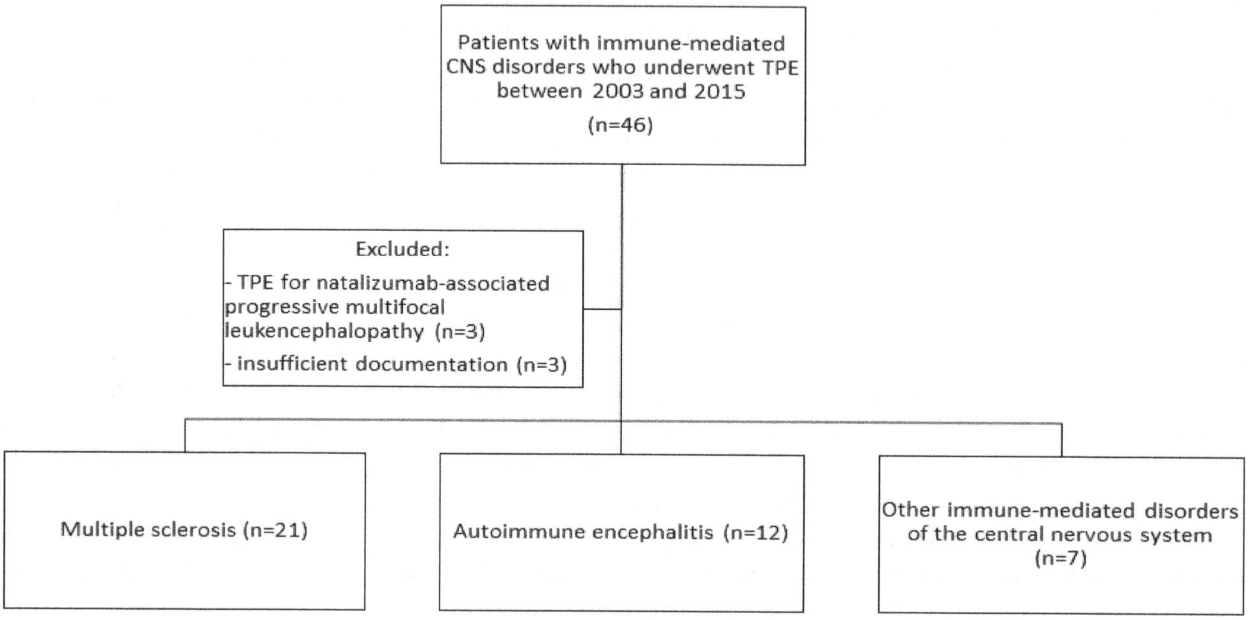

Figure 1. Flow chart for patient selection.

TPE was performed by experienced neurointensivists via a central venous access catheter. The clinical response to TPE was rated with a scoring system introduced by Magaña et al. [6,17,18], which proposes three different response categories; these were no, mild, and good improvement. Patients in the first group showed no recovery at all or even deterioration of symptoms. Mild recovery was defined as "improvement in neurological status without impacting function". Individuals with functionally relevant neurological recovery were considered to have a good improvement. We studied the outcome within six months from TPE. If patients were not seen regularly on follow-up at our center, we contacted individual patients or their caregivers to collect information on their recovery.

2.3. Statistical Analysis

All statistical analyses were conducted using IBM SPSS Version 21.0 (SPSS, Chicago, IL, USA). Descriptive statistics for clinical, demographic, and outcome data are provided. We report the median (interquartile range, IQR) for continuous variables and frequency (percent) for categorical variables. Intergroup comparisons were performed using Fisher's exact and Mann–Whitney U tests and one-way ANOVA where appropriate. All reported p-values were two-tailed and considered statistically significant at $p < 0.05$.

3. Results

3.1. Clinical and Demographic Characteristics

We identified a total of 40 patients with immune-mediated CNS disorders who underwent PLEX between 2003 and 2015. As shown in Figure 1, the most frequent condition was MS in 52.5% ($n = 21$), followed by AE in 30% ($n = 12$). The remaining disorders (summarized as "others" in the following) were CNS lupus ($n = 3$), optic neuritis (not otherwise specified, $n = 2$), ADEM ($n = 1$), and NMOSD ($n = 1$).

There was a general trend towards the increased utilization of TPE over time (Figure 2). Half ($n = 20$) of all patients received the treatment within the past four years, whereas in the period of 2003–2008, only eight patients were treated with TPE.

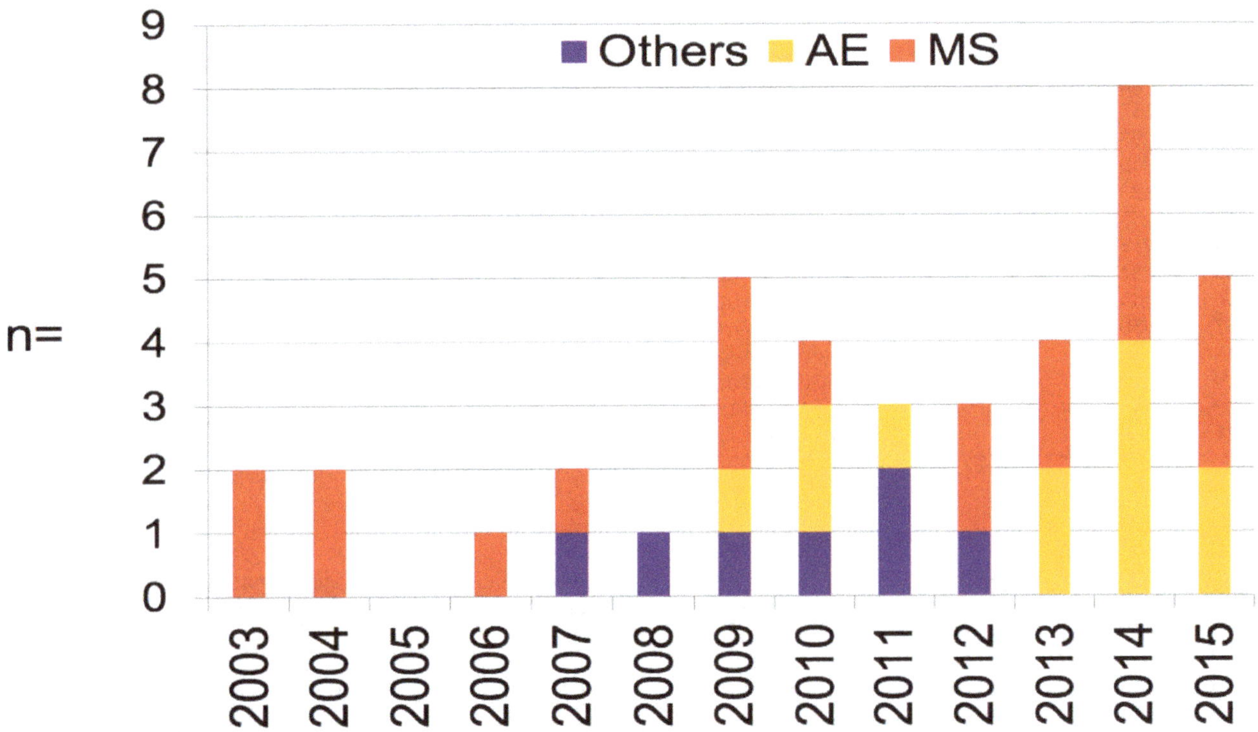

Figure 2. Time course of therapeutic plasma exchange (TPE) usage during the observation period.

The majority of patients were women ($n = 26$, 65%). In detail, women were more frequent in the MS group ($n = 15$, 71%), and the group of "other" immune-mediated CNS disorders comprised entirely women (100%). Of note, there were more male patients in the AE group ($n = 27$, 67%).

The mean age of patients with MS was 35.5 (standard deviation (SD) of 9.4). TPE was used in this group as second-line therapy except in one patient where steroids were contraindicated, as shown in Table 1. The most frequent indication was optic neuritis ($n = 9$), followed by pyramidal tract symptoms ($n = 6$). The mean number of TPE courses was 5.1 (range of 2–9). There were single patients with eight and nine TPE cycles, respectively.

Table 1. TPE in patients with multiple sclerosis.

No.	Age	Gender	Indication	GC Refractory	Courses of TPE	Clinical Response
1	42	M	GC contraindicated		5	good
2	37	F	optic neuritis	X	5	good
3	39	F	optic neuritis	X	5	good
4	44	F	optic neuritis	X	5	good
5	25	F	optic neuritis	X	5	mild
6	40	F	optic neuritis	X	5	mild
7	28	F	optic neuritis	X	5	mild
8	28	M	optic neuritis	X	5	mild
9	47	M	optic neuritis	X	5	no
10	33	F	optic neuritis	X	5	no
11	43	F	tetraparesis	X	2	good
12	23	M	tetraplegia	X	5	good
13	33	M	hemiparesis, dysarthria	X	5	good
14	17	M	hemiparesis	X	5	good
15	34	F	tetraparesis	X	5	mild
16	44	F	tetraplegia	X	8	no
17	50	M	tetrapresis, dysarthia, dysphagia	X	5	no
18	43	F	hemiparesis, ataxia	X	3	no
19	25	F	fulminant MRI, aphasia	X	5	good
20	29	F	fulminant MRI, natalizumab rebound	X	5	good
21	21	F	fulminant radiological findings	X	9	good

Legends: M, male; F, Female; MRI, magnetic resonance imaging; GC, glucocorticoid.

The mean age of patients with AE was 45.1 years (SD of 18.8), which was significantly higher than in MS ($p = 0.03$). The spectrum of clinical symptoms in patients with AE was broad, and the most frequent disturbances were psychiatric symptoms and epileptic seizures (Table 2). The average number of TPE cycles in patients with AE was 6.3 (SD of 2.7). Two patients had more than 10 cycles of TPE. In almost all patients, a prior treatment with intravenous immunoglobulins was performed. Some also received steroids prior to TPE. In the AE cohort ($n = 12$), eight (66%) patients had definite AE with positive antibodies (IgG for NMDA-R: $n = 4$, LGI1: $n = 2$, Ma 2: $n = 1$, and AMPA: $n = 1$). Six patients had inflammatory CSF and eight had pathologies on MRI. All except the patients with exclusively brainstem involvement developed neurocognitive signs, and seizures were common (60%). The four patients with anti-NMDAR-antibodies were women, two of whom had a histologically confirmed teratoma. All of the AE patients had additional treatments (surgery $n = 4$, steroids $n = 5$, IVIG $n = 11$, rituximab $n = 2$).

Table 2. TPE in patients with autoimmune encephalitis (AE).

n	Age	Gender	Details	Antibody	Memo	Epil	Psych	Move	Auto	Sleep	Pons	Detection of Lesion on MRI	CSF	Treatment	TPE Courses	Clinical Response
1	42	M	Paraneopl.AE	Ma1/Ma2	+	+	+			+		temporomesial	neg.	TPE/OP/Ritux	3	no
2	29	W	NMDAR-E	NMDAR		+	+	+				diffuse	IgG ↑	TPE/IVIG	10	good
3	26	W	NMDAR-E	NMDAR			+		+			none	33 cells	TPE/IVIG/OP	5	good
4	30	W	NMDAR-E	NMDAR		+	+					none	neg.	TPE/IVIG/OP	5	good
5	25	F	NMDAR-E	NMDAR		+	+	+				none	10 cells	TPE/IVIG/GC/OP	13	no
6	64	M	LE	LGI-1/VGKC	+	+	+					temporomesial	9 cells	TPE/IVIG/GC	5	mild
7	55	M	LE	none	+							temporomesial	21 cells	TPE/IVIG	5	mild
8	62	M	LE	AMPA-R1	+		+					temporomesial	16 cells	TPE/IVIG/Ritux	7	no
9	66	M	LE	LGI-1			+	+				none	neg.	TPE/ IVIG/ GC	4	good
10	24	F	probable LE	none		+	+			+		temperomesial	neg.	TPE/IVIG/GC	5	mild
11	71	M	Brainstem E	none							+	pons	neg.	TPE/IVIG	7	good
12	47	M	Brainstem E	none							+	pons	neg.	TPE/IVIG/GC	6	mild

Legends: LE: Limbic Encephalitis; NMDAR-E: NMDAR-Encephalitis; Brainstem E: Brainstem Encephalitis; memo: memory-deficit; epi: epileptic seizure; psych: psychiatric disorders; move: movement disorders; auto: autonomic dysfunction; sleep: sleep disturbance; pons: pontine signs; IVIG: intravenous immunoglobulins; GC: Glucocorticoids; OP: tumor surgery; Ritux: Rituximab.

The mean age of patients with other autoimmune CNS disorders was 50.7 years (SD 18.1). The mean number of TPE cycles was 5.7 (SD 2.1). Further details are presented in Table 3.

Table 3. TPE in patients with other immune-mediated disorders of the central nervous system (CNS).

No.	Age	Gender	Condition	TPE Courses (*n*)	Outcome
1	60	W	CNS-lupus	4	no
2	55	W	CNS-lupus	4	good
3	59	W	CNS-lupus	7	good
4	27	W	optic neuritis	5	good
5	47	W	optic neuritis	10	mild
6	78	W	NMOSD	5	no
7	29	W	ADEM	5	good

3.2. Time from Symptom Onset to Start of TPE

The time from relapse onset to the initiation of TPE was distinct among the three groups ($p = 0.03$). In detail, we calculated the median of 15 days (interquartile range (IQR) 10–27 days) for patients with MS, 77 days (24–203) for patients with AE, and 11 days (9–55) for patients with other immune-mediated disorders of the CNS.

3.3. Outcome

The overall rate of TPE responders was 75%. Further details are shown in Figure 3. A good or mild response was observed in 52.5% and 22.5% of the patients, respectively. The best outcome was observed within the "other CNS-ID" group, where 71% ($n = 5$) had a good recovery after PLEX, while only two patients showed no response (Table 3). The analysis of the MS and AE cohorts disclosed a functional improvement after plasma exchange treatment in 52% and 42%, respectively.

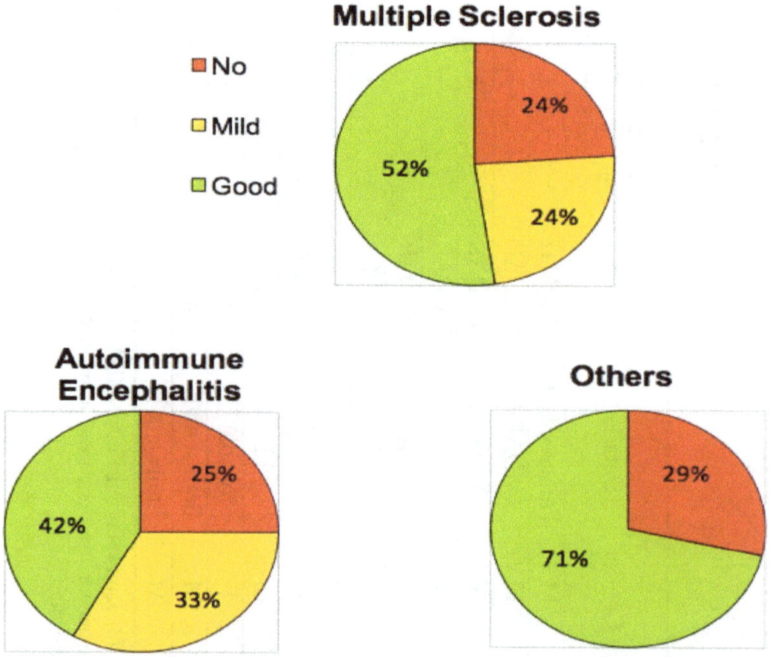

Figure 3. Clinical response to TPE across three subgroups of immune-mediated CNS disorders.

We also evaluated whether the period of symptom onset to the start of the TPE was distinct in patients with good response vs. mild/no response. In a pooled analysis of all three groups we did not find statistical differences (median of 16 days for the cohort with good response vs. 22 days for the cohort with mild or poor response).

3.4. Complications

In total, 219 TPEs were performed. Serious complications were found (1.8%): thrombosis of the subclavian vein, episode of bradycardia with transient loss of consciousness (one each), and two patients had impaired coagulation. No cases of death were reported.

4. Discussion

This study demonstrates that the majority of patients suffering from immune-mediated CNS disorders benefit from TPE, and the rate of non-responders is similar throughout the conditions. Moreover, the number of patients with AE treated with TPE is increasing over time, which reflects increased recognition of TPE as an effective treatment option. Of note, 50% of our patients with AE received TPE for intractable seizures and status epilepticus. Recent studies indicate that immune-mediated epilepsy such as in AE responds better to immunotherapies than to conventional epilepsy therapies [19]. Complications of TPE in our patient series was in the range of previously published studies in the real-life setting [3,20,21].

In our study, the rate of good recovery was higher in MS patients than in AE. This is could be related to the more complex pathogenesis and requirement of several lines of treatments for effective treatment of AE [10,22–24]. Thus, we cannot exclude the overlapping effects of prior treatment approaches. Among the patients with AE and no recovery after TPE, one suffered from a typical paraneoplastic syndrome with intracellular antibodies (MA1/2), which is to date believed to show no or limited response to TPE. In another patient with AE and poor response, the follow-up may have been too short. According to a study by Titulaer et al., almost half of the patients with NMDAR-encephalitis need a prolonged immune-suppressive treatment, and clinical improvement can be delayed [10]. Therefore, a delayed recovery cannot be excluded. Indeed, comparing two disorders with different pathogenesis is problematic. While AE may be monophasic, MS is mostly a relapsing-remitting disease. A B-cell-mediated pathogenesis is implicated in both AE and other CNS IDs, which backs the use of TPE, whereas this is the predominant process of acute inflammation in only a subset of MS patients [7,25]. Most importantly, time to TPE seems to be one of the most critical factors for observing an adequate treatment response [10,22,24]. Neurological involvement is relatively common in the majority of systemic autoimmune diseases and may lead to severe morbidity and mortality, if not treated promptly [26,27]. While our findings further support the use of TPE in neurological complications of systemic disease, our literature search revealed only a few case series for this indication [28,29]. Thus, prospective studies and establishment of registries are eagerly awaited. Open questions include the number of TPE cycles, definition of treatment goals and development of biomarkers. In addition, further studies should also elucidate the role of immunoadsorption as an alternative treatment option.

Moreover, the exact mechanism of action of TPE it is still incompletely understood. The removal of immunoglobulins seems to be a crucial factor. This process is likely to be followed by a shift from cerebral tissue towards systemic circulation [11]. TPE also modulates the immune system by changing the lymphocyte distribution, including changes in B and T cell numbers and activation, increased T suppressor function, and alteration in T-helper cell type 1/2 (Th1/Th2) ratio. In contrast, steroids alone often insufficiently resolve autoantibody-mediated pathologies [13]. A small retrospective review of 14 patients with NMDAR-encephalitis reports better outcomes in patients receiving TPE shortly after GCs than those with GC-treatment alone [12]. In our cohort, none of the 12 patients with AE were treated with TPE alone in the acute disease phase: 10 (83%) had additional IVIG and 6 (50%) had steroid treatment. Because adverse events are estimated to occur in about 6% of every single TPE procedure (the risk for the single individual is therefore multiplied by the number of exchanges), it was used as the ultima ratio treatment after failure of IVIG and/or GCs. Ehlers et al. studied a cohort of 37 GCS-unresponsive MS patients and reported a median time from symptom onset to begin of TPE of 44 days (range of 11–154) [30]. The median time in our MS cohort was 15 days, whereas 77 days had elapsed in patients with AE since the begin of clinical symptoms. This interval was even shorter for patient with other ID of the CNS (median 11 days). In the latter group were patients with known pathogenetic role of B-cells and humoral immunity including NMOSD and neurological manifestations of lupus. Moreover, due to this time lag, a delayed response to immunotherapies given prior to TPE is less likely. The long interval in AE is noteworthy and we assume that the approach for treatment escalation with TPE has changed over the recent years with knowledge about the key importance of an early TPE use in case of GCS-unresponsiveness and implementation in treatment guidelines [31]. In this regard, early initiation of TPE and lower patient age have been reported as predictors of a good response [22]. It also should be noted that none of our patients were treated with IA, which is an emerging treatment option in MS and CNS ID [2,15,32].

We report a low rate of adverse reactions. It should be noted that we exclusively used a central venous access which carries a significantly higher risk of complications than TPE via a peripheral line. In a recent study of complicated SLE and other autoimmune conditions (n = 66) using a central access device, the majority of complications were mild, with bleeding (25.8%) being the most common [28]. Electrolyte disturbances, hypotension, mild arrhythmia, and hypersensitivity were reported occasionally (6.1%, 9.1%, 3%, and 1.5%, respectively). Notably, 27.3% developed infections in the 14 days after TPE.

Improvement in function was achieved in 52.5% of all patients, which is in concert with TPE response rates found in literature ranging from 40% to 63%. Further subgroup analysis including analysis of predictors, however, could not be made due to the limited size of our cohort. Another limitation in this study is the retrospective character and the lack of a control-group.

5. Conclusions

Taken together we conclude that TPE shows similar response rates throughout different CNS IDs. Further studies should focus on the prediction of non-responders and development of alternative treatment strategies for these patients.

Author Contributions: Conceptualization, T.M. and J.S.; Data curation, G.H., A.K., F.O., C.B., M.L., V.C. and H.F.N.; Formal analysis, J.S.; Investigation, T.M. and J.S.; Methodology, T.M., G.H., Anush Karamyan and J.S.; Project administration, E.T. and J.S.; Resources, E.T. and J.S.; Writing—original draft, T.M. and J.S.; Writing—review & editing, G.H., A.K., F.O., C.B., M.L., V.C. and H.F.N.

Abbreviations

ADEM	Acute disseminated encephalomyelitis
AE	Autoimmune encephalitis
CNS-ID	Central nervous system-inflammatory disorders
GC	Glucocorticosteroids
IVIG	Intravenous immunoglobulins
LE	Limbic encephalitis
MS	Multiple sclerosis
NMDAR	N-methyl-D-aspartate-receptor encephalitis
NMOSD	Neuromyelitis optica spectrum disorder
NICU	Neurological intensive care unit
ON	Optic neuritis
TPE	Therapeutic plasma exchange

References

1. Mauch, E.; Zwanzger, J.; Hettich, R.; Fassbender, C.; Klingel, R.; Heigl, F. Immunoadsorption for steroid-unresponsive multiple sclerosis-relapses: clinical data of 14 patients. *Nervenarzt* **2011**, *82*, 1590–1595. [CrossRef] [PubMed]

2. Trebst, C.; Bronzlik, P.; Kielstein, J.T.; Schmidt, B.M.; Stangel, M. Immunoadsorption Therapy for Steroid-Unresponsive Relapses in Patients with Multiple Sclerosis. *Blood Purif.* **2012**, *33*, 1–6. [CrossRef] [PubMed]
3. Correia, I.; Sousa, L. Plasma exchange in severe acute relapses of multiple sclerosis—Results from a Portuguese cohort. *Mult. Scler. Relat. Disord.* **2018**, *19*, 148–152. [CrossRef] [PubMed]
4. Graus, F.; Titulaer, M.J.; Balu, R.; Benseler, S.; Bien, C.G.; Cellucci, T.; Cortese, I.; Dale, R.C.; Gelfand, J.M.; Geschwind, M.; et al. A clinical approach to diagnosis of autoimmune encephalitis. *Lancet Neurol.* **2016**, *15*, 391–404. [CrossRef]
5. Ehrlich, S.; Fassbender, C.M.; Blaes, C.; Finke, C.; Gunther, A.; Harms, L.; Hoffmann, F.; Jahner, K.; Klingel, R.; Kraft, A.; et al. Therapeutic apheresis for autoimmune encephalitis: A nationwide data collection. *Nervenarzt* **2013**, *84*, 498–507. [CrossRef]
6. Magana, S.M.; Keegan, B.M.; Weinshenker, B.G.; Erickson, B.J.; Pittock, S.J.; Lennon, V.A.; Rodriguez, M.; Thomsen, K.; Weigand, S.; Mandrekar, J.; et al. Beneficial plasma exchange response in central nervous system inflammatory demyelination. *Arch. Neurol.* **2011**, *68*, 870–878. [CrossRef]
7. Lindner, M.; Klotz, L.; Wiendl, H. Mechanisms underlying lesion development and lesion distribution in CNS autoimmunity. *J. Neurochem.* **2018**, *146*, 122–132. [CrossRef]
8. Rommer, P.S.; Milo, R.; Han, M.H.; Satyanarayan, S.; Sellner, J.; Hauer, L.; Illes, Z.; Warnke, C.; Laurent, S.; Weber, M.S.; et al. Immunological Aspects of Approved MS Therapeutics. *Front. Immunol.* **2019**, *10*, 207–220. [CrossRef]
9. Harutyunyan, G.; Hauer, L.; Dünser, M.W.; Karamyan, A.; Moser, T.; Pikija, S.; Leitinger, M.; Novak, H.F.; Trinka, E.; Sellner, J. Autoimmune Encephalitis at the Neurological Intensive Care Unit: Etiologies, Reasons for Admission and Survival. *Neurocrit. Care.* **2017**, *27*, 82–89. [CrossRef]
10. Titulaer, M.J.; McCracken, L.; Gabilondo, I.; Armangue, T.; Glaser, C.; Iizuka, T.; Honig, L.S.; Benseler, S.M.; Kawachi, I.; Martinez-Hernandez, E.; et al. Treatment and prognostic factors for long-term outcome in patients with anti-NMDA receptor encephalitis: an observational cohort study. *Lancet Neurol.* **2013**, *12*, 157–165. [CrossRef]
11. Reeves, H.M.; Winters, J.L. The mechanisms of action of plasma exchange. *Br. J. Haematol.* **2014**, *164*, 342–351. [CrossRef] [PubMed]
12. DeSena, A.D.; Noland, D.K.; Matevosyan, K.; King, K.; Phillips, L.; Qureshi, S.S.; Greenberg, B.M.; Graves, D. Intravenous methylprednisolone versus therapeutic plasma exchange for treatment of anti-n-methyl-d-aspartate receptor antibody encephalitis: A retrospective review. *J. Clin. Apher.* **2015**, *30*, 212–216. [CrossRef] [PubMed]
13. Norda, R.; Berséus, O.; Stegmayr, B. Adverse events and problems in therapeutic hemapheresis. A report from the Swedish registry. *Transfus. Apher. Sci.* **2001**, *25*, 33–41. [CrossRef]
14. Kleiter, I.; Gahlen, A.; Borisow, N.; Fischer, K.; Wernecke, K.D.; Hellwig, K.; Florence Pache, K.R.; Pache, F.; Ruprecht, K.; Havla, J.; et al. Apheresis therapies for NMOSD attacks: A retrospective study of 207 therapeutic interventions. *Neurol. Neuroimmunol. Neuroinflamm.* **2018**, *5*, e504. [CrossRef] [PubMed]
15. Lipphardt, M.; Mühlhausen, J.; Kitze, B.; Heigl, F.; Mauch, E.; Helms, H.-J.; Müller, G.A.; Koziolek, M.J. Immunoadsorption or plasma exchange in steroid-refractory multiple sclerosis and neuromyelitis optica. *J. Clin. Apher.* **2019**, *34*, 381–391. [CrossRef]
16. Thompson, A.J.; Banwell, B.L.; Barkhof, F.; Carroll, W.M.; Coetzee, T.; Comi, G.; Correale, J.; Fazekas, F.; Filippi, M.; Freedman, M.S.; et al. Diagnosis of multiple sclerosis: 2017 revisions of the McDonald criteria. *Lancet Neurol.* **2018**, *7*, 162–173. [CrossRef]
17. Weinshenker, B.G.; O'Brien, P.C.; Petterson, T.M.; Noseworthy, J.H.; Lucchinetti, C.F.; Dodick, D.W.; Pineda, A.A.; Stevens, L.N.; Rodriguez, M. A randomized trial of plasma exchange in acute central nervous system inflammatory demyelinating disease. *Ann. Neurol.* **1999**, *46*, 878–886. [CrossRef]
18. Keegan, M.; Pineda, A.A.; McClelland, R.L.; Darby, C.H.; Rodriguez, M.; Weinshenker, B.G. Plasma exchange for severe attacks of CNS demyelination: predictors of response. *Neurology* **2002**, *58*, 143–146. [CrossRef]
19. De Bruijn, M.A.A.M.; van Sonderen, A.; van Coevorden-Hameete, M.H.; Bastiaansen, A.E.M.; Schreurs, M.W.J.; Rouhl, R.P.W.; van Donselaar, C.A.; Majoie, M.H.J.M.; Neuteboom, V.O.R.C.I.D.P.F.; Smitt, P.A.E.S.; et al. Evaluation of seizure treatment in anti-LGI1, anti-NMDAR, and anti-GABA(B)R encephalitis. *Neurology* **2019**, *92*, e2185–e2196. [CrossRef]

20. Jiao, Y.; Cui, L.; Zhang, W.; Zhang, Y.; Wang, W.; Zhang, L.; Tang, W.; Jiao, J. Plasma Exchange for Neuromyelitis Optica Spectrum Disorders in Chinese Patients and Factors Predictive of Short-term Outcome. *Clin. Ther.* **2018**, *40*, 603–612. [CrossRef]
21. Manguinao, M.; Krysko, K.M.; Maddike, S.; Rutatangwa, A.; Francisco, C.; Hart, J.; Chong, J.; Graves, J.S.; Waubant, E. A retrospective cohort study of plasma exchange in central nervous system demyelinating events in children. *Mult. Scler. Relat. Disord.* **2019**, *35*, 50–54. [CrossRef] [PubMed]
22. Llufriu, S.; Castillo, J.; Blanco, Y.; Ramió-Torrentà, L.; Rio, J.; Valles, M.; Lozano, M.; Castellà, M.D.; Calabia, J.; Horga, A.; et al. Plasma exchange for acute attacks of CNS demyelination: Predictors of improvement at 6 months. *Neurology* **2009**, *73*, 949–953. [CrossRef] [PubMed]
23. Zhang, M.; Li, W.; Zhou, S.; Zhou, Y.; Yang, H.; Yu, L.; Wang, J.; Wang, Y.; Zhang, L. Clinical Features, Treatment, and Outcomes Among Chinese Children with Anti-methyl-D-aspartate Receptor (Anti-NMDAR) Encephalitis. *Front. Neurol.* **2019**, *10*, 596. [CrossRef] [PubMed]
24. Harutyunyan, G.; Hauer, L.; Dünser, M.W.; Moser, T.; Pikija, S.; Leitinger, M.; Novak, H.F.; Trinka, E.; Sellner, J. Risk Factors for Intensive Care Unit Admission in Patients with Autoimmune Encephalitis. *Front. Immunol.* **2017**, *28*, 835. [CrossRef] [PubMed]
25. Huda, S.; Whittam, D.; Bhojak, M.; Chamberlain, J.; Noonan, C.; Jacob, A. Neuromyelitis optica spectrum disorders. *Clin. Med.* **2019**, *19*, 169–176. [CrossRef]
26. Kivity, S.; Agmon-Levin, N.; Zandman-Goddard, G.; Chapman, J.; Shoenfeld, Y. Neuropsychiatric lupus: a mosaic of clinical presentations. *BMC Med.* **2015**, *13*, 43. [CrossRef]
27. Chessa, E.; Piga, M.; Floris, A.; Mathieu, A.; Cauli, A. Demyelinating syndrome in SLE: review of different disease subtypes and report of a case series. *Reumatismo* **2017**, *69*, 175–183. [CrossRef]
28. Aguirre-Valencia, D.; Naranjo-Escobar, J.; Posso-Osorio, I.; Macía-Mejía, M.C.; Nieto-Aristizábal, I.; Barrera, T.; Obando, M.A.; Tobón, G.J. Therapeutic Plasma Exchange as Management of Complicated Systemic Lupus Erythematosus and Other Autoimmune Diseases. *Autoimmune Dis.* **2019**, *2019*. [CrossRef]
29. Pons-Estel, G.J.; Salerni, G.E.; Serrano, R.M.; Gómez-Puerta, J.A.; Plasín, M.A.; Aldasoro, E.; Lozano, M.; Cid, J.; Cervera, R.; Espinosa, G. Therapeutic plasma exchange for the management of refractory systemic autoimmune diseases: Report of 31 cases and review of the literature. *Autoimmun. Rev.* **2011**, *10*, 679–684. [CrossRef]
30. Ehler, J.; Blechinger, S.; Rommer, P.S.; Koball, S.; Mitzner, S.; Hartung, H.-P.; Leutmezer, F.; Sauer, M.; Zettl, U.K. Treatment of the First Acute Relapse Following Therapeutic Plasma Exchange in Formerly Glucocorticosteroid-Unresponsive Multiple Sclerosis Patients—A Multicenter Study to Evaluate Glucocorticosteroid Responsiveness. *Int. J. Mol. Sci.* **2017**, *18*, 1749. [CrossRef]
31. Cortese, I.; Cornblath, D.R. Therapeutic plasma exchange in neurology: 2012. *J. Clin. Apher.* **2013**, *28*, 16–19. [CrossRef] [PubMed]
32. Faissner, S.; Nikolayczik, J.; Chan, A.; Hellwig, K.; Gold, R.; Yoon, M.-S.; Haghikia, A. Plasmapheresis and immunoadsorption in patients with steroid refractory multiple sclerosis relapses. *J. Neurol.* **2016**, *263*, 1092–1098. [CrossRef] [PubMed]

16

Streptococcus thermophilus ST285 Alters Pro-Inflammatory to Anti-Inflammatory Cytokine Secretion against Multiple Sclerosis Peptide in Mice

Narges Dargahi [1], John Matsoukas [2] and Vasso Apostolopoulos [1,*]

[1] Institute for Health and Sport, Victoria University, Melbourne VIC 3030, Australia; narges.dargahi@vu.edu.au

[2] NewDrug, Patras Science Park, 26500 Patras, Greece; imats1953@gmail.com

* Correspondence: vasso.apostolopoulos@vu.edu.au;

Abstract: Probiotic bacteria have beneficial effects to the development and maintenance of a healthy microflora that subsequently has health benefits to humans. Some of the health benefits attributed to probiotics have been noted to be via their immune modulatory properties suppressing inflammatory conditions. Hence, probiotics have become prominent in recent years of investigation with regard to their health benefits. As such, in the current study, we determined the effects of *Streptococcus thermophilus* to agonist $MBP_{83–99}$ peptide immunized mouse spleen cells. It was noted that *Streptococcus thermophilus* induced a significant increase in the expression of anti-inflammatory IL-4, IL-5, IL-10 cytokines, and decreased the secretion of pro-inflammatory IL-1β and IFN-γ. Regular consumption of *Streptococcus thermophilus* may therefore be beneficial in the management and treatment of autoimmune diseases such as multiple sclerosis.

Keywords: probiotics; *Streptococcus thermophilus*; ST285; $MBP_{83–99}$ peptide; mannan; immune modulation; multiple sclerosis; agonist peptide

---

1. Introduction

There is an increasing trend in immune-mediated disorders across the world that is believed to be in part, a result of intestinal dysbiosis. The imbalance in the intestinal ecosystem can lead to a dysfunctional immune system that consequently causes immune disorders including autoimmune diseases (multiple sclerosis, MS) and other inflammatory disorders [1,2]. Probiotics have long been implicated for the overall improvement of health and the management of a number of health conditions including infection, constipation, allergies, and autoimmune diseases, and are either consumed in the form of different fermented foods and dairy products or taken as capsules. In either case, there is strong evidence that suggests that the ingestion of probiotics can alter intestinal dysbiosis and relieve dysfunctionality complications, with subsequent improvements to health [3].

Probiotic bacteria have been evolved inside the human intestinal tract (GIT), and through this co-evolution, the gut and its microbiome have developed a symbiotic relationship that is of mutual benefit. While the GIT microflora relies on the gut's warm habitat and food content, in return, it not only provides numerous unique bioactive components such as vitamins B and K, minerals, short chain fatty acids (SCF), and miosins to the host, but it also assists in modulating the immune system [3]. In fact, probiotics are able to modulate monocytes, macrophages, B cells, T helper (h)1, Th2, Th17, regulatory T cells (Treg), natural killer (NK) cells, and dendritic cells (DC) [3–6].

Chronic inflammation is the pathophysiological condition involved in neuro-degenerative disorders including MS, Parkinson's disease, and Alzheimer's disease [7,8]. There is cross-talk between the gut microbiota and the central nervous system (CNS) [8–10], known as the gut–brain axis. An insufficient or imbalanced GIT microflora can also lead to dysfunctions in the gut–brain axis and the pathogenesis of a number of diseases inside the GIT (such as inflammatory bowel disease, IBD) and outside the GIT (such as the CNS). Experimental autoimmune encephalomyelitis (EAE) is an animal model of human MS that has been used to study the effects of probiotic bacteria on CNS [11,12]. One of the safe and appropriate ways to modulate T cells in MS is to orally administer specific autoantigens [13,14]. Administration of Bifidobacteria or Lactobacteria probiotic strains to mice has been shown to increase Treg cells and tumor growth factor (TGF)-β levels and reduce the severity of EAE clinical symptoms, in parallel with improvement in the regeneration of myelin in the spinal cord compared to the control [15,16]. Administration of both Bifidobacteria and Lactobacteria strains induce an additional significant delay in the onset of EAE and related clinical symptoms, together with a substantial reduction of mononuclear infiltration into the CNS, and increased level of Treg cells of the $CD4^+CD25^+Foxp3^+$ phenotype in mouse spleen and lymph nodes.

In SJL/J mice, immunization with the $MBP_{83\text{–}99}$ peptide mixed with mycobacterium stimulates autoimmune $CD4^+$ T cells in mice, and induces EAE [7,17]. Major histocompatibility complex (MHC) class II H-2^s haplotype in the SJL/J mouse strain resembles many clinical, histopathological, and immunological characteristics of human MS, thus the SJL/J mouse is regularly used for immunization studies. Different peptides are immunogenic in different mouse strains however, in the SJL/J mouse strain, the peptide $MBP_{81\text{–}100}$ binds to MHC class II H-2^s with high affinity with the minimum epitope being $MBP_{83\text{–}99}$ [7,17]. As such, the $MBP_{83\text{–}99}$ epitope has been used as an agonist peptide to immunize mice for the activation of $CD4^+$ T cells [7,17]. We have shown that injection of the $MBP_{83\text{-}99}$ peptide conjugated to the carrier mannan or mixed in complete Freund's adjuvant induces Th1 pro-inflammatory interferon-gamma (IFN γ-g) secreting $CD4^+$ T cells [18–25]. Studies have shown that there is a cross-reactivity between the MBP self-peptide and some microbial peptides (i.e., UL15, PMM) for Hy.1B11 T cell receptor (TCR), which has been isolated from a patient with MS. It has been highlighted that there are chemical interactions underlying the recognition mechanisms between TCR and the peptides presented by MHC proteins, as a critical constituent in adaptive immune responses to foreign antigens [26].

The Streptococcus genus constitutes over 100 species, amongst which *S. thermophilus* (ST) are non-pathogenic and food related bacteria that represent outstanding technological features in the food industry [27]. ST are commonly used as secondary starter cultures in dairy products to transform lactose into lactic acid and to acidify the pH of milk [27,28], contributing to both the fermentation and flavoring of dairy products [29]. Most probiotics belong to lactic acid bacteria (LAB); Gram-positive lactic acid producing bacteria that include lactobacilli, bifidobacterial, and enterococci [3]. As such, live LABs are not only used in foods for their health benefits, but exopolysaccharide-producing strains of ST such as ST1342, ST1275, and ST285 are generally used due to their beneficial properties (i.e., relieving lactose intolerance and suppressing acute conditions such as acute ulcerative colitis) [29]. Additionally, experimental studies designed to investigate the effect of VSL3 (Streptococcus, Bifidobacterium, and Lactobacillus species) on the peripheral immune system and the GIT microbiota in MS patients and healthy subjects showed improved abundance of many taxa with enriched taxa mainly consisting of Lactobacillus, Streptococcus, and Bifidobacterium. VSL3 also induced peripheral anti-inflammatory immune responses [30].

We recently showed that ST bacteria have anti-inflammatory properties [29]. U937 pro-monocytic cell line co-cultured with three ST bacteria (ST1342, ST1275 and ST285) induced an anti-inflammatory profile [29]. ST285 was further shown to have immune modulating effects via gene arrays to human peripheral blood mononuclear cells (PBMC) [31] and monocyte cells isolated from PBMC [32]. Herein, we immunized SJL/J mice with agonist $MBP_{83\text{–}99}$ peptide conjugated to mannan three times, isolated spleen cells, and after re-stimulation of spleen cells with the $MBP_{83\text{–}99}$ peptide, IFN-γ was secreted by spleen cells. Re-stimulation of spleen cells with the $MBP_{83\text{–}99}$ peptide in the presence of ST285 probiotics was able to downregulate IFN-γ responses and stimulate the Th2, IL-4, IL-5, and IL-10 cytokine profile. These studies show that probiotics are able to modulate and alter the immune profile of MBP_{83-99} specific cells to anti-inflammatory, which warrant in vivo EAE mouse experiments and hold promise as a therapeutic alternative approach to MS in human clinical trials.

2. Materials and Methods

2.1. Bacterial Strains

Pure bacterial cultures of *S. thermophilus* 285 (ST285) were obtained from the Victoria University culture collection (Werribee, Vic, Australia). Stock cultures were stored in cryobeads at −80 °C. Prior to each experiment, the cultures were propagated in M17 broth (Oxoid, Denmark) with 20 g/L lactose and incubated at 37 °C under aerobic conditions. Bacteria were also cultured on M17 agar (1.5% *w/v* agar) with 20 g/L lactose (Oxoid, Denmark) to assess the characteristics, morphology, purity, and Gram-positive confirmation [1].

2.2. Preparation of Live Bacterial Suspensions

Media were prepared and autoclaved at 121 °C for 15 min prior to the experiments. Bacterial cultures were grown three times in M17 broth with 20 g/L lactose at 37 °C aerobically for 18 h with a 1% inoculum transfer rate [33]. Cultures grow optimally at 37–42 °C for 24 h [29]. The growth period of cultures were consistent at 18 h (at the end of the exponential growth phase) and before the stationary growth phase to prevent cell lysis.

2.3. Enumeration of Bacterial Cells

For the actual experiment, bacteria were grown in broth media to the stationary phase at 37 °C aerobically, pelleted by centrifugation (6000× g) for 15 min at 4 °C, transferred, and resuspended in Dulbecco's phosphate-buffered saline, pH 7.4 (Invitrogen, Pty Ltd. Australia). The bacterial density in suspension was adjusted to 10^8 colony forming units (cfu)/mL for final concentration by determining the optical density at 600 nm, followed by two washes with Dulbecco's phosphate-buffered saline. These samples constituted the live-cell suspensions and were resuspended in the Roswell Park Memorial Institute (RPMI) 1640 culture media prior to co-culturing with spleen cells [1].

2.4. Mouse Experimental Procedures

2.4.1. Mice, Conjugates, and Immunization Schedule

Female SJL/J mice, aged 6–9 weeks, used in all experiments were purchased from the Animal Resources Center (ARC, Perth, Australia), and accommodated at the animal house (Victoria University, Werribee campus, Melbourne, Australia). All mice were ensured free access to water and food, and were housed in a temperature controlled room with a 12 h day 12 h night cycle. All immunizations were conducted according to the guidelines of the Australian Code of Practice for the Care and Use of Animals for Scientific Purposes and the study was approved by the Victoria University Animal Ethics Committee (AEC15/013) of Victoria University, Melbourne, Australia.

The MBP_{83-99} agonist peptide of over 99% purity with $(KG)_5$ at the C-terminus was conjugated to mannan via a method previously described [34–38]. Briefly, 14 mg of mannan (Sigma, VIC Australia) was oxidized in sodium carbonate buffer and 0.1 M sodium periodate at 4 °C after which ethylene glycol was added and incubated for 30 min at 4 °C. Oxidized mannan comprising aldehyde groups was passed through a PD-10 column (Sigma, VIC Australia) pre-equilibrated in carbonate-bicarbonate buffer pH 9.0 and 2 mL of oxidized mannan was collected and 1 mg of MBP_{83-99}-$(KG)_5$ peptide was added and allowed to react overnight at room temperature in the dark. The resultant MBP_{83-99}-$(KG)_5$-mannan conjugate was used to immunize the mice.

The MBP_{83-99} mannan peptide conjugate (50 μg/mouse) was injected in the SJL/J mice subcutaneously into the base of the tail, three times, every two weeks [17]. This conjugate has been shown to induce T cell proliferation and IFN-γ cytokine secretion to the agonist MBP_{83-99} peptide in SJL/J mice [17,19,23,24]. Ten to fourteen days after the three injections, spleen cells were isolated, red blood cells were lysed using 0.73% NH_4Cl, and counted.

2.4.2. Isolation of Spleen Cells and In Vitro Stimulation with ST285

Spleen cells were resuspended in RPMI 1640 media supplemented with 10% heat-inactivated fetal bovine serum (Invitrogen, Pty Ltd. Australia), 1% antibiotic-antimycotic solution, and 2 mM L-glutamine in T75 cm^2 cell culture flasks. Mouse spleen cells (1×10^7) in RPMI media only was used as the negative control, 5 µg/mL recall agonist MBP_{83-99} peptide was used as the recall control, or 1×10^8 ST285 bacteria were added together with the MBP_{83-99} peptide, and cultured at 37 °C, 5% CO_2 for 24 h [29]. We previously showed that 24 h co-culture was adequate for the stimulation of the monocyte/macrophage cell line, human peripheral blood mononuclear cells, and human monocytes isolated from peripheral blood mononuclear cells [29,32]. At the end of the culture period, cells were transferred into falcon tubes, and centrifuged for 5 min at 1200 rpm to pellet the cells. All cell-free supernatants were collected and frozen at −20 °C until cytokine analysis.

2.5. Cytokine Production Analysis

Cytokine secretion of the spleen cell culture supernatants was analyzed by commercially available capture and detection antibodies in a Bioplex multiplex bead assay for a panel of nine mouse cytokines and chemokines using a 9-plex kit (BioRad, Melbourne Australia) to measure Interleukin (IL)-1β, IL-2, IL-4, IL-5, IL-6, IL-10, GM-CSF, TNF-α, and IFN-γ. Cell-free supernatants were collected and the assay procedures were performed according to the manufacturer's instructions. Briefly, a flat bottom 96-well plate was coated with 1× coupled beads and washed twice, followed by adding the standard serial dilutions, blanks, and samples to assigned wells. Post incubation at shaking at room temperature, plates were washed twice, adequate 1× detection antibody was added, and incubated at room temperature. Plates were washed three times and 1× Streptavidin Phycoerythrin (SA-PE) stop solution was added to each well, followed by incubating at room temperature and washing. Data collection was repeated twice, data were expressed as the mean cytokine response minus background (pg/mL) of each treatment from three replicate wells, plus or minus the standard error of the mean.

2.6. Statistical Analysis

Significant differences between all treatment groups were tested by analysis of variance (ANOVA) using the Statistical Package for the Social Sciences for Windows 25.0 (SPSS; IBM Corp), followed by a comparison between treatments performed by Tukey's honest significance test/degree and Fisher's least significant difference method, with a level of significance defined as $p < 0.05$.

3. Results

3.1. ST285 Reduces Pro-Inflammatory TNF-α and IFN-γ Production by MBP_{83-99} Primed Mouse Splenocytes

Interferon gamma (IFN-γ) is a pro-inflammatory Th1 cytokine involved in macrophage activation and cellular immunity. IFN-γ promotes Th1 cells and inhibits Th2 anti-inflammatory cells. In MS, IFN-γ is induced following $CD4^+$ T cell activation by agonist peptide MBP_{83-99}. SJL/J mice immunized with MBP_{83-99}–mannan conjugates induced IFN-γ responses by spleen cells, following overnight MBP_{83-99} peptide re-stimulation (Figure 1A, $p < 0.01$). Spleen cells re-stimulated with the agonist MBP_{83-99} peptide in the presence of ST285 reduced IFN-γ cytokine secretion (Figure 1A, $p < 0.05$). TNF-α, a Th1 cytokine, was not secreted by spleen cells from immunized mice wither by re-stimulation of the MBP_{83-99} peptide or MBP_{83-99} peptide plus ST285 (Figure 1B).

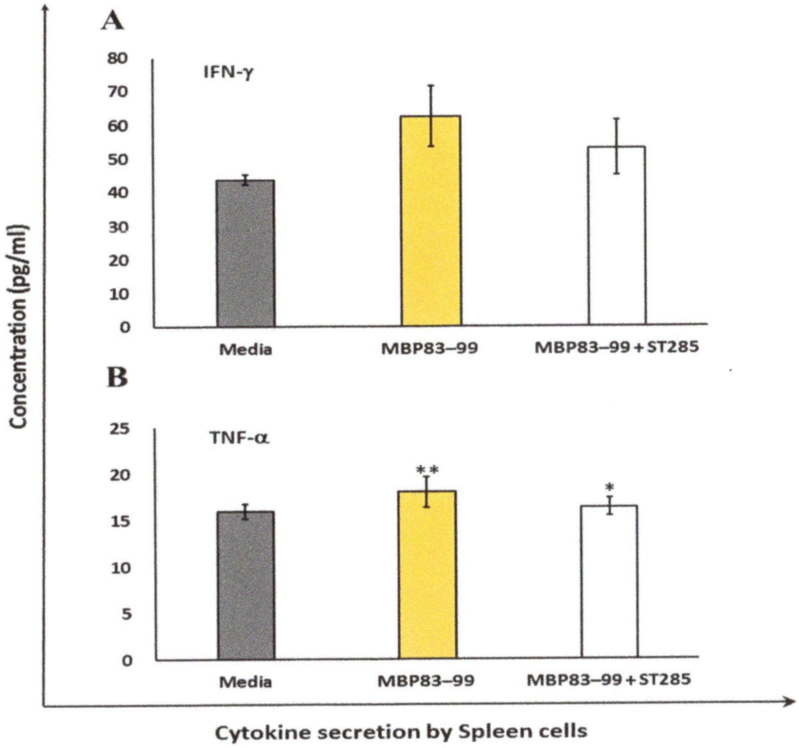

Figure 1. *S. thermophilus* 285 reduces pro-inflammatory cytokine production by mouse splenocytes. Spleen cells isolated from immunized mice ($n = 3$) were stimulated with *S. thermophilus* (ST) ST285 and recall agonist MBP_{83-99} peptide for 24 h and secretion of (**A**) IFN-γ and (**B**) TNF-α were measured. Recall MBP_{83-99} peptide was used as an internal positive control, and media refers to spleen cells from immunized mice ($n = 3$) without any additional recall peptide, or ST285 probiotic bacteria plus the MBP_{83-99} peptide. Means of two different readings of three replicate experiments were measured and analyzed. The means of readings for $n = 3$ mice were calculated and presented as plus or minus (±) the standard error of the mean. Symbols represent the p value for the Tukey test (one way ANOVA) where * $p < 0.05$ and ** $p < 0.01$.

3.2. ST285 Decreases Secretion of IL-1β, IL-2, and IL-6 by Mouse Spleen Cells

Secretion of IL-1β was slightly, but significantly reduced in immunized mouse spleen cells re-stimulated with the MBP_{83-99} peptide and ST285 compared to no re-stimulation, or the MBP_{83-99} peptide re-stimulation without ST285 ($p < 0.05$) (Figure 2A). IL-2 production was significantly increased in immunized spleen cells re-stimulated with the MBP_{83-99} peptide ($p < 0.01$), which was weakly but significantly decreased as a result of the co-stimulation of mouse spleen cells with the MBP_{83-99} peptide plus ST285 ($p < 0.05$) (Figure 2B). The production of IL-6 was profoundly increased by immunized mouse spleen cells upon co-culture of ST285 and the recall MBP_{83-99} peptide compared to the control media or MBP_{83-99} recall peptide ($p < 0.001$) (Figure 2C); spleen cells recalled with the MBP_{83-99} peptide alone also increased IL-6 secretion.

3.3. ST285 Induces Anti-Inflammatory Cytokine Profile by Mouse Splenocytes

Mice immunized with the MBP_{83-99} agonist peptide did not induce IL-4, IL-5, and IL-10 anti-inflammatory cytokines in the control (media alone) and recall agonist peptide MBP_{83-99} (Figure 3). However, the Th2 anti-inflammatory cytokine IL-4 was significantly ($p < 0.001$) increased by immunized mouse spleen cells when the MBP_{83-99} recall peptide was co-cultured with ST285 probiotic bacteria (Figure 3A). IL-5 was also increased by immunized spleen cells following co-culture with ST285 and the recall agonist MBP_{83-99} peptide (Figure 3B) ($p < 0.01$). The anti-inflammatory IL-10 cytokine was also significantly increased by immunized mouse spleen cells when co-cultured with ST285 and agonist recall $MBP_{83–99}$ peptide compared to the $MBP_{83–99}$ peptide alone or media control ($p < 0.001$) (Figure 3C).

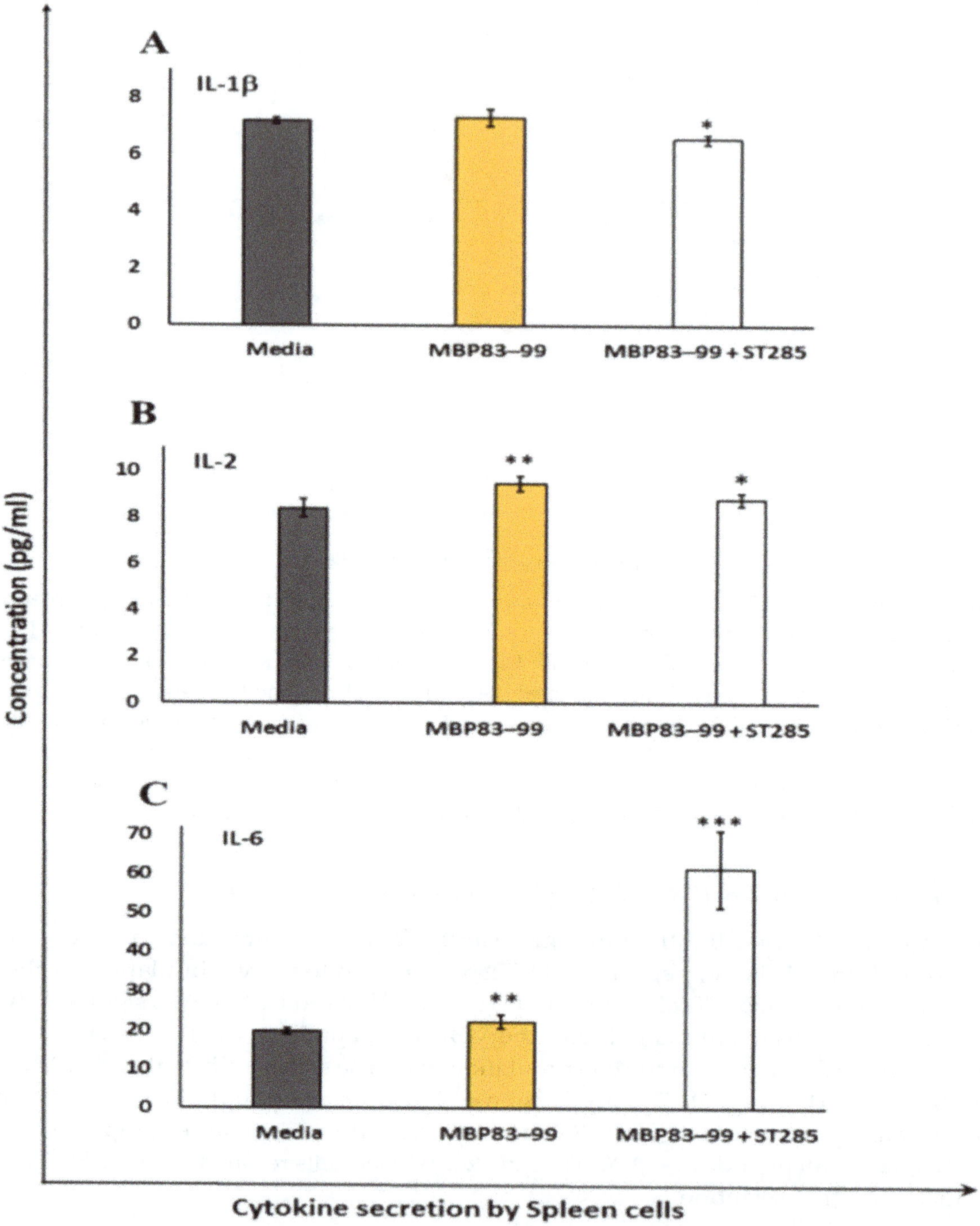

Figure 2. *S. thermophilus* 285 decreases expression of IL-1β, IL-2, and increases IL-6 by mouse spleen cells. Spleen cells isolated from immunized mice ($n = 3$) were stimulated with *S. thermophilus* (ST) ST285 and recall agonist $MBP_{83–99}$ peptide for 24 h and secretion of (**A**) IL-1β, (**B**) IL-2, and (**C**) IL-6 were measured. Recall $MBP_{83–99}$ peptide was used as the reference peptide, and media refers to spleen cells from immunized mice ($n = 3$) without any additional recall peptide or ST285 probiotic bacteria plus $MBP_{83–99}$ peptide. Means are shown as plus or minus (±) standard error of the means. Symbols represent the p value for the Tukey test (one way ANOVA) where * $p < 0.05$ and ** $p < 0.01$ and *** $p < 0.001$.

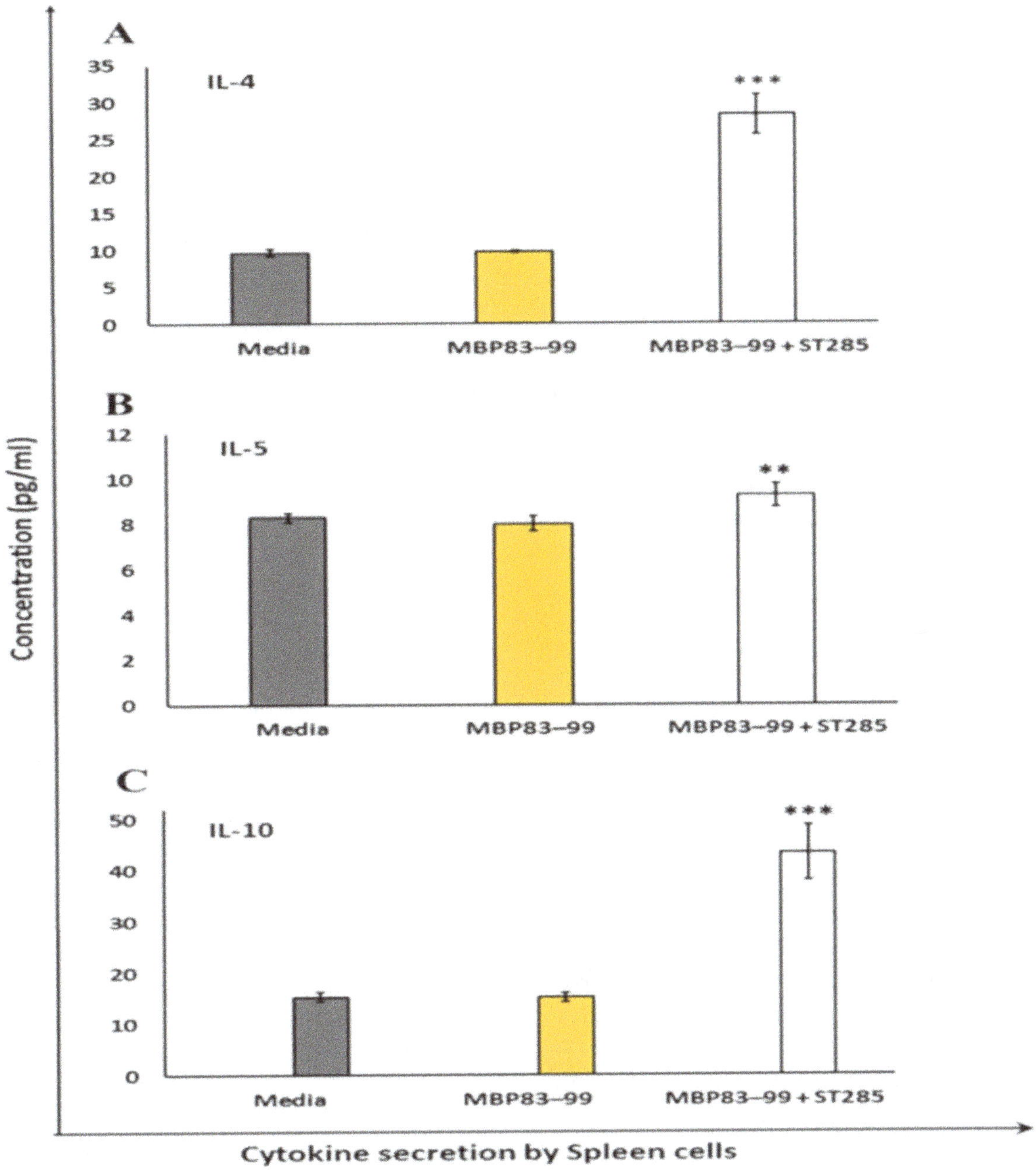

Figure 3. *S. thermophilus* 285 induces the anti-inflammatory cytokine profile by immunized mouse splenocytes. Spleen cells isolated from immunized mice ($n = 3$) were stimulated with *S. thermophilus* (ST) ST285 and the recall agonist $MBP_{83–99}$ peptide for 24 h and the secretion of (**A**) IL-4, (**B**) IL-5, and (**C**) IL-10 were measured. Recall $MBP_{83–99}$ peptide, media alone, or recall $MBP_{83–99}$ peptide plus ST285 are shown from immunized mice ($n = 3$). The means of readings for $n = 3$ mice were calculated and presented as plus or minus (±) the standard error of the mean. Symbols represent the p value for the Tukey test (one way ANOVA) where ** $p < 0.01$ and *** $p < 0.001$.

3.4. *ST285 Does Not Alter the Secretion of Granulocyte-macrophage Colony-stimulating Factor by Mouse Spleen Cells*

Secretion of granulocyte-macrophage colony-stimulating factor (GM-CSF) did not show any change by immunized mouse spleen cells upon co-culture with ST285 and agonist recall $MBP_{83–99}$ peptide compared to the negative control or $MBP_{83–99}$ peptide (Figure 4), despite significant upregulation of GM-CSF by ST285 on monocytes/macrophage cells [29].

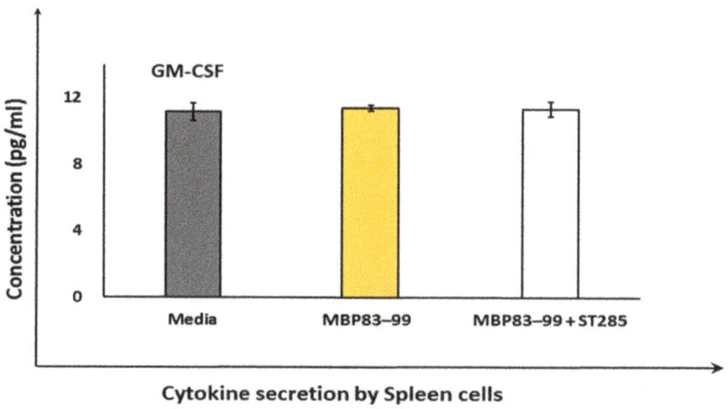

Figure 4. *S. thermophilus* 285 does not alter secretion of GM-CSF by mouse spleen cells. Spleen cells isolated from immunized mice ($n = 3$) were stimulated with *S. thermophilus* (ST) ST285 and the recall reference peptide for 24 hours and secretion of GM-CSF was measured. Recall $MBP_{83–99}$ peptide, media alone, or recall $MBP_{83–99}$ peptide plus ST285 are shown from immunized mice ($n = 3$). The means of readings for $n = 3$ mice were calculated and presented as plus or minus (±) the standard error of the mean.

4. Discussion

The Th1 pro-inflammatory cytokines IFN-γ and TNF-α are both involved in the defense against bacterial infections and in acute phase reactions. In MS, these two cytokines are implicated in the pathogenesis of disease by stimulating $CD4^+$ T cells against the myelin sheath. Mice immunized with the mannan $MBP_{83–99}$ peptide stimulated IFN-γ secretion, which was reduced in the presence of ST285. This reduction is very important in the context of inflamed situations such as autoimmune and inflammatory diseases, as any reduction in the amount of mediators that cause inflammation is imperative in the relief of symptoms. We previously noted that high levels of TNF-α and IFN-γ was secreted by the U937 monocytic cell line in the presence of ST285 [29]. However, the addition of ST285 to the $MBP_{83–99}$ recall peptide reduced IFN-γ secretion by mouse splenocytes. Spleen cells were populated with B, T, NK cells, macrophages, and monocytes, while the U937 cell line that we previously used were purely monocytic/macrophage cells. Additionally, the polarized inflammatory state of cytokines as a result of the immunization regimen and further exposure of spleen cells to the recall $MBP_{83–99}$ peptide that operate as inflammatory stimuli, compared to the U937 monoclonal cells only being exposed to ST285 bacteria, might give a clue as to the ability of ST285 probiotics to dampen the inflammatory immune response in the instance of exposure to polyclonal spleen cells.

Secretion of IL-1β by monocytes is involved in regulating the immune and inflammatory responses to infections and injuries; therefore, it has a role in innate immunity. IL-1β is also a major mediator in inflammatory responses associated with various cellular activities such as differentiation, proliferation, and apoptosis [39]. In addition, IL-1β is a regulator of inflammatory reactions and is involved in the stimulation of the central nervous system through cyclooxygenase-2 (PTGS2/COX2), which is involved in neurodegenerative disorders such as MS [33,40], Down's Syndrome, Alzheimer's disease, and HIV-associated dementia [41,42].

We noted the secretion of IL-1β by immunized mouse spleen cells was marginally, but significantly reduced in the presence of ST285 with the recall $MBP_{83–99}$ peptide. We previously noted that ST285 did not induce IL-1β cytokine to the U937 cell lines, however, significant upregulation of IL-1β mRNA was induced by human PBMC [31] and monocytes post co-culture with ST285 [32]. It is therefore clear that the immunized mouse spleens and the recall of T cells with the $MBP_{83–99}$ peptide in the presence of ST285 caused a reduction in IL-1β secretion. Likewise, IL-2 was marginally decreased in the presence of ST285 compared to the increased secretion caused by the $MBP_{83–99}$ peptide in the positive control. Co-culturing human PBMC with ST285 also downregulates IL-2 mRNA expression [31].

IL-6 is produced by activated immune cells including DC, B cells, and macrophages. Although IL-6 is associated with acute phase responses, it is also associated with a reduction of Th1 polarization, while promoting Th2 differentiation, B cell maturation, and macrophage differentiation. Proliferation and differentiation of Th2 cells changed the polarized Th1 environment and skewed the Th1/Th2 balance toward Th2, which is beneficial in relieving autoimmune conditions such as MS. IL-6 production was significantly higher (three times) in mouse splenocytes cultured with ST285 compared to the control, hence, it is likely that ST285 bacteria may potentially change the balance toward a healthier state in MS. We previously noted significant upregulation of IL-6 to human monocytes [manuscript submitted] and to bulk PBMC co-cultures [31] with ST285, which are also in accord with the increase in IL-6 levels by the U937 promonocytic cell line co-cultured with ST285 [29]. Likewise, the commercially used probiotic *L. paracasei* DG induces IL-6 cytokines to the THP-1 human monocyte cell line [43]. In contrast, ingestion of *B. bifidum* by mice did not increase the IL-6 levels, but boosted anti-oxidation activities in the spleen and thymus of mice and improved other immune functions by changing the gene expression of immune mediators [44].

It is likely that the constant-shifting in the equilibrium and the dynamics that exist between pro- and anti-inflammatory cytokines will lead to some controversy in the research findings regarding IL-6. On one hand, IL-6 may ease the autoimmune condition due to its downstream immunological effects. On the other hand, elevated levels of pro-inflammatory effector T cell cytokines such as IFN-γ, IL-17 as well as IL-6 are noted in patients with autoimmune myasthenia gravis and MS [45]. Thus, it might be likely that the role that cytokines such as IL-6 play may depend on their bio-environment and may be advantageous to the body, if probiotics such as ST285 are used for neutralization and/or reversing from a pro- to an anti-inflammatory state in the body.

IL-4 is one of the important cytokines required for anti-inflammatory responses against inflammatory conditions such as MS and allergies [29]. IL-4 production was significantly increased by mouse spleen cells in the presence of the recall MBP_{83-99} peptide and ST285 compared to either the MBP_{83-99} peptide alone or the negative control (media). Likewise, it was previously noted that ST285 induced U937 monocytic cells to produce IL-4, although no changes to mRNA expression levels of IL-4 were noted to human monocytes or to bulk human PBMC following co-cultures with ST285 [31]. In contrast, feeding BALB/c mice with *L. paracasei* BEJ01 alone or combined with aflatoxins B1 (AFB1) and fumonisin B1 (FB1) (known foodborne mycotoxins with immunomycotoxic effects on human health) was used to evaluate *L. paracasei* BEJ01 detoxification [46]. Assessing different splenic immunological factors indicated that exposure to these mycotoxins led to increased IL-4 mRNA levels, oxidative stress, and immunotoxicity in the spleen [46] whereas the combined LAB treatment with AFB1 or FB1 suppressed and normalized mRNA levels of IL-4, showing protective effects induced by LAB against AFB1 and FB1 via diminishing toxin adhesion and bioavailability [46]. In contrast, spleen cells isolated from BALB/c mice in vitro co-cultured individually with LAB strains (*L. casei* Lc2w (Lc), *L. plantarum* CCFM47 (Lp), and *L. acidophilus* CCFM137 (La)) showed reduced IL-4 production by spleen cells exposed to La only, while parallel animal studies displayed LAB-induced alleviation of inflammation post airway allergy for all strains through increased Treg cells and modulation of Th1/Th2 balance [47].

The anti-inflammatory cytokine IL-5 is produced by Th2 cells and mast cells. In the event of infection with helminth parasites, IL-5 leads to a lesser risk of autoimmune disorders, which is indirectly accredited to some therapeutic characteristics of IL-5 in autoimmune disorders. We noted a slight increase in the IL-5 production by spleen cells in response to ST285, whereas no changes to the mRNA expression levels of IL-5 were previously noted in ST285 co-cultures with human PBMC or human monocyte cells [manuscripts submitted]. A study showed that treating mice with *Fasciola hepatica* excretion/secretions (FHES) reduced EAE clinical signs due to a significant decrease in the infiltration of Th1 and Th17 cells into the brain and an increase in IL-5 (and IL-23) response, with subsequent increase in eosinophils [48]. It is likely that the small but significant increase of IL-5 may be beneficial to MS.

IL-10, an anti-inflammatory cytokine, is secreted by Th2 and Treg cells. Amongst all the anti-inflammatory cytokines and chemokines, anti-inflammatory properties of IL-10 are the most potent in suppressing inflammatory mediators by other activated immune cells (TNF-α, IFN-γ, IL-1, IL-17, and IL-23 cytokines) [49]. A significant amplification in the IL-10 levels secreted by the spleen cells in the presence of ST285 was noted, which was similarly shown for the U937 monocytic cell line in the presence of ST285 and to human PBMC, although no significant changes were shown in human monocyte cells [manuscripts submitted]. Likewise, oral administration of *L. reuteri* and *L. lactis* strains to mice stimulated the production of anti-inflammatory IL-10 and Treg cells [50,51]. In addition, sub-clinical studies of *L. salivarius* UCC118, *L. lactis* MG1363, and *L. plantarum* WCFS1 administered to mice and re-exposure of their isolated bone marrow cells to the three bacterial co-cultures showed all three strains differentially stimulated IL-10 production [52]. Correspondingly, when DC from spleen and mesenteric lymph nodes of mice were matured using *L. acidophilus* X37 and exposed to commensal gut *Bifidobacterium longum* Q46, *L. acidophilus* X37, and *Escherichia coli* Nissle 1917, increased IL-10 levels were noted [53]. Similarly, after BALB/c mice were fed with *L. paracasei* BEJ01 alone or combined with aflatoxins B1 and fumonisin B1, high IL-10 mRNA levels were induced [46]. In addition, mice fed with kefir-derived *Lactobacillus kefiri* CIDCA 8348 also increased IL-10 gene expression [54]. In the context of MS, the use of ST285 was shown to downregulate Th1 responses and upregulate Th2 responses, something of the utmost importance to patients with MS to alleviate MS symptoms and/or reversal of the disease [31].

5. Conclusions

Immunization of SJL/J mice with agonist $MBP_{83–99}$ peptide conjugated to mannan induces Th1 pro-inflammatory IFN-γ responses and no Th2 anti-inflammatory responses when spleen cells are co-cultured in vitro in the presence of the agonist recall $MBP_{83–99}$ peptide. However, stimulation of spleen cells with the recall $MBP_{83–99}$ peptide in the presence of ST285 significantly increased the secretion of IL-4, IL-6, and IL-10, along with mild upregulation in IL-2 and IL-5, suggesting a role for ST285 in the activation of immune response phenotypes toward a predominant anti-inflammatory profile, tolerance, and suppression of inflammation. In addition, ST285, downregulated the secretion of IL-1a and IFN-γ—the immune mediators involved in Th1 type responses—collectively pointing to a shift in immune responses from Th1 to a Th2 phenotype. More importantly, the significant increase of IL-10 could further contribute by the differentiation of naïve $CD4^+$ T cells and proliferation of Tregs, which can also drive the immune balance further toward a dominant anti-inflammatory phenotype. Additionally, given the drastic increase of GM-CSF in our previous studies of ST285 co-cultured with the U937 monocytic cell line, human PBMC, and human monocyte cells, and no change to the secretion of GM-CSF in spleen cells with GM-CSF being a major cytokine for proliferation and recruitment of the immune cells, this might indicate a deliberate and purposeful neutralization of GM-CSF by ST285. The effects of ST285 on the immune response could be used as a novel approach in modulating chronic inflammatory and autoimmune conditions such as MS. Further studies should involve the effects of ST285 in mice with EAE or be used to prevent EAE induction, which will pave the way for new modalities for the treatment of MS in human clinical trials.

Author Contributions: Conceptualization, N.D. and V.A.; Methodology, N.D and V.A.; Formal analysis, N.D.; Investigation, V.A and J.M.; Resources, V.A. and J.M.; Data curation, N.D.; Writing - original draft preparation, N.D.; Writing—review and editing, V.A and J.M.; Supervision, V.A.; Project administration, V.A.; Funding acquisition, V.A. All authors have read and agreed to the published version of the manuscript.

Acknowledgments: V.A and N.D would like to thank the Immunology and Translational Research Group, the Mechanisms and Interventions in Health and Disease Program, and the Institute of Health and Sport, Victoria University, Australia for their support.

References

1. De Palma, G.; Collins, S.M.; Bercik, P.; Verdu, E.F. The microbiota-gut-brain axis in gastrointestinal disorders: Stressed bugs, stressed brain or both? *J. Physiol.* **2014**, *592*, 2989–2997. [CrossRef] [PubMed]
2. Adamczyk-Sowa, M.; Medrek, A.; Madej, P.; Michlicka, W.; Dobrakowski, P. Does the Gut Microbiota Influence Immunity and Inflammation in Multiple Sclerosis Pathophysiology? *J. Immunol. Res.* **2017**, *2017*, 7904821. [CrossRef] [PubMed]
3. Dargahi, N.; Johnson, J.; Donkor, O.; Vasiljevic, T.; Apostolopoulos, V. Immunomodulatory effects of probiotics: Can they be used to treat allergies and autoimmune diseases? *Maturitas* **2019**, *119*, 25–38. [CrossRef] [PubMed]
4. Asarat, M.; Apostolopoulos, V.; Vasiljevik, T.; Donkor, O. Short-chain fatty acids produced by synbiotic mixtures in skim milk differentially regulate proliferation and cytokine production in peripheral blood mononuclear cells. *Int. J. Food Sci. Nutr.* **2015**, *66*, 755–765. [CrossRef]
5. Hardy, H.; Harris, J.; Lyon, E.; Beal, J.; Foey, A.D. Probiotics, prebiotics and immunomodulation of gut mucosal defences: Homeostasis and immunopathology. *Nutrients* **2013**, *5*, 1869–1912. [CrossRef]
6. Wolvers, D.; Antoine, J.M.; Myllyluoma, E.; Schrizenmeir, J.; Szajewska, H.; Rijkers, G.T. Guidance for substantiating the evidence for beneficial effects of probiotics: Prevention and management of infections by probiotics. *J. Nutr.* **2010**, *140*, 698S–712S. [CrossRef]
7. Dargahi, N.; Katsara, M.; Tselios, T.; Androutsou, M.E.; De Courten, M.; Matsoukas, J.; Apostolopoulos, V. Multiple sclerosis: Immunopathology and treatment update. *Brain Sci.* **2017**, *7*, 78. [CrossRef]
8. Mukherjee, A.; Biswas, A.; Das, S.K. Gut dysfunction in Parkinson's disease. *World J. Gastroenterol.* **2016**, *22*, 5742–5752. [CrossRef]
9. Catanzaro, R.; Anzalone, M.; Calabrese, F.; Milazzo, M.; Capuana, M.; Italia, A.; Occhipinti, S.; Marotta, F. The gut microbiota and its correlations with the central nervous system disorders. *Panminerva Med.* **2015**, *57*, 127–143.
10. Russo, R.; Cristiano, C.; Avagliano, C.; De Caro, C.; Rana, G.L.; Raso, G.M.; Canani, R.B.; Meli, R.; Calignano, A. Gut-brain axis: Role of lipids in the regulation of inflammation, pain and CNS diseases. *Curr. Med. Chem.* **2018**, *25*, 3930–3952. [CrossRef]
11. Kwon, H.K.; Kim, G.C.; Kim, Y.; Hwang, W.; Jash, A.; Sahoo, A.; Kim, J.E.; Nam, J.H.; Im, S.H. Amelioration of experimental autoimmune encephalomyelitis by probiotic mixture is mediated by a shift in T helper cell immune response. *Clin. Immunol.* **2013**, *146*, 217–227. [CrossRef] [PubMed]
12. Lavasani, S.; Dzhambazov, B.; Nouri, M.; Fak, F.; Buske, S.; Molin, G.; Thorlacius, H.; Alenfall, J.; Jeppsson, B.; Westrom, B. A novel probiotic mixture exerts a therapeutic effect on experimental autoimmune encephalomyelitis mediated by IL-10 producing regulatory T cells. *PLoS ONE* **2010**, *5*, e9009. [CrossRef] [PubMed]
13. Buerth, C.; Mausberg, A.K.; Heininger, M.K.; Hartung, H.P.; Kiesseier, B.C.; Ernst, J.F. Oral tolerance induction in experimental autoimmune encephalomyelitis with Candida utilis expressing the immunogenic MOG35-55 peptide. *PLoS ONE* **2016**, *11*, e0155082. [CrossRef] [PubMed]
14. Maassen, C.B.M.; Laman, J.D.; Van Holten-Neelen, C.; Hoogteijling, L.; Visser, L.; Schellekens, M.M.; Boersma, W.J.A.; Claassen, E. Reduced experimental autoimmune encephalomyelitis after intranasal and oral administration of recombinant lactobacilli expressing myelin antigens. *Vaccine* **2003**, *21*, 4685–4693. [CrossRef]
15. Consonni, A.; Cordiglieri, C.; Rinaldi, E.; Marolda, R.; Ravanelli, I.; Guidesi, E.; Eli, M.; Mantegaza, R.; Baggi, F. Administration of bifidobacterium and lactobacillus strains modulates experimental myasthenia gravis and experimental encephalomyelitis in Lewis rats. *Oncotarget* **2018**, *9*, 22269–22287. [CrossRef] [PubMed]
16. Salehipour, Z.; Haghmorad, D.; Sankian, M.; Nosratabdi, R.; Sotan Dallal, M.M.; Tabasi, N.; Khazee, M.; Nasirali, L.R.; Mahmoudi, M. Bifidobacterium animalis in combination with human origin of Lactobacillus plantarum ameliorate neuroinflammation in experimental model of multiple sclerosis by altering CD4+ T cell subset balance. *Biomed. Pharmacother.* **2017**, *95*, 1535–1548. [CrossRef] [PubMed]
17. Yannakakis, M.P.; Simal, C.; Tzoupis, H.; Rodi, M.; Dargahi, N.; Prakash, M.; Mouzaki, A.; Platts, J.A.; Apostolopoulos, V.; Tselios, T.V. Design and synthesis of non-peptide mimetics mapping the immunodominant myelin basic protein (MBP83–96) epitope to function as T-cell receptor antagonists. *Int. J. Mol. Sci.* **2017**, *18*, 1215. [CrossRef]

18. Katsara, M.; Apostolopoulos, V. Editorial: Multiple Sclerosis: Pathogenesis and Therapeutics. *Med. Chem.* **2018**, *14*, 104–105. [CrossRef]
19. Katsara, M.; Deraos, G.; Tselios, T.; Matsoukas, J.; Apostolopoulos, V. Design of novel cyclic altered peptide ligands of myelin basic protein MBP83-99 that modulate immune responses in SJL/J mice. *J. Med. Chem.* **2008**, *51*, 3971–3978. [CrossRef]
20. Katsara, M.; Deraos, G.; Tselios, T.; Matsoukas, M.T.; Friligou, I.; Matsoukas, J.; Apostolopoulos, V. Design and synthesis of a cyclic double mutant peptide (cyclo (87–99)[A91, A96] MBP87–99) induces altered responses in mice after conjugation to mannan: Implications in the immunotherapy of multiple sclerosis. *J. Med. Chem.* **2009**, *52*, 214–218. [CrossRef]
21. Katsara, M.; Deraos, S.; Tselios, T.; Pietersz, G.; Matsoukas, J.; Apostolopoulos, V. Immune responses of linear and cyclic PLP139-151 mutant peptides in SJL/J mice: Peptides in their free state versus mannan conjugation. *Immunotherapy* **2014**, *6*, 709–724. [CrossRef] [PubMed]
22. Katsara, M.; Matsoukas, J.; Deraos, G.; Apostolopoulos, V. Towards immunotherapeutic drugs and vaccines against multiple sclerosis. *Acta Biochim. Biophys. Sin.* **2008**, *40*, 636–642. [CrossRef] [PubMed]
23. Katsara, M.; Yuriev, E.; Ramsland, P.A.; Deraos, G.; Tselios, T.; Matsoukas, J.; Apostolopoulos, V. A double mutation of MBP83–99 peptide induces IL-4 responses and antagonizes IFN-γ responses. *J. Neuroimmunol.* **2008**, *200*, 77–89. [CrossRef] [PubMed]
24. Katsara, M.; Yuriev, E.; Ramsland, P.A.; Deraos, G.; Tselios, T.; Matsoukas, J.; Apostolopoulos, V. Mannosylation of mutated MBP83–99 peptides diverts immune responses from Th1 to Th2. *Mol. Immunol.* **2008**, *45*, 3661–3670. [CrossRef] [PubMed]
25. Katsara, M.; Yuriev, E.; Ramsland, P.A.; Tselios, T.; Deraos, G.; Lourbopoulos, A.; Grigoriadis, N.; Matsoukas, J.; Apostolopoulos, V. Altered peptide ligands of myelin basic protein (MBP87–99) conjugated to reduced mannan modulate immune responses in mice. *Immunology* **2009**, *128*, 521–533. [CrossRef] [PubMed]
26. Kumar, A.; Delogu, F. Dynamical footprint of cross-reactivity in a human autoimmune T-cell receptor. *Sci. Rep.* **2017**, *7*, 42496. [CrossRef] [PubMed]
27. Tarrah, A.; Treu, L.; Giaretta, S.; Duarte, V.; Corich, V.; Giacomini, A. Differences in Carbohydrates Utilization and Antibiotic Resistance Between Streptococcus macedonicus and Streptococcus thermophilus Strains Isolated from Dairy Products in Italy. *Curr. Microbiol.* **2018**, *75*, 1334–1344. [CrossRef]
28. Tarrah, A.; Noal, V.; Treu, L.; Giaretta, S.; da Silva Duarte, V.; Corich, V.; Giacomini, A. Short communication: Comparison of growth kinetics at different temperatures of Streptococcus macedonicus and Streptococcus thermophilus strains of dairy origin. *J. Dairy Sci.* **2018**, *101*, 7812–7816. [CrossRef]
29. Dargahi, N.; Johnson, J.; Donkor, O.; Vasiljevic, T.; Apostolopoulos, V. Immunomodulatory effects of Streptococcus thermophilus on U937 monocyte cell cultures. *J. Funct. Foods* **2018**, *49*, 241–249. [CrossRef]
30. Tankou, S.K.; Regev, K.; Healy, B.C.; Cox, L.M.; Tjon, E.; Kivisakk, P.; Vanande, I.P.; Cook, S.; Gandhi, R.; Glanz, B.; et al. Investigation of probiotics in multiple sclerosis. *Mult. Scler.* **2018**, *24*, 58–63. [CrossRef]
31. Dargahi, N.; Johnson, J.; Apostolopoulos, V. Streptococcus thermophilus alters the expression of genes associated with innate and adaptive immunity in human peripheral blood mononuclear cells. *PLoS ONE* **2020**, *15*, e0228531. [CrossRef]
32. Dargahi, N.; Johnson, J.; Apostolopoulos, V. Immune modulatory effects of probiotic Streptococcus thermophilus in human monocytes. 2020; in preparation.
33. McGuinness, M.C.; Powers, J.M.; Bias, W.B.; Schmeckpeper; Segal, A.H.; Gowda, V.C.; Wesselignh, S.L.; Berger, J.; Griffin, D.E.; Smith, K.D. Human leukocyte antigens and cytokine expression in cerebral inflammatory demyelinative lesions of X-linked adrenoleukodystrophy and multiple sclerosis. *J. Neuroimmunol.* **1997**, *75*, 174–182. [CrossRef]
34. Apostolopoulos, V.; Barnes, N.; Pietersz, G.A.; McKenzie, I.F. Ex vivo targeting of the macrophage mannose receptor generates anti-tumor CTL responses. *Vaccine* **2000**, *18*, 3174–3184. [CrossRef]
35. Apostolopoulos, V.; Pietersz, G.A.; Gordon, S.; Martinez-Pomares, L.; McKenzie, I.F. Aldehyde-mannan antigen complexes target the MHC class I antigen-presentation pathway. *Eur. J. Immunol.* **2000**, *30*, 1714–1723. [CrossRef]
36. Apostolopoulos, V.; Pietersz, G.A.; Loveland, B.E.; Sandrin, M.S.; McKenzie, I.F. Oxidative/reductive conjugation of mannan to antigen selects for T1 or T2 immune responses. *Proc. Natl. Acad. Sci. USA* **1995**, *92*, 10128–10132. [CrossRef]
37. Apostolopoulos, V.; Pietersz, G.A.; McKenzie, I.F. Cell-mediated immune responses to MUC1 fusion protein coupled to mannan. *Vaccine* **1996**, *14*, 930–938. [CrossRef]

38. Tselios, T.V.; Lamari, F.N.; Karathanasopoulos, I.; Katsara, M.; Apostolopoulos, V.; Pietersz, G.A.; Matsoukas, J.M.; Karamanos, N.K. Synthesis and study of the electrophoretic behavior of mannan conjugates with cyclic peptide analogue of myelin basic protein using lysine-glycine linker. *Anal. Biochem.* **2005**, *347*, 121–128. [CrossRef]
39. Masters, S.L.; Simon, A.; Aksentjevich, I.; Kastner, D.L. Horror autoinflammaticus: The molecular pathophysiology of autoinflammatory disease. *Annu. Rev. Immunol.* **2009**, *27*, 621–668. [CrossRef]
40. Paré, A.; Mailhot, B.; Levesque, S.A.; Juzwik, C.; Doss, P.M.I.A.; Lecuyer, M.A.; Prat, A.; Rangachari, M.; Fournier, A.; Lacroix, S. IL-1β enables CNS access to CCR2hi monocytes and the generation of pathogenic cells through GM-CSF released by CNS endothelial cells. *Proc. Natl. Acad. Sci. USA* **2018**, *115*, E1194–E1203. [CrossRef]
41. Griffin, W.S.T.; Stanley, L.C.; Ling, C.; White, L.; McLeod, V.; Perrot, L.J.; White Iii, C.L.; Araoz, C. Brain interleukin 1 and S-100 immunoreactivity are elevated in Down syndrome and Alzheimer disease. *Proc. Natl. Acad. Sci. USA* **1989**, *86*, 7611–7615. [CrossRef] [PubMed]
42. Shaftel, S.S.; Griffin, W.S.T.; Kerry, K.M. The role of interleukin-1 in neuroinflammation and Alzheimer disease: An evolving perspective. *J. Neuroinflamm.* **2008**, *5*, 7. [CrossRef] [PubMed]
43. Balzaretti, S.; Taverniti, S.; Guglielmetti, S.; Fiore, W.; Minuzzo, M.; Ngo, H.N.; Ngere, J.B.; Sadiq, S.; Humphreys, P.N.; Laws, A.P. A novel rhamnose-rich hetero-exopolysaccharide isolated from Lactobacillus paracasei DG activates THP-1 human monocytic cells. *Appl. Environ. Microbiol.* **2017**, *83*, e02702–e02716. [CrossRef] [PubMed]
44. Fu, Y.R.; Yi, Z.J.; Pei, J.L.; Guan, S. Effects of Bifidobacterium bifidum on adaptive immune senescence in aging mice. *Microbiol. Immunol.* **2010**, *54*, 578–583. [CrossRef] [PubMed]
45. Danikowski, K.M.; Jayaraman, S.; Prabhakar, B.S. Regulatory T cells in multiple sclerosis and myasthenia gravis. *J. Neuroinflamm.* **2017**, *14*, 117. [CrossRef] [PubMed]
46. Abbès, S.; Ben Salah-Abbes, J.; Jebali, R.; Younes, R.B.; Oueslati, R. Interaction of aflatoxin B1 and fumonisin B1 in mice causes immunotoxicity and oxidative stress: Possible protective role using lactic acid bacteria. *J. Immunotoxicol.* **2016**, *13*, 46–54. [CrossRef]
47. Ai, C.; Ma, N.; Zhang, Q.; Wang, G.; Liu, X.; Tian, F.; Chen, P.; Chen, W. Immunomodulatory effects of different lactic acid bacteria on allergic response and its relationship with in vitro properties. *PLoS ONE* **2016**, *11*, e0164697. [CrossRef]
48. Finlay, C.M.; Stefanska, A.M.; Walsh, K.P.; Kelly, P.J.; Boon, L.; Lavelle, E.C.; Walsh, P.T.; Mills, K.H.G. Helminth products protect against autoimmunity via innate type 2 cytokines IL-5 and IL-33, which promote eosinophilia. *J. Immunol.* **2016**, *196*, 703–714. [CrossRef]
49. Iyer, S.S.; Cheng, G. Role of interleukin 10 transcriptional regulation in inflammation and autoimmune disease. *Crit. Rev. Immunol.* **2012**, *32*, 23–63. [CrossRef]
50. Souza, B.M.; Preisser, T.M.; Pereira, V.B.; Zurita-Turk, M.; Castro, C.P.; Cunha, V.P.; Oliveira, R.P.; Gomes-Santos, A.C.; Faria, A.M.C.; Machado, D.C.C.; et al. Lactococcus lactis carrying the pValac eukaryotic expression vector coding for IL-4 reduces chemically-induced intestinal inflammation by increasing the levels of IL-10-producing regulatory cells. *Microb. Cell Fact.* **2016**, *15*, 150. [CrossRef]
51. Levkovich, T.; Poutahidis, T.; Smillie, C.; Varian, B.J.; Ibrahim, Y.M.; Lakritz, J.R.; Alm, E.J.; Erdman, S.E. Probiotic Bacteria Induce a 'Glow of Health'. *PLoS ONE* **2013**, *8*, e53867. [CrossRef] [PubMed]
52. Smelt, M.J.; de Haan, B.J.; Bron, P.A.; van Swam, I.; Meijerink, M.; Wells, J.M.; Faas, M.M.; de Vos, P.L. L. plantarum, L. salivarius, and L. lactis Attenuate Th2 Responses and Increase Treg Frequencies in Healthy Mice in a Strain Dependent Manner. *PLoS ONE* **2012**, *7*, e47244. [CrossRef] [PubMed]
53. Fink, L.N.; Frøkiær, H. Dendritic cells from Peyer's patches and mesenteric lymph nodes differ from spleen dendritic cells in their response to commensal gut bacteria. *Scand. J. Immunol.* **2008**, *68*, 270–279. [CrossRef] [PubMed]
54. Carasi, P.; Racedo, S.M.; Jacquot, C.; Romanin, D.E.; Serradell, M.A.; Urdaci, M.C. Impact of kefir derived lactobacillus kefiri on the mucosal immune response and gut microbiota. *J. Immunol. Res.* **2015**. [CrossRef]

Permissions

All chapters in this book were first published by MDPI; hereby published with permission under the Creative Commons Attribution License or equivalent. Every chapter published in this book has been scrutinized by our experts. Their significance has been extensively debated. The topics covered herein carry significant findings which will fuel the growth of the discipline. They may even be implemented as practical applications or may be referred to as a beginning point for another development.

The contributors of this book come from diverse backgrounds, making this book a truly international effort. This book will bring forth new frontiers with its revolutionizing research information and detailed analysis of the nascent developments around the world.

We would like to thank all the contributing authors for lending their expertise to make the book truly unique. They have played a crucial role in the development of this book. Without their invaluable contributions this book wouldn't have been possible. They have made vital efforts to compile up to date information on the varied aspects of this subject to make this book a valuable addition to the collection of many professionals and students.

This book was conceptualized with the vision of imparting up-to-date information and advanced data in this field. To ensure the same, a matchless editorial board was set up. Every individual on the board went through rigorous rounds of assessment to prove their worth. After which they invested a large part of their time researching and compiling the most relevant data for our readers.

The editorial board has been involved in producing this book since its inception. They have spent rigorous hours researching and exploring the diverse topics which have resulted in the successful publishing of this book. They have passed on their knowledge of decades through this book. To expedite this challenging task, the publisher supported the team at every step. A small team of assistant editors was also appointed to further simplify the editing procedure and attain best results for the readers.

Apart from the editorial board, the designing team has also invested a significant amount of their time in understanding the subject and creating the most relevant covers. They scrutinized every image to scout for the most suitable representation of the subject and create an appropriate cover for the book.

The publishing team has been an ardent support to the editorial, designing and production team. Their endless efforts to recruit the best for this project, has resulted in the accomplishment of this book. They are a veteran in the field of academics and their pool of knowledge is as vast as their experience in printing. Their expertise and guidance has proved useful at every step. Their uncompromising quality standards have made this book an exceptional effort. Their encouragement from time to time has been an inspiration for everyone.

The publisher and the editorial board hope that this book will prove to be a valuable piece of knowledge for researchers, students, practitioners and scholars across the globe.

List of Contributors

Maria-Eleni Androutsou
Vianex S.A., Tatoiou Str., 18th km Athens-Lamia National Road, 14671 Athens, Greece

Agathi Nteli, Areti Gkika and Theodore Tselios
Department of Chemistry, University of Patras, 26504 Patras, Greece

Maria Avloniti, Anastasia Dagkonaki and Lesley Probert
Laboratory of Molecular Genetics, Hellenic Pasteur Institute, 127 Vasilissis Sophias Ave., 11521 Athens, Greece

Simona Golič Grdadolnik
Laboratory for Molecular Structural Dynamics, National Institute of Chemistry, Hajdrihova 19, 1001 Ljubljana, Slovenia

Michalina Rzepka, Mateusz Toś, Katarzyna Gibas and Ewa Krzystanek
Department of Neurology, Faculty of Medical Sciences in Katowice, Medical University of Silesia, 40-752 Katowice, Poland

Michał Boroń
Department of Gynecology and Obstetrics, Faculty of Medical Sciences in Katowice, Medical University of Silesia, 40-752 Katowice, Poland

Simon Thebault and Mark S. Freedman
Department of Medicine and the Ottawa Hospital Research Institute, The University of Ottawa, Ottawa, ON K1H8L6, Canada

Ronald A. Booth
Department of Pathology and Laboratory Medicine, Eastern Ontario Regional Laboratory Association and Ottawa Hospital Research Institute, University of Ottawa & The Ottawa Hospital, Ottawa, ON K1H8L6, Canada

Natalia V. Voge and Enrique Alvarez
Rocky Mountain Multiple Sclerosis Center at the University of Colorado, Department of Neurology, University of Colorado School of Medicine, Academic Office 1, Mail Stop B-185, 12631 East 17th Avenue, Aurora, CO 80045, USA

Craig D. Workman
Department of Health and Human Physiology, University of Iowa, Iowa City, IA 52242, USA

Laura L. Boles Ponto
Department of Radiology, University of Iowa Hospitals and Clinics, Iowa City, IA 52242, USA

John Kamholz
Department of Neurology, University of Iowa Hospitals and Clinics, Iowa City, IA 52242, USA

Thorsten Rudroff
Department of Health and Human Physiology, University of Iowa, Iowa City, IA 52242, USA
Department of Neurology, University of Iowa Hospitals and Clinics, Iowa City, IA 52242, USA

Stanley Cohan, Elisabeth Lucassen, Kyle Smoot, Justine Brink and Chiayi Chen
Providence Multiple Sclerosis Center, Providence Brain and Spine Institute, Providence St, Vincent Medical Center, Portland, OR 97225, USA

Navzer D. Sachinvala
United States Department of Agriculture, Agricultural Research Service, USDA-ARS, New Orleans, Home 2261 Brighton Place, Harvey, LA 70058, USA

Angeline Stergiou
Department of Medicine, Fairfield Medical Center, 401 North Ewing, Lancaster, OH 43130, USA

Duane E. Haines
Department of Neurobiology and Anatomy, Wake Forest School of Medicine, 1 Medical Center Boulevard, Winston-Salem, NC 27157, USA
Department of Neurology, Wake Forest School of Medicine, 1 Medical Center Boulevard, Winston-Salem, NC 27157, USA
Department of Neurobiology and Anatomy, The University of Mississippi Medical Center, Jackson, MS 39216, USA

Armen Kocharian
Department of Radiology, Houston Methodist Hospital, 6565 Fannin Street, Houston, TX 77030, USA

Andrew Lawton
Department of Ophthalmology, Ochsner Hospital, 1514 Jefferson Highway, New Orleans, 70121, USA

Catherine Koukoulitsa, Eleni Chontzopoulou, Sofia Kiriakidi and Thomas Mavromoustakos
Department of Chemistry, National and Kapodistrian University of Athens, Zographou, 15784 Athens, Greece

Andreas G. Tzakos
Department of Chemistry, Section of Organic Chemistry and Biochemistry, University of Ioannina, 45110e Ioannina, Greece

Gabrielle Macaron and Daniel Ontaneda
Mellen Center for Multiple Sclerosis, Neurological Institute, Cleveland Clinic Foundation, Cleveland, OH 44195, USA

Maria Chountoulesi and Costas Demetzos
Section of Pharmaceutical Technology, Department of Pharmacy, School of Health Sciences, National and Kapodistrian University of Athens, Panepistimioupolis Zografou, 15771 Athens, Greece

Giulia Cardamone and Elvezia Maria Paraboschi
Department of Biomedical Sciences, Humanitas University, Via Rita Levi Montalcini 4, 20090 Pieve Emanuele, Milan, Italy

Giulia Soldà, Stefano Duga and Rosanna Asselta
Department of Biomedical Sciences, Humanitas University, Via Rita Levi Montalcini 4, 20090 Pieve Emanuele, Milan, Italy
Humanitas Clinical and Research Center, Via Manzoni 56, 20089 Rozzano, Milan, Italy

Janna Saarela
Institute for Molecular Medicine Finland, Helsinki Institute of Life Science (HiLIFE), University of Helsinki, 00290 Helsinki, Finland

Maria Chiara Buscarinu, Arianna Fornasiero, Alessandro Bozzao and Giovanni Ristori
Department of Neurosciences, Mental Health and Sensory Organs, Centre for Experimental Neurological Therapies (CENTERS), Faculty of Medicine and Psychology, Sapienza University, 00189 Rome, Italy

Giulia Pellicciari, Roberta Reniè and Anna Chiara Landi
Faculty of Medicine and Psychology, Sapienza University, 00189 Rome, Italy

Cristina Cappelletti and Pia Bernasconi
Neurology IV–Neuroimmunology and Neuromuscular Diseases Unit, Fondazione IRCCS Istituto Neurologico Carlo Besta, 20133 Milan, Italy

Marco Salvetti
Department of Neurosciences, Mental Health and Sensory Organs, Centre for Experimental Neurological Therapies (CENTERS), Faculty of Medicine and Psychology, Sapienza University, 00189 Rome, Italy
IRCCS Istituto Neurologico Mediterraneo (INM) Neuromed, 86077 Pozzilli, Italy

Valentina Gatta
Department of Psychological, Health and Territorial Sciences, School of Medicine and Health Sciences, "G. d'Annunzio" University, 66100 Chieti, Italy

Guadalupe Mengod
IIBB-CSIC, IDIBAPS, CIBERNED, 08036 Barcelona, Spain

Marcella Reale
Department of Medical, Oral and Biotechnological Science, University "G. d'Annunzio" Chieti-Pescara, 66100 Chieti, Italy

Ada Maria Tata
Department of Biology and Biotechnologies C. Darwin, "Sapienza" University of Rome, 00185 Rome, Italy
Research Center of Neurobiology Daniel Bovet, "Sapienza" University of Rome, 00185 Rome, Italy

Stanley L. Cohan, Elisabeth B. Lucassen and Meghan C. Romba
Providence Multiple Sclerosis Center, Providence Brain and Spine Institute, Portland, OR 97225, USA

Stefanie N. Linch
Providence Health and Services, Regional Research Department, Portland, OR 97213, USA

Tobias Moser, Gayane Harutyunyan, Anush Karamyan, Ferdinand Otto, Carola Bacher, Vaclav Chroust, Markus Leitinger, Helmut F. Novak and Eugen Trinka
Department of Neurology, Christian Doppler Medical Center, Paracelsus Medical University, 5020 Salzburg, Austria

Johann Sellner
Department of Neurology, Christian Doppler Medical Center, Paracelsus Medical University, 5020 Salzburg, Austria
Department of Neurology, Klinikum rechts der Isar, Technische Universität München, 81675 München, Germany
Department of Neurology, Landesklinikum Mistelbach-Gänserndorf, 2130 Mistelbach, Austria

Narges Dargahi and Vasso Apostolopoulos
Institute for Health and Sport, Victoria University, Melbourne VIC 3030, Australia

John Matsoukas
New Drug, Patras Science Park, 26500 Patras, Greece

Index

www.ingramcontent.com/pod-product-compliance
Lightning Source LLC
LaVergne TN
LVHW060530210926
848485LV00005B/1175